ESAP™ 2

Endocrine Society's
Endocrine Self-Assessment Program
Questions, Answers, and Discussions

Lisa R. Tannock, MD, Program Chair
Professor of Medicine
Chief, Division of Endocrinology
and Molecular Medicine
University of Kentucky and
Department of Veterans Affairs

Kristien Boelaert, MD
Reader in Endocrinology Center for
Endocrinology, Diabetes, and Metabolism
University of Birmingham

Barbara Gisella Carranza Leon, MD
Assistant Professor of Medicine
Division of Diabetes, Endocrinology,
and Metabolism
Vanderbilt University Medical Center

Stephen Clement, MD
Medical Director, Endocrine Services
Inova Fairfax Hospital

Kathryn McCrystal Dahir, MD
Assistant Professor of Medicine
Division of Endocrinology
Vanderbilt University Medical Center

Thomas W. Donner, MD
Associate Professor of Medicine
Division of Endocrinology,
Diabetes, and Metabolism
Johns Hopkins University

Marie Freel, MB, ChB, PhD
Consultant Endocrinologist
Queen Elizabeth University Hospital
Glasgow, United Kingdom

Mimi Hu, MD
Associate Professor
Department of Endocrine Neoplasia
and Hormonal Disorders
University of Texas MD Anderson
Cancer Center

Michael S. Irwig, MD
Associate Professor
George Washington University

Jacqueline Jonklaas, MD, PhD
Professor
Division of Endocrinology and Metabolism
Georgetown University

Steven Magill, MD, PhD
Associate Clinical Professor of Medicine
Endocrinology, Diabetes, and Metabolism
Medical College of Wisconsin

Deepika Reddy, MD
Assistant Professor
Division of Diabetes, Endocrinology,
and Metabolism
University of Utah Healthcare

Roberto Salvatori, MD
Professor of Medicine
Medical Director,
Johns Hopkins Pituitary Center
Johns Hopkins University

Savitha Subramanian, MD
Associate Professor of Medicine
University of Washington

Anand Vaidya, MD, MMSC
Assistant Professor of Medicine
Brigham and Women's Hospital
Harvard Medical School

Corrine Welt, MD
Professor of Medicine
University of Utah School of Medicine

Abbie L. Young, MS, CGC, ELS(D)
Medical Editor

Endocrine Society
2055 L Street NW, Suite 600, Washington, DC 20036
1-888-ENDOCRINE • www.endocrine.org

ENDOCRINE
SOCIETY
Hormone Science to Health

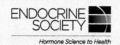

The Endocrine Society is the world's largest, oldest, and most active organization working to advance the clinical practice of endocrinology and hormone research. Founded in 1916, the Society now has more than 18,000 global members across a range of disciplines. The Society has earned an international reputation for excellence in the quality of its peer-reviewed journals, educational resources, meetings, and programs that improve public health through the practice and science of endocrinology.

Visit us at:
education.endocrine.org
endocrine.org

Other Publications:
https://www.endocrine.org/publications

ISBN: 978-1-879225-49-7
Library of Congress Control Number: 2019951424

On the Cover:
Left: X-ray of the right femur showing areas of lateral cortical thickening that cause a "beaking" or "flaring" effect adjacent to areas of transverse fracture lines, which eventually evolve and propagate medially and ultimately lead to a complete fracture.
Middle: PET-CT showing fluorodeoxyglucose-avid skeletal metastatic disease in the right scapula, several ribs, thoracolumbar vertebra, pelvis, the right vertebral body of L5, and the sacrum in a patient with radioiodine-refractory differentiated thyroid cancer.
Right: Unenhanced CT of the adrenal glands showing multiple nonpigmented nodules larger than 10 mm in diameter in both adrenals in a patient with bilateral macronodular adrenal hyperplasia.

OVERVIEW

The Endocrine Self-Assessment Program (ESAP™) is a self-study curriculum aimed at physicians wanting a self-assessment and a broad review of endocrinology. The ESAP Reference Edition consists of 120 brand-new multiple-choice questions in all areas of endocrinology, diabetes, and metabolism. There is extensive discussion of each correct answer, a comprehensive syllabus, and references. ESAP is updated annually with new questions.

The ESAP reference book is intended primarily for consultation and self-assessment of knowledge relating to endocrinology. As a reference book, educational credits are not available upon completion of the multiple-choice questions included. For information on educational products that include educational credit, please visit endocrine.org/store.

LEARNING OBJECTIVES

ESAP 2018 will allow learners to assess their knowledge of all aspects of endocrinology, diabetes, and metabolism.

Upon completion of this educational activity, learners will be able to:

- Recognize clinical manifestations of endocrine and metabolic disorders and select among current options for diagnosis, management, and therapy.
- Identify risk factors for endocrine and metabolic disorders and develop strategies for prevention.
- Evaluate endocrine and metabolic manifestations of systemic disorders.
- Use existing resources pertaining to clinical guidelines and treatment recommendations for endocrine and related metabolic disorders to guide diagnosis and treatment.

TARGET AUDIENCE

ESAP is a self-study curriculum aimed at physicians seeking initial certification or recertification in endocrinology, program directors interested in a testing and training instrument, and clinicians simply wanting a self-assessment and a broad review of endocrinology.

STATEMENT OF INDEPENDENCE

The Endocrine Society has a policy of ensuring that the content and quality of this educational activity are balanced, independent, objective, and scientifically rigorous. The scientific content of this activity was developed under the supervision of the Endocrine Society's ESAP Faculty Working Group.

DISCLOSURE POLICY

The faculty, committee members, and staff who are in position to control the content of this activity are required to disclose to the Endocrine Society and to learners any relevant financial relationship(s) of the individual or spouse/partner that have occurred within the last 12 months with any commercial interest(s) whose products or services are related to the content. Financial relationships are defined by remuneration in any amount from the commercial interest(s) in the form of grants; research support; consulting fees; salary; ownership interest (eg, stocks, stock options, or ownership interest excluding diversified mutual funds); honoraria or other payments for participation in speakers' bureaus, advisory boards, or boards of directors; or other financial benefits. The intent of this disclosure is not to prevent planners with relevant financial relationships from planning or delivering content, but rather to provide learners with information that allows them to make their own judgments of whether these financial relationships may have influenced the educational activity with regard to exposition or conclusion. The Endocrine Society has reviewed all disclosures and resolved or managed all identified conflicts of interest, as applicable.

The following faculty reported relevant financial relationship(s): **Thomas W. Donner, MD**, is a study site principal investigator for Novo Nordisk. **Mimi Hu, MD**, is a primary investigator for AstraZeneca. **Michael Irwig, MD**, served as male hypogonadism faculty for Medscape. **Roberto Salvatori, MD**, receives grant support from National Institutes of Health and the Department of Defense; is a reviewer for the National Institutes of Health; and is an investigator for Pfizer Novartis, Chiasma, Millendo Therapeutics, and Strongbridge Biopharma. **Savitha Subramanian, MD**, receives grant support from Ionis Pharmaceuticals. **Anand Vaidya, MD**, received grant support from the National Institutes of Health and the Doris Duke Charitable Foundation. **Corrine Welt, MD**, is a writer for UpToDate and a consultant for Takeda.

The following faculty members reported no relevant financial relationships **Kristien Boelaert, MD**; **Barbara Gisella Carranza Leon, MD**; **Stephen Clement, MD**; **Kathryn Dahir, MD**; **Marie Freel, MD**; **Jacqueline Jonklaas, MD, PhD**; **Steven Magill, MD**; **Deepika Reddy, MD**; and **Lisa R. Tannock, MD**.

The medical editor for this program, **Abbie L. Young, MS, CGC, ELS(D)**, reported no relevant financial relationships.

The Endocrine Society staff associated with the development of content for this activity reported no relevant financial relationships.

DISCLAIMERS

The information presented in this activity represents the opinion of the faculty and is not necessarily the official position of the Endocrine Society.

USE OF PROFESSIONAL JUDGMENT:

The educational content in this self-assessment test relates to basic principles of diagnosis and therapy and does not substitute for individual patient assessment based on the health care provider's examination of the patient and consideration of laboratory data and other factors unique to the patient. Standards in medicine change as new data become available.

DRUGS AND DOSAGES:

When prescribing medications, the physician is advised to check the product information sheet accompanying each drug to verify conditions of use and to identify any changes in drug dosage schedule or contraindications.

POLICY ON UNLABELED/OFF-LABEL USE

The Endocrine Society has determined that disclosure of unlabeled/off-label or investigational use of commercial product(s) is informative for audiences and therefore requires this information to be disclosed to the learners at the beginning of the presentation. Uses of specific therapeutic agents, devices, and other products discussed in this educational activity may not be the same as those indicated in product labeling approved by the Food and Drug Administration (FDA). The Endocrine Society requires that any discussions of such "off-label" use be based on scientific research that conforms to generally accepted standards of experimental design, data collection, and data analysis. Before recommending or prescribing any therapeutic agent or device, learners should review the complete prescribing information, including indications, contraindications, warnings, precautions, and adverse events.

ACKNOWLEDGMENT OF COMMERCIAL SUPPORT

This activity is not supported by educational grant(s) or other funds from any commercial supporter.

PUBLICATION DATE: September 2017

Laboratory Reference Ranges

Reference ranges vary among laboratories. Conventional units are listed first with SI units in parentheses.

Lipid Values

High-density lipoprotein (HDL) cholesterol

    Optimal ----------------------------------- >60 mg/dL (>1.55 mmol/L)

    Normal---------------------------- 40-60 mg/dL (1.04-1.55 mmol/L)

    Low -------------------------------------- <40 mg/dL (<1.04 mmol/L)

Low-density lipoprotein (LDL) cholesterol

    Optimal----------------------------------<100 mg/dL (<2.59 mmol/L)

    Low ---------------------------- 100-129 mg/dL (2.59-3.34 mmol/L)

    Borderline-high ---------------- 130-159 mg/dL (3.37-4.12 mmol/L)

    High---------------------------- 160-189 mg/dL (4.14-4.90 mmol/L)

    Very high --------------------------------- ≥190 mg/dL (≥4.92 mmol/L)

Non-HDL cholesterol

    Optimal----------------------------------<130 mg/dL (<3.37 mmol/L)

    Borderline-high ---------------- 130-159 mg/dL (3.37-4.12 mmol/L)

    High--- ≥240 mg/dL (≥6.22 mmol/L)

Total cholesterol

    Optimal----------------------------------<200 mg/dL (<5.18 mmol/L)

    Borderline-high ----------------- 200-239 mg/dL (5.18-6.19 mmol/L)

    High--- ≥240 mg/dL (≥6.22 mmol/L)

Triglycerides

    Optimal----------------------------------<150 mg/dL (<3.88 mmol/L)

    Borderline-high ---------------- 150-199 mg/dL (3.88-5.15 mmol/L)

    High-------------------------- 200-499 mg/dL (5.18-12.92 mmol/L)

    Very high --------------------------------- ≥500 mg/dL (≥12.95 mmol/L)

Lipoprotein (a) ------------------------------- ≤30 mg/dL (≤1.07 µmol/L)

Apolipoprotein B -----------------------------50-110 mg/dL (0.5-1.1 g/L)

Hematologic Values

Erythrocyte sedimentation rate ------------------------------- 0-20 mm/h

Haptoglobin -----------------------------30-200 mg/dL (300-2000 mg/L)

Hematocrit----------------------------------41%-50% (0.41-0.51) (male);

    35%-45% (0.35-0.45) (female)

Hemoglobin A$_{1c}$---------------------------- 4.0%-5.6% (20-38 mmol/mol)

Hemoglobin----------------------- 13.8-17.2 g/dL (138-172 g/L) (male);

    12.1-15.1 g/dL (121-151 g/L) (female)

International normalized ratio -------------------------------------0.8-1.2

Mean corpuscular volume (MCV) -------------- 80-100 µm³ (80-100 fL)

Platelet count---------------------- 150-450 × 10³/µL (150-450 × 10⁹/L)

Protein (total) ---------------------------------- 6.3-7.9 g/dL (63-79 g/L)

Reticulocyte count -------- 0.5%-1.5% of red blood cells (0.005-0.015)

White blood cell count--------------- 4500-11,000/µL (4.5-11.0 × 10⁹/L)

Thyroid Values

Thyroglobulin --- 3-42 ng/mL (3-42 µg/L) (after surgery and radioactive

    iodine treatment: <1.0 ng/mL [<1.0 µg/L])

Thyroglobulin antibodies ------------------------ ≤4.0 IU/mL (≤4.0 kIU/L)

Thyrotropin (TSH) --------------------------------------- 0.5-5.0 mIU/L

Thyroid-stimulating immunoglobulin ----------- ≤120% of basal activity

Thyroperoxidase (TPO) antibodies-------------- <2.0 IU/mL (<2.0 kIU/L)

Thyroxine (T$_4$) (free)----------------- 0.8-1.8 ng/dL (10.30-23.17 pmol/L)

Thyroxine (T$_4$) (total) -------------- 5.5-12.5 µg/dL (94.02-213.68 nmol/L)

Free thyroxine (T$_4$) index --- 4-12

Triiodothyronine (T$_3$) (free) ------------ 2.3-4.2 pg/mL (3.53-6.45 pmol/L)

Triiodothyronine (T$_3$) (total)------------ 70-200 ng/dL (1.08-3.08 nmol/L)

Triiodothyronine (T$_3$), reverse ----------- 10-24 ng/dL (0.15-0.37 nmol/L)

Triiodothyronine uptake, resin--------------------------------25%-38%

Radioactive iodine uptake--- 3%-16% (6 hours); 15%-30% (24 hours)

Endocrine Values

Serum

Aldosterone---------------------------- 4-21 ng/dL (111.0-582.5 pmol/L)

Alkaline phosphatase ----------------------50-120 U/L (0.84-2.00 µkat/L)

Alkaline phosphatase (bone-specific) ------------ ≤20 µg/L (adult male);

    ≤14 µg/L (premenopausal female); ≤22 µg/L (postmenopausal female)

Androstenedione --------65-210 ng/dL (2.27-7.33 nmol/L) (adult male);

    80-240 ng/dL (2.79-8.38 nmol/L) (adult female)

Antimullerian hormone-------------- 0.7-19.0 ng/mL (5.0-135.7 pmol/L)

    (male, >12 years);

    0.9-9.5 ng/mL (6.4-67.9 pmol/L) (female, 13-45 years);

    <1.0 ng/mL (<7.1 pmol/L) (female, >45 years)

Calcitonin ---------------------- <16 pg/mL (<4.67 pmol/L) (basal, male);

    <8 pg/mL (<2.34 pmol/L) (basal, female);

    ≤130 pg/mL (≤37.96 pmol/L) (peak calcium infusion, male);

    ≤90 pg/mL (≤26.28 pmol/L) (peak calcium infusion, female)

Carcinoembryonic antigen ---------------------- <2.5 ng/mL (<2.5 µg/L)

Chromogranin A------------------------------------<93 ng/mL (<93 µg/L)

Corticosterone--------- 53-1560 ng/dL (1.53-45.08 nmol/L) (>18 years)

Corticotropin (ACTH)-------------------- 10-60 pg/mL (2.2-13.2 pmol/L)

Cortisol (8 AM)------------------------- 5-25 µg/dL (137.9-689.7 nmol/L)

Cortisol (4 PM)-------------------------2-14 µg/dL (55.2-386.2 nmol/L)

C-peptide ------------------------------0.9-4.3 ng/mL (0.30-1.42 nmol/L)

C-reactive protein ---------------------0.8-3.1 mg/L (7.62-29.52 nmol/L)

Cross-linked N-telopeptide of type 1 collagen ---------------------------

    5.4-24.2 nmol BCE/mmol creat (male);

    6.2-19.0 nmol BCE/mmol creat (female)

Dehydroepiandrosterone sulfate (DHEA-S)

Patient Age	Female	Male
18-29 years	44-332 µg/dL	89-457 µg/dL
	(1.19-9.00 µmol/L)	(2.41-12.38 µmol/L)
30-39 years	31-228 µg/dL	65-334 µg/dL
	(0.84-6.78 µmol/L)	(1.76-9.05 µmol/L)
40-49 years	18-244 µg/dL	48-244 µg/dL
	(0.49-6.61 µmol/L)	(1.30-6.61 µmol/L)

Patient Age	Female	Male
50-59 years	15-200 µg/dL	35-179 µg/dL
	(0.41-5.42 µmol/L)	(0.95-4.85 µmol/L)
≥60 years	15-157 µg/dL	25-131 µg/dL
	(0.41-4.25 µmol/L)	(0.68-3.55 µmol/L)

Deoxycorticosterone------------- <10 ng/dL (<0.30 nmol/L) (>18 years)

1,25-Dihydroxyvitamin D_3 ------------16-65 pg/mL (41.6-169.0 pmol/L)

Estradiol ---------------------- 10-40 pg/mL (36.7-146.8 pmol/L) (male);
   10-180 pg/mL (36.7-660.8 pmol/L) (follicular, female);
   100-300 pg/mL (367.1-1101.3 pmol/L) (midcycle, female);
   40-200 pg/mL (146.8-734.2 pmol/L) (luteal, female);
   <20 pg/mL (<73.4 pmol/L) (postmenopausal, female)

Estrone----------------------- 10-60 pg/mL (37.0-221.9 pmol/L) (male);
   17-200 pg/mL (62.9-739.6 pmol/L) (premenopausal female);
   7-40 pg/mL (25.9-147.9 pmol/L) (postmenopausal female)

α-Fetoprotein--------------------------------------<6 ng/mL (<6 µg/L)

Follicle-stimulating hormone (FSH) -----------------------------------
   1.0-13.0 mIU/mL (1.0-13.0 IU/L) (male);
   <3.0 mIU/mL (<3.0 IU/L) (prepuberty, female);
   2.0-12.0 mIU/mL (2.0-12.0 IU/L) (follicular, female);
   4.0-36.0 mIU/mL (4.0-36.0 IU/L) (midcycle, female);
   1.0-9.0 mIU/mL (1.0-9.0 IU/L) (luteal, female);
   >30 mIU/mL (>30 IU/L) (postmenopausal, female)

Free fatty acids ------------------------10.6-18.0 mg/dL (0.4-0.7 nmol/L)

Gastrin --- <100 pg/mL (<100 ng/L)

Growth hormone (GH) ------- 0.01-0.97 ng/mL (0.01-0.97 µg/L) (male);
   0.01-3.61 ng/mL (0.01-3.61 µg/L) (female)

Homocysteine ---------------------------------≤1.76 mg/L (≤13 µmol/L)

β-Human chorionic gonadotropin (β-hCG)-----------------------------------
   <3.0 mIU/mL (<3.0 IU/L) (nonpregnant female);
   >25 mIU/mL (>25 IU/L) indicates a positive pregnancy test

β-Hydroxybutyrate ----------------------------<3.0 mg/dL (<300 µmol/L)

17-Hydroxypregnenolone ------------ 29-189 ng/dL (0.87-5.69 nmol/L)

17α-Hydroxyprogesterone ----<220 ng/dL (<6.67 nmol/L) (adult male);
   <80 ng/dL (<2.42 nmol/L) (follicular, female);
   <285 ng/dL (<8.64 nmol/L) (luteal, female);
   <51 ng/dL (1.55 nmol/L) (postmenopausal, female)

25-Hydroxyvitamin D -- <10 ng/mL (<25.0 nmol/L) (severe deficiency);
   10-24 ng/mL (25.0-59.9 nmol/L) (mild to moderate deficiency);
   25-80 ng/mL (62.4-199.7 nmol/L) (optimum levels);
   >80 ng/mL (>199.7 nmol/L) (toxicity possible)

Inhibin B ------------------------------ 15-300 pg/mL (15-300 ng/L)

Insulinlike growth factor 1 (IGF-1)

Patient Age	Female	Male
18 years	162-541 ng/mL	170-640 ng/mL
	(21.2-70.9 nmol/L)	(22.3-83.8 nmol/L)
19 years	138-442 ng/mL	147-527 ng/mL
	(18.1-57.9 nmol/L)	(19.3-69.0 nmol/L)
20 years	122-384 ng/mL	132-457 ng/mL
	(16.0-50.3 nmol/L)	(17.3-59.9 nmol/L)
21-25 years	116-341 ng/mL	116-341 ng/mL
	(15.2-44.7 nmol/L)	(15.2-44.7 nmol/L)
26-30 years	117-321 ng/mL	117-321 ng/mL
	(15.3-42.1 nmol/L)	(15.3-42.1 nmol/L)
31-35 years	113-297 ng/mL	113-297 ng/mL
	(14.8-38.9 nmol/L)	(14.8-38.9 nmol/L)
36-40 years	106-277 ng/mL	106-277 ng/mL
	(13.9-36.3 nmol/L)	(13.9-36.3 nmol/L)
41-45 years	98-261 ng/mL	98-261 ng/mL
	(12.8-34.2 nmol/L)	(12.8-34.2 nmol/L)
46-50 years	91-246 ng/mL	91-246 ng/mL
	(11.9-32.2 nmol/L)	(11.9-32.2 nmol/L)
51-55 years	84-233 ng/mL	84-233 ng/mL
	(11.0-30.5 nmol/L)	(11.0-30.5 nmol/L)
56-60 years	78-220 ng/mL	78-220 ng/mL
	(10.2-28.8 nmol/L)	(10.2-28.8 nmol/L)
61-65 years	72-207 ng/mL	72-207 ng/mL
	(9.4-27.1 nmol/L)	(9.4-27.1 nmol/L)
66-70 years	67-195 ng/mL	67-195 ng/mL
	(8.8-25.5 nmol/L)	(8.8-25.5 nmol/L)
71-75 years	62-184 ng/mL	62-184 ng/mL
	(8.1-24.1 nmol/L)	(8.1-24.1 nmol/L)
76-80 years	57-172 ng/mL	57-172 ng/mL
	(7.5-22.5 nmol/L)	(7.5-22.5 nmol/L)
≥80 years	53-162 ng/mL	53-162 ng/mL
	(6.9-21.2 nmol/L)	(6.9-21.2 nmol/L)

Insulinlike growth factor binding protein 3 ------------------ 2.5-4.8 mg/L

Insulin --------------------------------1.4-14.0 µIU/mL (9.7-97.2 pmol/L)

Islet-cell antibody assay--------- 0 Juvenile Diabetes Foundation units

Luteinizing hormone (LH)---------1.0-9.0 mIU/mL (1.0-9.0 IU/L) (male);
   <1.0 mIU/mL (<1.0 IU/L) (prepuberty, female);
   1.0-18.0 mIU/mL (1.0-18.0 IU/L) (follicular, female);
   20.0-80.0 mIU/mL (20.0-80.0 IU/L) (midcycle, female);
   0.5-18.0 mIU/mL (0.5-18.0 IU/L) (luteal, female);
   >30 mIU/mL (>30 IU/L) (postmenopausal, female)

Metanephrines (plasma fractionated)

Metanephrine----------------------------------<57 pg/mL (<289 pmol/L)

Normetanephrine----------------------------- <148 pg/mL (<808 pmol/L)

75-g oral glucose tolerance test--60-100 mg/dL (3.3-5.6 mmol/L) (fasting)
   Blood glucose values ---------<200 mg/dL (<11.1 mmol/L) (1 hour);
      <140 mg/dL (<7.8 mmol/L) (2 hour)
   Between 140-200 mg/dL (7.8-11.1 mmol/L) is considered
   impaired glucose tolerance or prediabetes. Greater than
   200 mg/dL (11.1 mmol/L) is a sign of diabetes mellitus.

50-g oral glucose tolerance test for gestational diabetes --------------
   <140 mg/dL (<7.8 mmol/L) (1 hour)

100-g oral glucose tolerance test for gestational diabetes --------------
   <95 mg/dL (<5.3 mmol/L) (fasting);
   <180 mg/dL (<10.0 mmol/L) (1 hour);
   <155 mg/dL (<8.6 mmol/L) (2 hour);
   <140 mg/dL (<7.8 mmol/L) (3 hour)

Osteocalcin -----------------------------9.0-42.0 ng/mL (9.0-42.0 µg/L)

Parathyroid hormone, intact (PTH)----------- 10-65 pg/mL (10-65 ng/L)

Parathyroid hormone–related protein (PTHrP) 14-27 pg/mL (14-27 ng/L)

Progesterone -------------------------≤1.2 ng/mL (≤3.8 nmol/L) (male);

≤1.0 ng/mL (≤3.2 nmol/L) (follicular, female);

2.0-20.0 ng/mL (6.4-63.6 nmol/L) (luteal, female);

≤1.1 ng/mL (≤3.5 nmol/L) (postmenopausal, female);

>10.0 ng/mL (>31.8 nmol/L) (evidence of ovulatory adequacy)

Proinsulin --------------------------26.5-176.4 pg/mL (3.0-20.0 pmol/L)

Prolactin ------------------------ 4-23 ng/mL (0.17-1.00 nmol/L) (male);

4-30 ng/mL (0.17-1.30 nmol/L) (nonlactating female);

10-200 ng/mL (0.43-8.70 nmol/L) (lactating female)

Prostate-specific antigen-----------<2.0 ng/mL (<2.0 µg/L) (≤40 years);

<2.8 ng/mL (<2.8 µg/L) (≤50 years);

<3.8 ng/mL (<3.8 µg/L) (≤60 years);

<5.3 ng/mL (<5.3 µg/L) (≤70 years);

<7.0 ng/mL (<7.0 µg/L) (≤79 years);

<7.2 ng/mL (<7.2 µg/L) (≥80 years)

Renin activity, plasma, sodium replete, ambulatory --0.6-4.3 ng/mL per h

Renin, direct concentration----------------30-40 pg/mL (0.7-1.0 pmol/L)

Sex hormone–binding globulin---1.1-6.7 µg/mL (10-60 nmol/L) (male);

2.2-14.6 µg/mL (20-130 nmol/L) (female)

α-Subunit of pituitary glycoprotein hormones -- <1.2 ng/mL (<1.2 µg/L)

Testosterone (bioavailable) ---------- 0.8-4.0 ng/dL (0.03-0.14 nmol/L)

(20-50 years, female on oral estrogen);

0.8-10.0 ng/dL (0.03-0.35 nmol/L)

(20-50 years, female not on oral estrogen);

83.0-257.0 ng/dL (2.88-8.92 nmol/L) (male 20-29 years);

72.0-235.0 ng/dL (2.50-8.15 nmol/L) (male 30-39 years);

61.0-213.0 ng/dL (2.12-7.39 nmol/L) (male 40-49 years);

50.0-190.0 ng/dL (1.74-6.59 nmol/L) (male 50-59 years);

40.0-168.0 ng/dL (1.39-5.83 nmol/L) (male 60-69 years)

Testosterone (free) -----------9.0-30.0 ng/dL (0.31-1.04 nmol/L) (male);

0.3-1.9 ng/dL (0.01-0.07 nmol/L) (female)

Testosterone (total)-----------300-900 ng/dL (10.4-31.2 nmol/L) (male);

8-60 ng/dL (0.3-2.1 nmol/L) (female)

Vitamin B$_{12}$------------------------------ 180-914 pg/mL (180-914 ng/L)

Chemistry Values

Alanine aminotransferase------------------- 10-40 U/L (0.17-0.67 µkat/L)

Albumin ------------------------------------- 3.5-5.0 g/dL (35-50 g/L)

Amylase---------------------------------26-102 U/L (0.43-1.70 µkat/L)

Aspartate aminotransferase--------------- 20-48 U/L (0.33-0.80 µkat/L)

Bicarbonate-----------------------------------21-28 mEq/L (21-28 mmol/L)

Bilirubin (total) ------------------------- 0.3-1.2 mg/dL (5.1-20.5 µmol/L)

Blood gases

Po$_2$, arterial blood ------------------ 80-100 mm Hg (10.6-13.3 kPa)

Pco$_2$, arterial blood ------------------------35-45 mm Hg (4.7-6.0 kPa)

Blood pH---7.35-7.45

Calcium -------------------------------- 8.2-10.2 mg/dL (2.1-2.6 mmol/L)

Calcium (ionized)----------------------- 4.60-5.08 mg/dL (1.2-1.3 mmol/L)

Carbon dioxide ------------------------------22-28 mEq/L (22-28 mmol/L)

CD$_4$ cell count --------------------------500-1400/µL (0.5-1.4 × 10⁹/L)

Chloride---------------------------------96-106 mEq/L (96-106 mmol/L)

Creatine kinase-------------------------50-200 U/L (0.84-3.34 µkat/L)

Creatinine -------------------- 0.7-1.3 mg/dL (61.9-114.9 µmol/L) (male);

0.6-1.1 mg/dL (53.0-97.2 µmol/L) (female)

Ferritin------------------------------ 15-200 ng/mL (33.7-449.4 pmol/L)

Folate ---≥4.0 ng/mL (≥4.0 µg/L)

Glucose ----------------------------------- 70-99 mg/dL (3.9-5.5 mmol/L)

γ-Glutamyltransferase ------------------------2-30 U/L (0.03-0.50 µkat/L)

Iron --------------------------------50-150 µg/dL (9.0-26.8 µmol/L) (male);

35-145 µg/dL (6.3-26.0 µmol/L) (female)

Lactate dehydrogenase -------------------- 100-200 U/L (1.7-3.3 µkat/L)

Lactic acid ------------------------------ 5.4-20.7 mg/dL (0.6-2.3 mmol/L)

Lipase------------------------------------ 10-73 U/L (0.17-1.22 µkat/L)

Magnesium ------------------------------1.5-2.3 mg/dL (0.6-0.9 mmol/L)

Osmolality -----------------------275-295 mOsm/kg (275-295 mmol/kg)

Phosphorus----------------------------2.3-4.7 mg/dL (0.7-1.5 mmol/L)

Potassium -----------------------------3.5-5.0 mEq/L (3.5-5.0 mmol/L)

Prothrombin time--- 8.3-10.8 s

Serum urea nitrogen -----------------------8-23 mg/dL (2.9-8.2 mmol/L)

Sodium------------------------------136-142 mEq/L (136-142 mmol/L)

Transferrin saturation ---------------------------------------14%-50%

Troponin I ----------------------------------- <0.6 ng/mL (<0.6 µg/L)

Tryptase--<11.5 ng/mL (<11.5 µg/L)

Uric acid ----------------------------3.5-7.0 mg/dL (208.2-416.4 µmol/L)

Urine

Albumin -------------------- 30-300 µg/mg creat (3.4-33.9 µg/mol creat)

Albumin-to-creatinine ratio ------------------------------- <30 mg/g creat

Aldosterone-------------------------------3-20 µg/24 h (8.3-55.4 nmol/d)

(should be <12 µg/24 h [<33.2 nmol/d] with oral sodium loading—

confirmed with 24-hour urinary sodium >200 mEq)

Calcium ------------------------------ 100-300 mg/24 h (2.5-7.5 mmol/d)

Catecholamine fractionation

Normotensive normal ranges:

Dopamine -------------------------- <700 µg/24 h (<4567 nmol/d)

Epinephrine --------------------------- <35 µg/24 h (<191 nmol/d)

Norepinephrine-------------------- <170 µg/24 h (<1005 nmol/d)

Cortisol-----------------------------------4-50 µg/24 h (11-138 nmol/d)

Cortisol following dexamethasone suppression test-------<10 µg/24 h

(<27.6 nmol/d) (low-dose: 2 day, 2 mg daily)

Creatinine ------------------------------ 1.0-2.0 g/24 h (8.8-17.7 mmol/d)

Glomerular filtration rate (estimated) ---------- >60 mL/min per 1.73 m²

5-Hydroxyindole acetic acid -----------2-9 mg/24 h (10.5-47.1 µmol/d)

Iodine (random)--->100 µg/L

17-Ketosteroids -----------6.0-21.0 mg/24 h (20.8-72.9 µmol/d) (male);

4.0-17.0 mg/24 h (13.9-59.0 µmol/d) (female)

Metanephrine fractionation

Metanephrine -------------------------- <400 µg/24 h (<2028 nmol/d)

Normetanephrine --------------------- <900 µg/24 h (<4914 nmol/d)

Total metanephrine ------------------ <1000 µg/24 h (<5260 nmol/d)

Osmolality --------------------150-1150 mOsm/kg (150-1150 mmol/kg)

Oxalate--<40 mg/24 h (<456 mmol/d)

Phosphate --------------------------- 0.9-1.3 g/24 h (29.1-42.0 mmol/d)

Potassium ----------------------------17-77 mEq/24 h (17-77 mmol/d)

Sodium ----------------------------- 40-217 mEq/24 h (40-217 mmol/d)

Uric acid --------------------------------- <800 mg/24 h (<4.7 mmol/d)

Saliva

Cortisol (salivary), midnight------------------- <0.13 µg/dL (<3.6 nmol/L)

Semen

Semen analysis------------------- >20 million sperm/mL; >50% motility

Abbreviations

ACTH--- corticotropin

ACE inhibitor ------------------ angiotensin-converting enzyme inhibitor

ALT --- alanine aminotransferase

AST-- aspartate aminotransferase

BMI--- body mass index

CNS -- central nervous system

CT --- computed tomography

DHEA--dehydroepiandrosterone

DHEA-S ---------------------------- dehydroepiandrosterone sulfate

DNA --deoxyribonucleic acid

DXA ---------------------------------- dual-energy x-ray absorptiometry

FDA----------------------------------- Food and Drug Administration

FNAB---fine-needle aspiration biopsy

FSH-- follicle-stimulating hormone

GH--growth hormone

GHRH ----------------------------- growth hormone–releasing hormone

GnRH----------------------------------- gonadotropin-releasing hormone

hCG -------------------------------------human chorionic gonadotropin

HDL --high-density lipoprotein

HIV -------------------------------------- human immunodeficiency virus

HMG-CoA reductase inhibitor --------------3-hydroxy-3-methylglutaryl
    coenzyme A reductase inhibitor

IGF-1 -- insulinlike growth factor 1

LDL--low-density lipoprotein

LH -- luteinizing hormone

MCV--- mean corpuscular volume

MRI---magnetic resonance imaging

NPH insulin ------------------------ neutral protamine Hagedorn insulin

PET--------------------------------------- positron emission tomography

PTH--parathyroid hormone

PTHrP ----------------------------- parathyroid hormone–related protein

T_3 --triiodothyronine

T_4 --- thyroxine

TPO antibodies----------------------------------thyroperoxidase antibodies

TRH -------------------------------------- thyrotropin-releasing hormone

TSH--- thyrotropin

VLDL --------------------------------------- very low-density lipoprotein

ENDOCRINE SELF-ASSESSMENT PROGRAM 2018

Part I

1 A 59-year-old man with an 18-year history of diabetes mellitus is being treated with insulin glargine and metformin. He has had longstanding hypertension, hyperlipidemia, and renal insufficiency, but no previous heart attack or stroke. His review of systems is negative. He stopped smoking cigarettes 2 years ago. He asks for recommendations to help him reduce his risk of a cardiovascular event. Both his father and paternal uncle have diabetes and developed coronary artery disease requiring stenting.

His medication regimen is as follows: insulin glargine, 36 units at bedtime; metformin, 500 mg twice daily; atorvastatin; lisinopril; hydrochlorothiazide; and amlodipine.

On physical examination, his blood pressure is 138/82 mm Hg and pulse rate is 88 beats/min. His height is 73.5 in (186.7 cm), and weight is 247 lb (112 kg) (BMI = 32.1 kg/m^2). Eye examination reveals bilateral retinal microaneurysms. On cardiac examination, he has a regular rate and rhythm, a loud S$_4$, no S$_3$, and no murmurs. There are no carotid bruits. His abdomen is obese with no striae or renal bruits. On neurologic examination, there is symmetric decreased light touch and vibration sense in both feet.

Laboratory test results:

  Hemoglobin A$_{1c}$ = 8.3% (4.0%-5.6%) (67 mmol/mol [20-38 mmol/mol])
  Fasting glucose = 142 mg/dL (70-99 mg/dL) (SI: 7.9 mmol/L [3.9-5.5 mmol/L])
  Serum urea nitrogen = 31 mg/dL (8-23 mg/dL) (SI: 11.1 mmol/L [2.9-8.2 mmol/L])
  Creatinine = 1.8 mg/dL (0.7-1.3 mg/dL) (SI: 159.1 μmol/L [61.9-114.9 μmol/L])
  Estimated glomerular filtration rate = 40 mL/min per 1.73 m^2 (>60 mL/min per 1.73 m^2)
  Liver function, normal

You decide to add therapy. Which of the following is the best agent for this patient?
  A. Premeal aspart insulin
  B. Glipizide
  C. Acarbose
  D. Sitagliptin
  E. Liraglutide

2 You are asked to evaluate a 24-year-old man who collapsed during an outdoor music festival 3 days earlier. Since his arrival at the hospital, he has developed intractable hypoglycemia, which has required a continuous 10% dextrose infusion. He has no notable medical history. He takes no regular prescribed medications, but he did consume amphetamines while at the music festival. His mother has type 2 diabetes mellitus treated with glibenclamide and metformin.

On physical examination, he is alert and oriented. He is centrally obese with some purple striae over his abdominal wall and inner thighs. His height is 70 in (177.8 cm), and weight is 224 lb (101.8 kg) (BMI = 32.1 kg/m^2). His blood pressure is 148/99 mm Hg, and pulse rate is 90 beats/min.

Laboratory test results (on 10% dextrose infusion):

  Sodium = 135 mEq/L (136-142 mEq/L) (SI: 135 mmol/L [136-142 mmol/L])
  Potassium = 4.2 mEq/L (3.5-5.0 mEq/L) (SI: 4.2 mmol/L [3.5-5.0 mmol/L])
  Serum urea nitrogen = 14 mg/dL (8-23 mg/dL) (SI: 5.0 mmol/L [2.9-8.2 mmol/L])
  Creatinine = 0.9 mg/dL (0.7-1.3 mg/dL) (SI: 79.6 μmol/L [61.9-114.9 μmol/L])
  Glucose = 53 mg/dL (70-99 mg/dL) (SI: 2.9 mmol/L [3.9-5.5 mmol/L])
  Insulin = 0.2 μIU/mL (1.4-14.0 μIU/mL) (SI: 1.4 pmol/L [9.7-97.2 pmol/L])
  C-peptide = 0.1 ng/mL (0.9-4.3 ng/mL) (SI: 0.03 nmol/L [0.30-1.42 nmol/L])
  β-Hydroxybutyrate= 0.12 mg/dL (<3 mg/dL) (SI: 11.5 μmol/L [<300 μmol/L])
  TSH = 1.4 mIU/L (0.5-5.0 mIU/L)
  Free T$_4$ = 1.2 ng/dL (0.8-1.8 ng/dL) (SI: 15.4 pmol/L [10.30-23.17 pmol/L])
  Early morning serum cortisol = 24 μg/dL (5-25 μg/dL) (SI: 662.1 nmol/L [137.9-689.7 nmol/L])

CT of the abdomen is shown (*see image*).

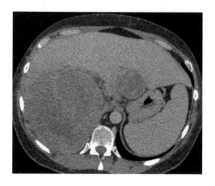

Which of the following tests is most likely to reveal the cause of this patient's hypoglycemia?
 A. ACTH stimulation test
 B. Arterial calcium stimulation test
 C. Urinary toxicology screen
 D. Plasma sulfonylurea screen
 E. Serum IGF-2 to IGF-1 ratio

3 You are asked to consult on a 43-year-old woman with a history of hypocalcemia. Sensorineural hearing loss was diagnosed at birth. This has progressed to 90% hearing loss and she requires multiple hearing aids. During evaluation for a syncopal event 10 years ago, she was noted to have hypocalcemia. At that time, her total calcium concentration was 5.3 mg/dL (8.2-10.2 mg/dL) (SI: 1.3 mmol/L [2.1-2.6 mmol/L]). She has since been on calcium and calcitriol supplementation.

When she is fatigued or when she forgets to take her calcium supplements, she occasionally notes diffuse pedal spasms and "Charlie horses" running up and down her legs. She has no perioral numbness or other paresthesias and she has had no seizures or arrhythmias since she has been on supplementation. Other medical problems include hypothyroidism and a history of ovarian cysts. Ultrasonography has documented that she has small kidneys. Both her daughter and her granddaughter have renal anomalies. She also reports a stillborn birth at 26 weeks' gestation due to renal dysplasia.

On physical examination, she is well nourished. Her height is 63 in (160 cm), and weight is 141 lb (64.1 kg) (BMI = 25 kg/m²). Her blood pressure is 108/60 mm Hg, and pulse rate is 83 beats/min. Neck examination reveals a small, firm thyroid gland. She has brisk reflexes. Her examination findings are otherwise unremarkable.

Her current medications include calcitriol, 0.25 mcg daily; calcium carbonate, 1000 mg twice daily; and levothyroxine, 75 mcg daily.

Laboratory test results:
 Serum total calcium = 8.0 mg/dL (8.2-10.2 mg/dL) (SI: 2.0 mmol/L [2.1-2.6 mmol/L])
 Ionized calcium = 3.73 mg/dL (4.60-5.08 mg/dL) (SI: 0.93 mmol/L [1.2-1.3 mmol/L])
 Phosphate = 4.0 mg/dL (2.3-4.7 mg/dL) (SI: 1.3 mmol/L [0.7-1.5 mmol/L])
 Serum creatinine = 0.99 mg/dL (0.6-1.1 mg/dL) (SI: 87.5 µmol/L [53.0-97.2 µmol/L])
 Alkaline phosphatase = 77 U/L (50-120 U/L) (SI: 1.3 µkat/L [0.84-2.00 µkat/L])
 PTH = 16 pg/mL (10-65 pg/mL) (SI: 16 ng/L [10-65 ng/L])
 Urinary calcium = 35 mg/24 h (100-300 mg/24 h) (SI: 0.9 mmol/d [2.5-7.5 mmol/d])

Which of the following is the most likely cause of her hypocalcemia?
 A. Abnormality in the calcium-sensing receptor
 B. Abnormal parathyroid development
 C. PTH resistance
 D. Autoimmune destruction of the parathyroid glands
 E. Wilson disease

4 A 43-year-old woman with a history of hypertension and gastroesophageal reflux disease returns to see you 1 year after sleeve gastrectomy. You initially met her 2 years ago for evaluation and management of her medically complicated obesity. After a complete evaluation, you recommended she undergo bariatric surgery. The patient was reluctant to have Roux-en-Y gastric bypass because her sister had multiple complications after the same procedure. The patient instead elected to have a sleeve gastrectomy, and her BMI decreased from 44 to 28 kg/m². The patient is pleased with her weight loss, but reports dysphagia with solids and epigastric pain. Also, she frequently feels nauseated and has had 1 episode of vomiting.

On physical examination, her vital signs are stable, abdomen is soft, bowel sounds are present, and there is no focal tenderness.

Given her symptoms, which of the following should be performed next?
  A. Esophageal pH testing
  B. Upper gastrointestinal series
  C. Abdominal ultrasonography
  D. Abdominal CT
  E. Gastric emptying study

5 A 22-year-old woman comes to you for follow-up of androgen insensitivity. The patient was found to have female genitalia at birth despite amniocentesis demonstrating a 46,XY karyotype. An elevated testosterone level was documented. At age 12 years, she underwent vaginal reconstruction/dilatation. The family elected not to have the patient undergo orchiectomy and the gonadal tissue remained in the abdomen. As an adult, the patient has not chosen to undergo orchiectomy based on her fear of decreased libido and her belief that the risks of malignancy are lower than those reported.

On physical examination, her blood pressure is 110/80 mm Hg. Her height is 69 in (175.3 cm), and weight is 147 lb (66.8 kg) (BMI = 21.7 kg/m²). On skin examination, she has no axillary or pubic hair. Her breasts are Tanner stage 5. No masses are noted on abdominal examination. Pelvic examination reveals a vaginal length of 1.5 cm.

Which of the following tests is the most important for follow-up in this patient who does not desire gonadectomy?
  A. Abdominal ultrasonography
  B. α-Fetoprotein measurement
  C. hCG measurement
  D. Testosterone measurement
  E. Bone density scan

6 A 67-year-old woman who was diagnosed with Hashimoto thyroiditis 3 years ago presents to the clinic with a 4-week history of progressive confusion and cognitive decline. Her husband reports dramatic deterioration in her symptoms over the preceding 5 days with disorientation, falls, and inability to perform routine tasks. Her appetite has been poor and she has lost 11 lb (5 kg). Her medical history includes celiac disease and hypertension. She smokes 20 cigarettes daily but does not drink alcohol. She follows a gluten-free diet, and her medications include levothyroxine, 100 mcg daily; aspirin; sertraline; and a thiazide diuretic.

On physical examination, her height is 66 in (167.6 cm) and weight is 123 lb (55.8 kg) (BMI = 19.9 kg/m²). Her blood pressure is 124/78 mm Hg, and pulse rate is 92 beats/min. She is afebrile. She is disorientated and agitated. She has a coarse tremor of the upper and lower limbs. There is no palpable thyroid enlargement. Neurologic examination reveals tremor and ankle clonus with bilateral hyperreflexia and normal plantar responses. Her gait is unsteady and her speech is slurred.

Laboratory test results:
  Complete blood cell count, normal
  Renal, liver, and calcium profile, normal
  C-reactive protein = <3.0 mg/L (0.8-3.1 mg/L) (SI: <28.57 nmol/L [7.62-29.52 nmol/L])
  TSH = 2.3 mIU/L (0.5-5.0 mIU/L)
  Free T$_4$ = 1.4 ng/dL (0.8-1.8 ng/dL) (SI: 18.02 pmol/L [10.30-23.17 pmol/L])
  TPO antibodies = 260 IU/mL (<2.0 IU/mL) (SI: 260 kIU/L [<2.0 kIU/L])
  Urine dipstick and microscopy: normal
  Cerebrospinal fluid examination: elevated protein concentration, no oligoclonal bands, otherwise normal
  Urine and blood bacterial cultures: no growth after 48 hours
  Cerebrospinal fluid bacterial cultures: no growth

Cerebrospinal fluid viral PCR: negative for herpes simplex types 1 and 2, varicella zoster, cytomegalovirus, Epstein-Barr virus, adenovirus, enterovirus, and polyoma virus

Serology for HIV and syphilis: negative

Vasculitis screen: negative

Chest radiography and brain CT do not reveal any abnormalities. She is admitted to the hospital and started empirically on broad-spectrum antibiotics and acyclovir. Twenty-four hours following admission, she has 3 brief tonic-clonic seizures, and electroencephalography shows diffuse slow-wave activity. Brain MRI is unremarkable. Anticonvulsant agents are initiated. She remains confused with periods of agitation after 72 hours.

Which of the following is the best next step?
   A. Increase the levothyroxine dosage to 125 mcg daily
   B. Start high-dosage glucocorticoid treatment
   C. Recommend treatment with plasmapheresis
   D. Start treatment with intravenous immunoglobulins
   E. Start treatment with liothyronine (T_3)

7 A 20-year-old man presents to the emergency department with diabetic ketoacidosis. Type 1 diabetes mellitus was diagnosed at age 10 years, and he has a history of moderate glycemic control. His insulin regimen consists of insulin glargine, 30 units each morning, and insulin aspart, 8 to 10 units with each meal. He uses insulin pens for both glargine and aspart. He keeps his insulin aspart pen on his person. The unused box of insulin aspart pens, as well as his insulin glargine, is kept in the refrigerator at his house. His blood glucose values usually range from 150 to 200 mg/dL (8.3-11.1 mmol/L).

One week before admission, he noticed that his blood glucose started to increase to the range of 250 to 300 mg/dL (13.9-16.7 mmol/L), with no change in his diet or his usual insulin doses. Over the next 5 days, he took multiple additional doses of insulin aspart, 10 units at a time. His glucose transiently dropped by 20 to 30 mg/dL (1.1-1.7 mmol/L) with each dose, but would return to the range of 250 to 300 mg/dL within 3 hours. On the day before admission, he noticed worsening fatigue, polyuria, and polydipsia. He never tests his urine for ketones.

There is no sign of infection or other precipitant. He had a previous episode of diabetic ketoacidosis 7 months ago for which no cause was found. He states that he does not use recreational drugs and has not recently consumed alcohol. He was under the care of a pediatric endocrinologist until age 18 years, but he has not seen an endocrinologist since then. His primary care physician prescribes his insulin.

Which of the following is the most important next step?
   A. Identify an endocrinologist who takes the patient's insurance and is willing to see him
   B. Initiate insulin pump therapy
   C. Initiate continuous glucose monitoring
   D. Change from insulin glargine to insulin detemir
   E. Ask the patient how the insulin was initially stored after picking it up from the pharmacy

8 A 67-year-old man with a history of prostate cancer is referred for evaluation of osteoporosis. He underwent prostatectomy 6 years ago and started leuprolide. One year ago, leuprolide was stopped and abiraterone with prednisone, 5 mg daily, was started because of progression to lymph nodes. He has no history of fractures or height loss. He does not eat much dairy, nor does he take calcium or vitamin D supplements.

On physical examination, his blood pressure is 119/67 mm Hg and pulse rate is 55 beats/min. His height is 71 in (180 cm), and weight is 257 lb (116.8 kg) (BMI = 35.8 kg/m^2). There is no evidence of cushingoid features or kyphosis.

Laboratory test results:
   Serum urea nitrogen = 39 mg/dL (8-23 mg/dL) (SI: 13.9 mmol/L [2.9-8.2 mmol/L])
   Creatinine = 1.8 mg/dL (0.7-1.3 mg/dL) (SI: 159.1 µmol/L [61.9-114.9 µmol/L])

Estimated glomerular filtration rate = 28 mL/min per 1.73 m^2 (>60 mL/min per 1.73 m^2)

Calcium = 9.6 mg/dL (8.2-10.2 mg/dL) (SI: 2.4 mmol/L [2.1-2.6 mmol/L])

Phosphate = 4.0 mg/dL (2.3-4.7 mg/dL) (SI: 1.3 mmol/L [0.7-1.5 mmol/L])

Albumin = 3.9 g/dL (3.5-5.0 g/dL) (SI: 39 g/L [35-50 g/L])

Total testosterone = <20 ng/dL (300-900 ng/dL) (SI: 0.7 nmol/L [10.4-31.2 nmol/L])

25-Hydroxyvitamin D = 16 ng/mL (25-80 ng/mL [optimal]) (SI: 39.9 nmol/L [62.4-199.7 nmol/L])

Bone mineral density as determined by DXA is shown (*see table*).

Region	T Score
L1-L4 spine	–2.8
Left total hip	–1.7
Left femoral neck	–1.7
Right total hip	–2.0
Right femoral neck	–2.2

Bone scan is negative for bone metastases.

After repleting vitamin D stores and recommending calcium supplementation, which of the following is the best recommendation now?

A. Stop prednisone

B. Initiate denosumab

C. Initiate teriparatide

D. Initiate alendronate

E. Initiate zoledronic acid

9 A previously healthy 20-year-old African American man comes to clinic for a follow-up visit. He was hospitalized for treatment of diabetic ketoacidosis 4 months ago.

Laboratory test results at hospital admission:

Plasma glucose = 748 mg/dL (70-99 mg/dL) (SI: 41.5 mmol/L [3.9-5.5 mmol/L])

Bicarbonate = 10 mEq/L (21-28 mEq/L) (SI: 10 mmol/L [21-28 mEq/L])

Anion gap = 22 mEq/L (3-11 mEq/L)

Creatinine = 2.2 mg/dL (0.7-1.3 mg/dL) (SI: 194.5 μmol/L [61.9-114.9 μmol/L])

Estimated glomerular filtration rate = 34 mL/min per 1.73 m^2 (>60 mL/min per 1.73 m^2)

Moderate ketones present in the serum

No obvious cause of the diabetic ketoacidosis was found. He was treated with intravenous fluids and a continuous insulin infusion. The acidosis resolved and he was discharged on basal-bolus insulin. The total insulin dose at the time of discharge was 1.0 units/kg per day.

He received diabetes education and has modified his diet. He has lost 22 lb (10 kg) since hospital discharge. The insulin doses have been gradually reduced over time. He is now administering 12 units of insulin glargine at bedtime and 3 units of insulin aspart before breakfast and dinner (he only eats 2 meals per day). The 2-week average glucose value is 107 mg/dL (5.9 mmol/L). The fasting glucose values range from 79 to 106 mg/dL (4.4-5.9 mmol/L).

He has no other medical problems. He does not have hypertension or dyslipidemia. He does not drink alcohol or smoke cigarettes. His mother, 2 of his 4 siblings, and other maternal relatives have a history of diabetes.

On physical examination, his height is 73 in (185 cm) and weight is 242 lb (110 kg) (BMI = 31.9 kg/m^2). His blood pressure is 122/83 mm Hg, and pulse rate is 82 beats/min. He has central weight distribution. There is evidence of acanthosis nigricans. The cardiac, lung, abdominal, and neurologic findings on examination are all normal.

Current laboratory test results (fasting):

Hemoglobin A$_{1c}$ = 5.8% (4.0%-5.6%) (40 mmol/mol [20-38 mmol/mol])

Creatinine = 1.3 mg/dL (0.7-1.3 mg/dL) (SI: 114.9 μmol/L [61.9-114.9 μmol/L])

Estimated glomerular filtration rate = >60 mL/min per 1.73 m^2 (>60 mL/min per 1.73 m^2)

Electrolytes, normal

TSH, normal

C-peptide = 3.2 ng/mL (0.9-4.3 ng/mL) (SI: 1.06 nmol/L [0.30-1.42 nmol/L])

Glucose = 124 mg/dL (70-99 mg/dL) (SI: 6.9 mmol/L [3.9-5.5 mmol/L])

Glutamic acid decarboxylase antibodies, undetectable

Which of the following is the best next step in treating this patient's diabetes?

A. Stop insulin aspart and start empagliflozin

B. Stop insulin aspart and start glimepiride

C. Stop all insulin and start metformin

D. Stop all insulin and instruct the patient to continue diet treatment alone

E. Continue the current insulin regimen

10 You are asked to consult on a 69-year-old woman with a history of high serum calcium noted on routine laboratory testing over the past 2 years. She reports a progressive decline in her health, including an unintentional 25-lb (11.4-kg) weight loss, constipation, and joint pain. She had a dry cough for the last few years, which improved with steroid nasal spray. She takes no over-the-counter supplements, specifically no calcium or vitamin D. She has been avoiding dairy products. Her other medical problems include gastrointestinal reflux and hypertension. There is no family history of calcium or parathyroid disorders.

Her current medications include valsartan, carvedilol, amlodipine, pantoprazole, and furosemide.

On physical examination, she is a thin woman. Her height is 66.5 in (168.9 cm), and weight is 137 lb (62.3 kg) (BMI = 21.8 kg/m^2). Her blood pressure is 148/61 mm Hg, and pulse rate is 62 beats/min.

Laboratory test results:

Serum total calcium = 12.2 mg/dL (8.2-10.2 mg/dL)
    (SI: 3.1 mmol/L [2.1-2.6 mmol/L])

Ionized calcium = 6.17 mg/dL (4.60-5.08 mg/dL)
    (SI: 1.5 mmol/L [1.2-1.3 mmol/L])

Phosphate = 3.5 mg/dL (2.3-4.7 mg/dL)
    (SI: 1.1 mmol/L [0.7-1.5 mmol/L])

Serum creatinine = 2.39 mg/dL (0.6-1.1 mg/dL)
    (SI: 211.3 μmol/L [53.0-97.2 μmol/L])

Estimated glomerular filtration rate = 32 mL/min per 1.73 m^2
    (>60 mL/min per 1.73 m^2)

PTH = 12 pg/mL (10-65 pg/mL) (SI: 12 ng/L [10-65 ng/L])

PTHrP = 2.9 pg/mL (14-27 pg/mL) (SI: 2.9 ng/L [14-27 ng/L])

Magnesium = 2.7 mg/dL (1.5-2.3 mg/dL)
    (SI: 1.1 mmol/L [0.6-0.9 mmol/L])

25-Dihydroxyvitamin D = 30 ng/mL (25-80 ng/mL [optimal])
    (SI: 74.9 nmol/L [62.4-199.7 nmol/L])

1,25-Dihydroxyvitamin D = 84.9 pg/mL (16-65 pg/mL)
    (SI: 221.7 pmol/L [41.6-169.0 pmol/L])

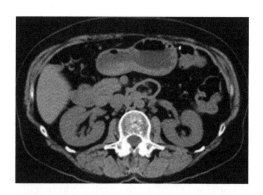

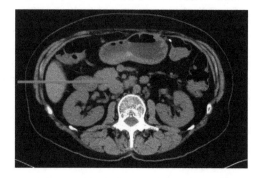

CT of the abdomen and chest shows chronic-appearing interstitial lung disease and scattered lymph nodes most pronounced in the abdomen (*see images*).

In addition to intravenous fluids, which of the following should be prescribed?
   A. Cinacalcet
   B. Denosumab
   C. Zoledronate
   D. Prednisone
   E. Raloxifene

11 A 45-year-old woman presents with hypertension (180/100 mm Hg), hirsutism, and hypokalemia (potassium = 3.1 mEq/L [3.1 mmol/L]). A 7-cm adrenocortical carcinoma with invasion of the inferior vena cava is identified. She has numerous metastases to the liver and lungs, hypercortisolism causing Cushing syndrome, and biochemical hyperandrogenism.

Laboratory test results:
   Urinary free cortisol = 1750 μg/24 h (4-50 μg/24 h) (SI: 4830 nmol/d [11-138 nmol/d])
   Plasma renin activity = <0.6 ng/mL per h (0.6-4.3 ng/mL per h)
   Serum aldosterone = <4.0 ng/dL (4.0-21.0 ng/dL) (SI: <111.0 pmol/L [111.0-582.5 pmol/L])

The patient is prescribed mifepristone (a glucocorticoid and progesterone receptor antagonist).

Which of the following is the most likely consequence of mifepristone treatment in this patient?

Answer	Blood Pressure	Potassium	Uterine Endometrium
A.	Hypotension	Hypokalemia	Thin
B.	Hypotension	Hyperkalemia	Thin
C.	Hypertension	Hypokalemia	Thick
D.	Hypertension	Hyperkalemia	Thin
E.	Hypertension	Hyperkalemia	Thick

12 A 28-year-old woman of South Asian ancestry is seen at week 25 of her second pregnancy. She did not have gestational diabetes mellitus with her first pregnancy 3 years ago. She reports both her parents have type 2 diabetes. She undergoes a 75-g oral glucose tolerance test with the following results:

   Blood glucose at baseline = 120 mg/dL (6.7 mmol/L)
   1 hour = 195 mg/dL (10.8 mmol/L)
   2 hours = 149 mg/dL (8.3 mmol/L)

Gestational diabetes is diagnosed. In addition to lifestyle modification, metformin and sulfonylurea are prescribed. She has good glycemic control, with fasting blood glucose values less than 90 mg/dL (<5.0 mmol/L) and 2-hour postprandial blood glucose values less than 120 mg/dL (<6.7 mmol/L) more than 80% of the time.
   On physical examination, her blood pressure is 111/62 mm Hg, pulse rate is 88 beats/min, and BMI is 28.3 kg/m³. Her examination findings are normal.

Which of the following factors is the strongest predictor of future development of type 2 diabetes in this patient?
   A. Parity
   B. Gestational fasting blood glucose level
   C. South Asian ethnicity
   D. BMI
   E. Family history of type 2 diabetes

13 A 64-year-old woman is referred for possible lipid-lowering therapy. She notes that "high cholesterol" was detected 15 years ago. Medical nutrition therapy was offered, and she was prescribed atorvastatin at that time (dosage unknown) but she did not start it. She has a history of biopsy-proven primary biliary cirrhosis that is treated with ursodiol and has been stable over many years. She takes no other medications. She walks 3 to 4 miles several times a week and does Pilates twice a week. She does not smoke cigarettes, and she drinks 3 alcoholic beverages weekly. In reviewing her family history, you learn that her father had a myocardial infarction and 2-vessel coronary artery bypass grafting at age 51 years and died after his second myocardial infarction at age 64 years. A paternal uncle died at age 42 years after a massive myocardial infarction. The patient has 2 adult daughters who are reportedly healthy.

On physical examination, her blood pressure is 120/72 mm Hg. Her height is 64 in (162.5 cm), and weight is 128 lb (58.2 kg) (BMI = 22 kg/m^2). There are no xanthomas or other remarkable findings.

Laboratory test results (sample drawn while fasting):
Total cholesterol = 270 mg/dL (<200 mg/dL [optimal]) (SI: 6.99 mmol/L [<5.18 mmol/L])
LDL cholesterol = 163 mg/dL (<100 mg/dL [optimal]) (SI: 4.22 mmol/L [<2.59 mmol/L])
Triglycerides = 89 mg/dL (<150 mg/dL [optimal]) (SI: 1.01 mmol/L [<3.88 mmol/L])
HDL cholesterol = 89 mg/dL (>60 mg/dL [optimal]) (SI: 2.31 mmol/L [>1.55 mmol/L])
Non–HDL-cholesterol = 181 mg/dL (<130 mg/dL [optimal]) (SI: 4.69 mmol/L [<3.37 mmol/L])
Apolipoprotein B = 132 mg/dL (50-110 mg/dL) (SI: 1.32 g/L [0.5-1.1 g/L])
Lipoprotein(a) = 14 mg/dL (≤30 mg/dL) (SI: 5.14 μmol/L [≤1.07 μmol/L])
Hemoglobin A$_{1c}$ = 5.9% (4.0%-5.6%) (41 mmol/mol [20-38 mmol/mol])
TSH = 3.2 mIU/L (0.5-5.0 mIU/L)
Liver function, normal

According to the 2013 American College of Cardiology/American Heart Association atherosclerotic cardiovascular disease risk calculator, her calculated 10-year risk is 4.2%.

Which of the following should you recommend as the best next step in this patient's management?
A. No medication needed, recommend low-fat diet
B. Colesevelam
C. Ezetimibe
D. A statin
E. Metformin

14 A 54-year-old man is referred to you after a low serum testosterone concentration (120 ng/dL [4.2 nmol/L]) was identified during the workup of new-onset erectile dysfunction. He has noted no change in weight and no new headache pattern. He has no history of hypertension or diabetes mellitus.

On physical examination, his blood pressure is 128/75 mm Hg. His height is 69 in (175.3 cm), and weight is 177 lb (80.5 kg) (BMI = 26.1 kg/m^2). Examination findings are normal. Testes are 10 mL bilaterally. Formal visual field testing shows a mild bitemporal defect.

Laboratory test results:
LH = 2.0 mIU/mL (1.0-9.0 mIU/mL) (SI: 2.0 IU/L [1.0-9.0 IU/L])
FSH = 4.2 mIU/mL (1.0-13.0 mIU/mL) (SI: 4.2 IU/L [1.0-13.0 IU/L])
Prolactin = 81 ng/mL (4-23 ng/mL) (SI: 3.5 nmol/L [0.17-1.00 nmol/L])
Cortisol (8 AM) = 21 μg/dL (5-25 μg/dL) (SI: 579.3 nmol/L [137.9-689.7 nmol/L])
Free T$_4$, normal
TSH, normal
IGF-1, normal

Pituitary MRI shows a 2.3 × 2.2-cm solid mass with suprasellar extension (*see image*). The optic chiasm is displaced upwards.

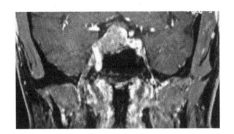

Which of the following is the most appropriate next management step?
- A. Measure macroprolactin
- B. Start therapy with bromocriptine or cabergoline
- C. Refer to neurosurgery
- D. Start testosterone therapy
- E. Measure α subunit

15 You are asked to see a 25-year-old man with a history of intermittent hypercalcemia and kidney stones. He was first noted to have high calcium levels on routine blood work as a teenager, but this resolved on subsequent testing. Over the last 8 years, his serum calcium has ranged from 10.2 to 11.3 mg/dL (2.6-2.8 mmol/L). Although he states that he currently takes no calcium, vitamin A, or vitamin D, he does frequent health food stores for other supplements. He reports at least 5 episodes of kidney stones in the last 2 years. Otherwise he feels well, his weight has been stable, and he has not experienced night sweats or fatigue. A recent chest x-ray was normal. His medical history is otherwise unremarkable and he takes no medications. There is no family history of calcium disorders.

Laboratory test results:
Serum total calcium = 10.7 mg/dL (8.2-10.2 mg/dL) (SI: 2.7 mmol/L [2.1-2.6 mmol/L])
Ionized calcium = 5.1 mg/dL (4.60-5.08 mg/dL) (SI: 1.3 mmol/L [1.2-1.3 mmol/L])
Phosphate = 2.9 mg/dL (2.3-4.7 mg/dL) (SI: 0.9 mmol/L [0.7-1.5 mmol/L])
Magnesium = 2.4 mg/dL (1.5-2.3 mg/dL) (SI: 1.0 mmol/L [0.6-0.9 mmol/L])
Serum creatinine = 1.94 mg/dL (0.6-1.1 mg/dL) (SI: 171.5 μmol/L [53.0-97.2 μmol/L])
PTH = 7 pg/mL (10-65 pg/mL) (SI: 7 ng/L [10-65 ng/L])
PTHrP = <1.5 pg/mL (14-27 pg/mL) (SI: <1.5 ng/L [14-27 ng/L])
25-Hydroxyvitamin D = 24 ng/mL ([optimal] 25-80 ng/mL) (SI: 59.9 nmol/L [62.4-199.7 nmol/L])
1,25-Dihydroxyvitamin D = 112 pg/mL (16-65 pg/mL) (SI: 291.2 pmol/L [41.6-169.0 pmol/L])
24,25-Dihydroxyvitamin D = <0.3 ng/mL (1.6-9.1 ng/mL)
Angiotensin-converting enzyme = 11 U/L (9-67 U/L)

Which of the following is most likely the cause of this patient's hypercalcemia?
- A. Overingestion of over-the-counter cholecalciferol
- B. Sarcoidosis
- C. Lymphoma
- D. Inactivating mutation in the *CYP24A1* gene
- E. Inactivating mutation in the *CASR* gene

16 A 57-year-old man with a history of hypertension, severe osteoarthritis, chronic fatigue, hypothyroidism, type 2 diabetes mellitus, and obesity comes to see you for assistance with weight loss. His diabetes is managed with a multiple daily injection regimen, and his last hemoglobin A_{1c} measurement was 7.0% (53 mmol/mol). The patient has severe osteoarthritis in both knees, which limits his activity. For the past 12 months he has been using an electric wheelchair because of severe pain when he stands.

On physical examination, his height is 67 in (170 cm) and weight is 273 lb (124 kg) (BMI = 42.8 kg/m²). His blood pressure is 130/85 mm Hg, and pulse rate is 84 beats/min. Pulmonary and cardiovascular examination findings are unremarkable. He has reduced range of motion and crepitus bilaterally on knee examination.

Given his current BMI, an orthopedic surgeon deemed that he was not a surgical candidate for knee replacement at this time. The surgeon has agreed to operate once his BMI is below 40 kg/m², which corresponds to a body weight less than 253 lb (<115 kg). During your evaluation, the patient tells you he is interested in a weight-loss program that will help him quickly achieve weight loss, so he can proceed with knee replacement as soon as possible.

Which of the following treatment recommendations would you suggest?
- A. Very low-calorie diet
- B. Low-carbohydrate diet
- C. Lorcaserin
- D. Phentermine
- E. Liraglutide

17 A 48-year-old woman with a 26-year history of type 1 diabetes mellitus follows a basal-bolus insulin injection regimen with insulin glargine at bedtime and premeal insulin lispro. She asks whether one of the newer long-acting insulins would improve her glycemic control. She adjusts insulin lispro doses on the basis of the carbohydrate content of her meals and her measured glucose level. She has tried to maintain tight control since her diagnosis. Diabetes complications have been limited to stable, mild background retinopathy. She measures glucose levels 6 to 8 times daily, always boluses before meals, and closely assesses the carbohydrate content of her meals.

Her hemoglobin A_{1c} measurement today is 7.3% (4.0%-5.6%) (SI: 56 mmol/mol [20-38 mmol/mol]).

Data downloaded from her glucose meter for the past 2 weeks show average premeal glucose levels of 132 mg/dL (7.3 mmol/L) and average postmeal glucose levels of 168 mg/dL (9.3 mmol/L), with moderate glucose variability. Seven percent of the readings are below 70 mg/dL (<3.9 mmol/L).

Switching her regimen from insulin glargine to insulin degludec would be expected to result in reduced:
- A. Postmeal glucose
- B. Hemoglobin A_{1c}
- C. Nocturnal hypoglycemia
- D. Frequency of injections
- E. Microvascular complications

18 A 21-year-old woman presents to the adult clinic for transition of care with a history of congenital adrenal hyperplasia. She has no medical records but reports that she was diagnosed at age 2 months when she required genitoplasty for fused labia. She has been maintained on hydrocortisone, 15 mg in the morning and 10 mg in the evening. She has never required mineralocorticoids. She underwent menarche at age 12 years and has had regular menstrual cycles.

On physical examination, her blood pressure is 148/90 mm Hg and pulse rate is 63 beats/min. Her height is 62 in (157.5 cm), and weight is 172 lb (78.2 kg) (BMI = 31.5 kg/m²). She has acne scars and hyperpigmentation, but no hirsutism. She has no supraclavicular or dorsal cervical adiposity. Breast development is Tanner stage 5. Abdominal examination reveals no striae. Pelvic examination reveals Tanner stage 5 pubic hair development and no masses.

Laboratory test results:
Testosterone = 183 ng/dL (8-60 ng/dL) (SI: 6.35 nmol/L [0.3-2.1 nmol/L])
Androstenedione = 1090 ng/dL (80-240 ng/dL) (SI: 38.06 nmol/L [2.79-8.38 nmol/L])
DHEA-S = 165 μg/dL (44-332 μg/dL) (SI: 4.47 μmol/L [1.19-9.00 μmol/L])
17-Hydroxyprogesterone = 857 ng/dL (<285 ng/dL) (SI: 26.0 nmol/L [<8.64 nmol/L])
11-Deoxycortisol = 22,400 ng/dL (≤33 ng/dL) (SI: 647.4 nmol/L [≤0.95 nmol/L])
11-Deoxycorticosterone = 484 ng/dL (<10 ng/dL) (SI: 14.6 nmol/L [<0.30 nmol/L])
Progesterone = 1.5 ng/mL (≤1.0 ng/mL) (SI: 4.8 nmol/L [≤3.2 nmol/L])

Which of the following is the most likely diagnosis?
- A. Nonclassic 21-hydroxylase deficiency
- B. Classic 21-hydroxylase deficiency
- C. 3β-Hydroxysteroid dehydrogenase deficiency
- D. 11β-hydroxylase deficiency
- E. 17-hydroxylase deficiency

19 A 35-year-old woman is referred with a 6-month history of fatigue, general malaise, and dizziness. She reports intermittent abdominal pain and nausea. Her appetite is poor and she has lost 4.5 lb (2 kg). Type 1 diabetes mellitus was diagnosed at age 11 years and autoimmune hypothyroidism was diagnosed at age 23 years. Her diabetes is controlled with once-daily basal long-acting insulin injection and fixed doses of rapid-acting insulin analogue at mealtimes. In view of frequent episodes of hypoglycemia over the past 3 months, the doses of long- and short-acting insulin have been reduced. Two years ago, celiac disease was diagnosed by small-bowel biopsy. She has 1 daughter (age 6) and has no plans for further pregnancies. She takes levothyroxine, 100 mcg daily, and an ACE-inhibitor. She reports strict adherence to a gluten-free diet.

On physical examination, her height is 64 in (162.6 cm) and weight is 120 lb (54.4 kg) (BMI = 20.6 kg/m^2). When sitting, her blood pressure is 115/63 mm Hg, and pulse rate is 68 beats/min. When standing, her blood pressure is 92/51 mm Hg, and pulse rate is 75 beats/min. She has patches of hyperpigmentation in her mouth, as well as on her elbows and knees. There is no palpable thyroid enlargement in her neck. Findings on systems examination are otherwise unremarkable.

Laboratory test results:
  Sodium = 130 mEq/L (136-142 mEq/L) (SI: 136 mmol/L [136-142 mmol/L])
  Potassium = 5.2 mEq/L (3.5-5.0 mEq/L) (SI: 5.2 mmol/L [3.5-5.0 mmol/L])
  TSH = 1.8 mIU/L (0.5-5.0 mIU/L)
  Free T$_4$ = 1.6 ng/dL (0.8-1.8 ng/dL) (SI: 20.6 pmol/L [10.30-23.17 pmol/L])
  TPO antibodies = 300 IU/mL (<2.0 IU/mL) (SI: 300 kIU/L [<2.0 kIU/L])
  Hemoglobin A$_{1c}$ = 4.3% (4.0%-5.6%) (22.4 mmol/mol [20-38 mmol/mol])
  Random cortisol = 1.8 µg/dL (2-14 µg/dL) (SI: 49.6 nmol/L [55.2-386.2 nmol/L])
  ACTH = 500 pg/mL (10-60 pg/mL) (SI: 110 pmol/L [2.2-13.2 pmol/L])

For which of the following is this patient most at risk?
  A. Chronic candidiasis
  B. Sjogren syndrome
  C. Hypogonadism
  D. Hypoparathyroidism
  E. Alopecia areata

20 You are asked to evaluate a 56-year-old woman with an adrenal mass. Breast cancer (T2 N1 M0) was diagnosed 1 year ago and she is currently on letrozole therapy. She has no other notable health problems and takes no other medications.

On physical examination, she appears well. Her blood pressure is 112/78 mm/Hg. Her height is 65 in (165 cm), and weight is 135 lb (61.4 kg) (BMI = 22.5 kg/m^2). No abnormalities are noted.

Laboratory test results:
  Cortisol (8 AM, after 1 mg overnight dexamethasone suppression
    test) = 1.1 µg/dL (SI: 30.3 nmol/L)
  Metanephrines (plasma fractionated)
    Metanephrine = 22 pg/mL (<57 pg/mL)
      (SI: 111.5 pmol/L [<289 pmol/L])
    Normetanephrine = 112 pg/mL (<148 pg/mL)
      (SI: 611.5 pmol/L [<808 pmol/L])
  Aldosterone = 10 ng/dL (4-21 ng/dL)
    (SI: 277.4 pmol/L [111.0-582.5 pmol/L])
  Plasma renin activity = 1.4 ng/mL per h (0.6-4.3 ng/mL per h)

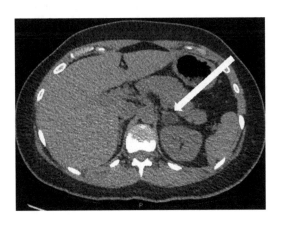

CT of adrenal glands is shown (*see noncontrast image*).

The CT is interpreted as showing a 2.7-cm adrenal adenoma (*arrow*) with a density of –10 Hounsfield units and greater than 50% washout 10 minutes after contrast.

Which of the following is the best step in the management of this patient's adrenal mass?
   A. No further investigation required
   B. Adrenal biopsy
   C. Laparoscopic adrenalectomy
   D. Fluorodeoxyglucose PET CT
   E. Adrenal MRI

21 A 25-year-old man with a history of congenital hypogonadotropic hypogonadism is transferring his endocrine care to your practice. Hypogonadism was diagnosed at age 15 years when he demonstrated no signs of pubertal development. At that time, his testicular volumes were 5 mL each and he had a normal sense of smell. Genetic testing revealed a mutation in the *GNRHR* gene. Puberty was induced with GnRH therapy, which he received for several years. He has been self-administering intramuscular testosterone esters since starting college.

The patient is sexually active with a female partner. He reports a normal libido and erectile function and has no gynecomastia. He is somewhat bothered by changes in his mood several days before his scheduled testosterone injection. He is curious as to whether he is fertile but does not desire children in the next few years.

His only current medication is testosterone cypionate, 150 mg intramuscularly every 2 weeks.

Laboratory test result:
   Total testosterone 7 days after an injection = 380 ng/dL (300-900 ng/dL) (SI: 13.2 nmol/L [10.4-31.2 nmol/L])

On physical examination, his blood pressure is 110/67 mm Hg. His height is 71 in (180 cm), and weight is 170 lb (77.3 kg) (BMI = 23.7 kg/m^2). Testes are 8 mL bilaterally without any masses, and he is well virilized.

Which of the following would you recommend next?
   A. Obtain a baseline semen analysis
   B. Increase the dosage of the testosterone cypionate
   C. Reassess his reproductive axis after stopping testosterone for 4 months
   D. Switch to transdermal testosterone
   E. Switch to hCG therapy

22 A 29-year-old man presented with severe thyrotoxicosis 1 year ago. His presentation was complicated by severe orbitopathy and underlying schizophrenia for which he had recently stopped taking his prescribed medications. His endocrinologist recommended that he undergo thyroidectomy, but he elected to be treated with antithyroid medications. He initially required 60 mg of methimazole daily to control his hyperthyroidism. His thyroid status has varied considerably while on treatment with periods of both undertreatment and overtreatment. However, recently he has been euthyroid while taking 5 mg of methimazole daily. The patient would now like to begin a trial off antithyroid agents to see if he can remain euthyroid. He currently has no symptoms of hyperthyroidism, except for some anxiety. He takes risperidone for his schizophrenia. He takes cholecalciferol for vitamin D deficiency, but he often forgets doses.

On physical examination, his height is 69 in (175.3 cm) and weight is 136 lb (61.8 kg) (BMI = 20.1 kg/m^2). His blood pressure is 108/76 mm Hg, and pulse rate is 88 beats/min. He has moderate proptosis, but no signs of active ophthalmopathy. His thyroid gland is slightly enlarged, but he has no bruit. His deep tendon reflexes are normal. He exhibits restlessness and paces the room during his visit.

His thyroid function test results at the time of diagnosis and current values are shown (*see table*).

Measurement	Time of Assessment	
	At Diagnosis	Now
TSH	<0.001 mIU/L	1.6 mIU/L
Free T$_4$	>7.0 ng/dL (90.1 pmol/L)	1.5 ng/dL (19.3 pmol/L)
Total T$_3$	>800 ng/dL (12.3 nmol/L)	140 ng/dL (2.2 nmol/L)
Thyroid-stimulating immunoglobulin	400%	290%

Reference ranges: TSH, 0.5-5.0 mIU/L; free T$_4$, 0.8-1.8 ng/dL (SI: 10.30-23.17 pmol/L); total T$_3$, 70-200 ng/dL (SI: 1.08-3.08 nmol/L); thyroid-stimulating immunoglobulin, ≤120% of basal activity.

Which of the following factors most directly predicts the likelihood that this patient will experience relapse of his Graves disease while off antithyroid medication?
   A. Vitamin D deficiency
   B. Initial requirement for 60 mg methimazole
   C. Variable adherence to taking medications
   D. Orbitopathy
   E. Current thyroid-stimulating immunoglobulin titer

23 A 32-year-old man has a 12-year history of type 1 diabetes mellitus. Insulin pump therapy was initiated 7 years ago. He has had reasonable glycemic control, with hemoglobin A$_{1c}$ levels ranging from 6.6% to 7.5% (49-58 mmol/mol) over the last 4 years. He has background retinopathy. The total insulin dose per day is 32.6 units; 34% is basal insulin and 66% is bolus and correctional insulin. He takes simvastatin, 20 mg daily. He has 4 to 6 beers per week and does not smoke cigarettes.

He is training for a half marathon, scheduled in 3 months. He runs between 5 and 12 miles in the late afternoon, 6 days per week. He usually leaves his insulin pump on when he trains and does not adjust the rate during the activity. His glucose values are in the range of 113 to 160 mg/dL (6.3-8.9 mmol/L) immediately after most of his runs. He has noted that hypoglycemia occurs 5 to 12 hours after some of the more strenuous runs. He does not have hypoglycemia unawareness, and there has never been a paramedic call to treat severe hypoglycemia. He is able to treat these nocturnal hypoglycemic episodes, but he would like to avoid them if possible.

On physical examination, his height is 72 in (183 cm) and weight is 174 lb (79.1 kg) (BMI = 23.6 kg/m^2). His blood pressure is 112/72 mm Hg, and pulse rate is 56 beats/min. Examination findings are normal except for several tiny dot hemorrhages noted in the left eye.

Laboratory test results:
   Hemoglobin A$_{1c}$ = 7.1% (4.0%-5.6%) (54 mmol/mol [20-38 mmol/mol])
   Creatinine = 1.0 mg/dL (0.7-1.3 mg/dL) (SI: 88.4 μmol/L [61.9-114.9 μmol/L])
   Estimated glomerular filtration rate = >90 mL/min per 1.73 m^2 (>60 mL/min per 1.73 m^2)
   Electrolytes, normal

Which of the following is the best treatment option for this patient?
   A. Ingest carbohydrates to increase glucose to >170 mg/dL (>9.4 mmol/L) before each strenuous run
   B. Lower the basal insulin rate by 50% before each strenuous run
   C. Skip the premeal bolus for the meal after the run
   D. Lower the basal rate for 7 hours after each strenuous run, starting at bedtime
   E. Remove the pump before each run and restart the pump after the run

24 You are asked to evaluate a 60-year-old postmenopausal woman for osteoporosis, which has worsened despite pharmacotherapy. Her first fracture was an elbow fracture in elementary school when she fell on the playground. Her medical history is remarkable for back pain secondary to degenerative disease. Her dental history is extensive. She lost her first baby tooth at age 4 years, and she has recently had loosening of her permanent teeth. She has had significant dental work for caries, abscesses, and cracked teeth. At age 55 years, a screening bone density assessment showed a femoral neck T score of –2.7 and an invalid result in the spine due to artifact from her arthritis and slight scoliosis. She was prescribed weekly risedronate because of additional risk factors for fracture, including a family history of hip fracture and personal history of spontaneous and recurrent metatarsal stress fractures. Follow-up bone densitometry 2 years later showed a 3% decline in hip bone mineral density despite reported adherence to the medication. Daily teriparatide injections were prescribed, and despite adherence to the regimen for the past 18 months, she has sustained additional metatarsal fractures, an ulnar styloid fracture, and a humerus fracture from lifting her infant granddaughter. Her bone pain has worsened and she now requires a cane.

Her current medications include teriparatide, 20 mg daily; calcium carbonate, 600 mg twice daily; and cholecalciferol, 800 IU daily.

Laboratory test results:
Calcium = 10.2 mg/dL (2.55 mmol/L) (8.2-10.2 mg/dL) (SI: 2.6 mmol/L [2.1-2.6 mmol/L])
Phosphate = 4.0 mg/dL (2.3-4.7 mg/dL) (SI: 1.3 mg/dL [0.7-1.5 mmol/L])
PTH = 55 pg/mL (10-65 pg/mL) (SI: 55 ng/L [10-65 ng/L])
Alkaline phosphatase = 27 U/L (50-120 U/L) (SI: 0.5 μkat/L [0.84-2.00 μkat/L])
25-Hydroxyvitamin D = 32 ng/mL (25-80 ng/mL [optimal]) (SI: 79.9 nmol/L [62.4-199.7 nmol/L])
Creatinine = 0.9 mg/dL (0.6-1.1 mg/dL) (SI: 79.6 μmol/L [53.0-97.2 μmol/L])
Urinary N-telopeptide = 18 nmol BCE/mmol creat

Given her worsening clinical scenario on teriparatide, which of the following options would you recommend now?
A. Subcutaneous asfotase alfa
B. Subcutaneous denosumab
C. Intravenous zoledronate
D. Oral raloxifene
E. Nasal calcitonin spray

25 A 47-year-old woman presents to the emergency department with ketoacidosis. Diabetes mellitus was diagnosed at age 35 years. She was initially treated with oral agents, and this regimen was continued with good glycemic control until age 45 years. At that time, she was injured in a motor vehicle crash. Her exercise was subsequently limited, leading to a 20-lb (9.1-kg) weight gain and worsening glycemic control. Insulin was recommended, but she refused. Despite maximum dosages of metformin, glipizide, and sitagliptin, her hemoglobin A_{1c} level remained greater than 9% (>75 mmol/mol). Five days ago, her physician prescribed canagliflozin, 100 mg daily. In addition to the new medication, the patient initiated a low-carbohydrate diet (<50 g per day).

In the emergency department, she has tachycardia, dyspnea, a cough, and mild sinus congestion. On physical examination, her height is 66 in (167.5 cm) and weight is 171.5 lb (78 kg) (BMI = 27.7 kg/m²). Her blood pressure is 134/62 mm Hg, pulse rate is 130 beats/min, respiratory rate is 18 breaths/min, and temperature is 98°F (36.7°C). Her examination findings are normal.

Laboratory test results:
Serum bicarbonate = 8 mEq/L (21-28 mEq/L) (SI: 8 mmol/L [21-28 mmol/L])
Anion gap = 25
Blood glucose = 252 mg/dL (70-99 mg/dL) (SI: 14.0 mmol/L [3.9-5.5 mmol/L])
Urinalysis, strongly positive for ketones and glucose

She is admitted to the hospital and treated with intravenous fluids and intravenous insulin. Canagliflozin is discontinued. This is her first hospital admission for ketoacidosis.

Which of the following is the best next step in this patient's management?
A. Inhaled insulin with meals
B. Once-weekly glucagonlike peptide 1 agonist
C. Insulin via an insulin pump
D. Long-acting basal insulin once daily
E. Acarbose

26 A 45-year-old man is referred by his primary care physician for lipid management after presenting to the emergency department with atypical chest pain a few weeks ago. Workup was negative for a cardiac etiology of chest pain. He has only recently reinitiated health care after not seeing a physician for 8 years. He recalls being told he had low HDL cholesterol 10 years ago, but he was never prescribed therapy. His primary care physician recently diagnosed hypertension and prescribed nifedipine. He takes no other medications or supplements. The patient does not smoke cigarettes and drinks 1 alcoholic beverage per week. He is adopted and therefore no family history is known.

On physical examination, his blood pressure is 130/70 mm Hg. His height is 65.5 in (166.5 cm), and weight is 154 lb (70 kg) (BMI = 25.2 kg/m^2). No hepatosplenomegaly or xanthomas are noted on examination.

Laboratory test results (sample drawn while fasting):
   Total cholesterol = 137 mg/dL (<200 mg/dL [optimal]) (SI: 3.55 mmol/L [<5.18 mmol/L])
   Triglycerides = 212 mg/dL (<150 mg/dL [optimal]) (SI: 2.40 mmol/L [<3.88 mmol/L])
   HDL cholesterol = 15 mg/dL (>60 mg/dL [optimal]) (SI: 0.39 mmol/L [>1.55 mmol/L])
   LDL cholesterol = 80 mg/dL (<130 mg/dL [optimal]) (SI: 2.07 mmol/L [<3.37 mmol/L])
   Non-HDL cholesterol = 122 mg/dL (<130 mg/dL [optimal]) (SI: 3.16 mmol/L [<3.37 mmol/L])
   Hemoglobin A$_{1c}$ = 6.7% (4.0%-5.6%) (50 mmol/mol [20-38 mmol/mol])
   TSH = 2.1 mIU/L (0.5-5.0 mIU/L)
   Plasma glucose = 120 mg/dL (70-99 mg/dL) (SI: 6.7 mmol/L [3.9-5.5 mmol/L])

Which of the following should be recommended now?
A. A statin
B. A fibrate
C. Niacin
D. Pioglitazone
E. No therapy

27 A 34-year-old woman is referred for evaluation of possible Cushing syndrome. She has gained 15 lb (6.8 kg) over the last year and has new-onset hypertension.

On physical examination, her blood pressure is 150/94 mm Hg, her face is plethoric, and she has evidence of retrocervical fat accumulation and facial hirsutism. Her height is 65 in (165 cm), and weight is 196 lb (89 kg) (BMI = 32.6 kg/m^2). Some purple striae are present on her abdomen.

Laboratory test results:
   Urinary free cortisol = 270 μg/24 h (4-50 μg/24 h) (SI: 745.2 nmol/d [11-138 nmol/d])
   Potassium = 3.2 mEq/L (3.5-5.0 mEq/L) (SI: 3.2 mmol/L [3.5-5.0 mmol/L])
   Sodium = 138 mEq/L (136-142 mEq/L) (SI: 138 mmol/L [136-142 mmol/L])
   ACTH = 59 pg/mL (10-60 pg/mL) (SI: 13.0 pmol/L [2.2-13.2 pmol/L])

Which of the following is the most appropriate next diagnostic step?
A. Inferior petrosal sinus sampling
B. Bedtime salivary cortisol measurement
C. Combined dexamethasone–corticotropin-releasing hormone test
D. Low-dose dexamethasone suppression test
E. Pituitary MRI

28 A 62-year-old woman presents to the emergency department with a 2-month history of progressively declining appetite, nausea with occasional vomiting, and unintentional weight loss of 20 lb (9.1 kg). She has debilitating arthralgias and bone pain that have limited her activity such that for the last week, she has barely been able to get out of bed. She feels lethargic and thirsty. She has had constipation, and her last bowel movement was about 1 week ago. She has had no syncopal episodes but does feel light-headed. She has smoked 1 pack of cigarettes per day for the last 40 years.

On physical examination, she is an ill-appearing woman who looks older than her stated age. She is afebrile, blood pressure is 98/58 mm Hg, pulse rate is 116 beats/min, and respiratory rate is 20 breaths/min. Her weight is 171.5 lb (78 kg), and height is not measured because she is unable to stand. She has dry mucous membranes and skin tenting. Palpation of the neck reveals a 2-cm mass on the left lower neck. Cardiac examination is notable only for sinus tachycardia. There are no active bowel sounds, and she has a diffusely tender abdomen with no fluid wave.

Laboratory test results:
Electrolytes, normal
Serum urea nitrogen = 36 mg/dL (8-23 mg/dL) (SI: 12.9 mmol/L [2.9-8.2 mmol/L])
Creatinine = 1.9 mg/dL (0.6-1.1 mg/dL) (SI: 168.0 µmol/L [53.0-97.2 µmol/L])
Estimated glomerular filtration rate = 34 mL/min per 1.73 m^2 (>60 mL/min per 1.73 m^2)
Calcium = 14.0 mg/dL (8.2-10.2 mg/dL) (SI: 3.5 mmol/L [2.1-2.6 mmol/L])
Phosphate = 2.3 mg/dL (2.3-4.7 mg/dL) (SI: 0.7 mmol/L [0.7-1.5 mmol/L])
Albumin = 4.2 g/dL (3.5-5.0 g/dL) (SI: 42 g/L [35-50 g/L])

Chest x-ray is negative for any lung masses or consolidations. CT of the neck without contrast shows a 3-cm mass inferior to the left lobe of the thyroid (*see image*).

You admit the patient to the hospital for continuous intravenous fluid hydration and medical management of hypercalcemia.

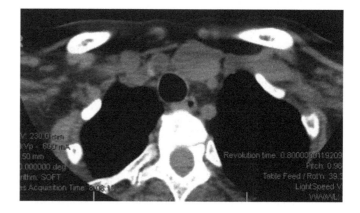

Which of the following is the best test to order next to identify the underlying cause of her hypercalcemia?
A. Serum protein electrophoresis
B. Intact PTH measurement
C. Sestamibi scintigraphy
D. 25-Hydroxyvitamin D measurement
E. FNAB of the left lower neck mass

29 A 54-year-old woman presents with weight gain, muscle weakness, and insomnia. She describes gaining 25 lb (11.4 kg) over the last 3 months despite dieting and exercise. During this time, she has also noted difficulty sleeping and not having the strength to climb stairs.

On physical examination, her blood pressure is 154/92 mm Hg and pulse rate is 90 beats/min. Her height is 64 in (162.6 cm), and weight is 200 lb (90.9 kg) (BMI = 34.3 kg/m²). She has truncal obesity, moon facies, a dorsocervical fat pad, abdominal striae, and proximal muscle weakness.

Laboratory test results:
   Urinary free cortisol = 241 µg/24 h (4-50 µg/24 h) (SI: 665.2 nmol/d [11-138 nmol/d]).
   Morning ACTH = 75 pg/mL (10-60 pg/mL) (SI: 16.5 pmol/L [2.2-13.2 pmol/L])
   Morning serum cortisol = 43 µg/dL (5-25 µg/dL) (SI: 1186.3 nmol/L [137.9-689.7 nmol/L])
   1-mg dexamethasone suppression test, AM cortisol = 8.9 µg/dL (245.5 nmol/L)
   8-mg dexamethasone suppression test, AM cortisol = 2.1 µg/dL (57.9 nmol/L)

Review of her records shows that she underwent an abdominal CT 4 months earlier when she presented with abdominal pain. A 2.4-cm right adrenal mass (5 Hounsfield units on unenhanced attenuation) consistent with an adrenal adenoma was noted at that time.

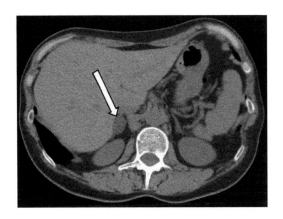

Which of the following is the most appropriate next step?
   A. Abdominal CT with adrenal washout protocol
   B. Chest CT
   C. Octreotide scan
   D. Brain MRI
   E. Adrenal venous sampling

30 You are consulted regarding a 56-year-old woman with a 10-year history of type 2 diabetes mellitus. She has a history of chronic pancreatitis for which she recently underwent partial pancreatectomy. Following the procedure, she continued to experience nausea and epigastric pain with ingestion of food. There is no evidence of gastric outlet obstruction, small-bowel obstruction, or other etiology for her symptoms.

Jejunal tube feeds via a gastrostomy-jejunostomy tube are initiated around the clock. She is tolerating this well, and she has reached the goal rate in 24 hours. She is treated with a combination of insulin glargine, 20 units, and supplemental scale (with regular insulin) every 6 hours. The regular insulin daily dose totals 10 to 14 units daily. With this regimen, her blood glucose measurements are in the range of 130 to 160 mg/dL (7.2-8.9 mmol/L). You are consulted regarding insulin management as the surgical team plans to change her to a nighttime tube feeding regimen from 8 PM to 8 AM. Total calories in the nocturnal feeding regimen will be 80% of that in the 24-hour regimen. The surgical team is hoping to discharge her home on this regimen.

Which of the following regimens would be most appropriate for treating hyperglycemia associated with tube feeds in this patient?
   A. Maintain the current regimen of insulin glargine and supplemental scale with regular insulin every 6 hours
   B. Switch to NPH insulin at the start of tube feeds and use supplemental scale with regular insulin every 6 hours
   C. Maintain insulin glargine, 20 units, but use supplemental scale with insulin aspart every 6 hours
   D. Stop long-acting insulin and use only insulin aspart every 4 hours
   E. Stop long-acting insulin and use only supplemental scale with regular insulin every 6 hours

31 A 32-year-old man seeks further management of advanced papillary thyroid cancer. At age 11 years, he was treated for Hodgkin lymphoma with chemotherapy and mantle radiotherapy. Papillary thyroid carcinoma with neck node involvement was diagnosed 2 years ago (American Joint Committee on Cancer stage T3 N1b M0), and he underwent total thyroidectomy and left lateral compartment neck node dissection followed by radioactive iodine remnant ablation with a 100-mCi dose of ^{131}I. Six months after treatment, he developed recurrent left cervical and mediastinal lymphadenopathy, as well as low-volume lung metastases. He has received 3 doses of radioiodine therapy in the last 18 months and has been given a total ^{131}I dose of 550 mCi. He takes levothyroxine, 175 mcg daily, and nonsteroidal anti-inflammatory agents for increasing back and left-sided hip pain.

On physical examination, his height is 71 in (180.3 cm) and weight is 172 lb (78.2 kg) (BMI = 24 kg/m^2). His blood pressure is 128/74 mm Hg, and pulse rate is 68 beats/min. He has a visible thyroidectomy scar but no palpable thyroid enlargement and no palpable cervical lymphadenopathy. Lung fields are clear to auscultation, and he has tenderness over his lumbar spine and pelvic bones.

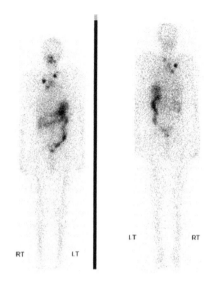

Laboratory test results:
  TSH = <0.01 mIU/L (0.5-5.0 mIU/L)
  Free T$_4$ = 2.1 ng/dL (27 pmol/L) (0.8-1.8 ng/dL)
    (SI: 27.0 pmol/L [10.30-23.17 pmol/L])
  Unstimulated thyroglobulin = 738 ng/mL (<0.1 ng/mL)
    (SI: 738 µg/L) [<0.1 µg/L])

A ^{131}I whole-body single-photon emission CT shows several areas of marked iodine accumulation in the left supraclavicular fossa, the right side of the mediastinum, the right hilum, and the right upper lung (*see image*). PET-CT shows fluorodeoxyglucose-avid skeletal metastatic disease in the right scapula, several ribs, thoracolumbar vertebra, pelvis, the right vertebral body of L5, and the sacrum (*see image*).

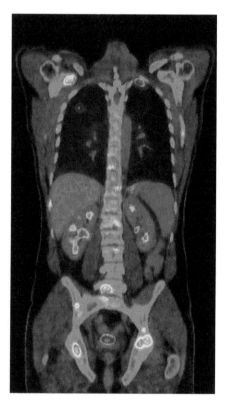

Which of the following is the best next step?
  A. An additional 150 mCi dose of ^{131}I
  B. Systemic chemotherapy with doxorubicin and cisplatin
  C. High-dosage glucocorticoids
  D. Tyrosine kinase inhibitor therapy
  E. Thalidomide therapy

32 A 22-year-old woman seeks treatment for infertility. She and her husband have been trying to conceive for the past year without success. She had axillary and pubic hair development at age 11 years, but had no breast development and never had spontaneous menses. Subsequently, she was treated with hormone replacement therapy (estradiol and progesterone) starting at age 16 years, which induced breast development and menses. She has no anosmia, hirsutism, acne, galactorrhea, headaches, or vasomotor flushes. She does not exercise and has no history of an eating disorder.

On physical examination, her blood pressure is 110/60 mm Hg. Her height is 62.5 in (158.8 cm), and weight is 114 lb (51.8 kg) (BMI = 20.5 kg/m^2). Her breast development is Tanner stage 5, and she has no masses or galactorrhea. Pelvic examination demonstrates Tanner stage 5 pubic hair, a small uterus, and nonpalpable ovaries.

Laboratory test results:

LH = <1.0 mIU/mL (1.0-18.0 mIU/mL) (SI: <1.0 IU/L [1.0-18.0 IU/L])
FSH = <2.0 mIU/mL (2.0-12.0 mIU/mL) (SI: <2.0 IU/L [2.0-12.0 IU/L])
Estradiol = <10 pg/mL (10-180 pg/mL) (SI: <36.7 pmol/L [36.7-660.8 pmol/L])
Prolactin = 10 ng/mL (4-30 ng/mL) (SI: 0.43 nmol/L [0.17-1.30 nmol/L])
TSH = 1.2 mIU/L (0.5-5.0 mIU/L)
Free T_4 = 0.9 ng/dL (0.8-1.8 ng/dL) (SI: 11.6 pmol/L [10.30-23.17 pmol/L])
Cortisol (8 AM) = 19.9 μg/dL (>18 μg/dL) (SI: 549.0 nmol/L [>496.6 nmol/L])

MRI of the pituitary and hypothalamus is normal.

Which of the following is the best treatment for this patient's infertility?
A. Estradiol and progesterone
B. Letrozole
C. Clomiphene citrate
D. Recombinant FSH
E. Human menopausal gonadotropin

33 A 43-year-old man is referred to you for management of obesity. Despite attempting lifestyle modification for 6 months, he has not lost weight. His primary care physician prescribed phentermine, 37.5 mg daily, and he has been taking this medication for 12 weeks. He reports a 12-lb (5.5-kg) weight loss since starting phentermine and is happy with the response. His only complaint has been increased insomnia. He has a history of depression and hypertension but is otherwise healthy. His medications include lisinopril, 20 mg daily, and fluoxetine, 20 mg daily.

On physical examination, his blood pressure is 148/92 mm Hg and pulse rate is 84 beats/min. His height is 69.7 in (177 cm), and weight is 264 lb (120 kg) (BMI = 38.2 kg/m²). He is healthy appearing. He does not have a rounded face, but he does have acanthosis nigricans on neck examination. There are no abdominal striae. The rest of his examination findings are normal. His last hemoglobin A_{1c} measurement at his primary care clinic 2 days ago was 6.9% (52 mmol/mol).

In addition to continuing healthful eating and regular exercise, which of the following is the best recommendation now?
A. Continue phentermine at the same dosage
B. Continue phentermine at the same dosage and add metoprolol, 50 mg twice daily
C. Stop phentermine and continue lifestyle modification
D. Stop phentermine and start lorcaserin, 10 mg twice daily
E. Stop phentermine and start liraglutide, increasing the dosage as tolerated to 3 mg daily

34 A 33-year-old man presents to discuss his androgen levels. Two years ago, he began a weight-lifting program but was not satisfied with his muscle growth. He did some reading online and spoke with several bodybuilders and fitness trainers. He decided to begin a compounded mixture of trenbolone, nandrolone, and testosterone cypionate that he obtained online from another country. He administers this regimen via intramuscular injection once weekly in addition to intramuscular hCG. While on this regimen, the patient has noticed increased muscle mass, less fat mass, and increased libido. His significant other has commented that he is more aggressive at times. The patient goes to the gym 5 to 6 days per week and drinks 4 alcoholic beverages per week.

He takes no prescription medications but does take several supplements for bodybuilding.

On physical examination, his blood pressure is 137/85 mm Hg. His height is 67 in (170 cm), and weight is 202 lb (92 kg) (BMI = 31.6 kg/m²). He is very muscular and has no gynecomastia. Testes are 15 mL bilaterally without masses.

Laboratory test results:

Total testosterone = 918 ng/dL (300-900 ng/dL) (SI: 31.9 nmol/L [10.4-31.2 nmol/L])
Bioavailable testosterone = 767 ng/dL (128-430 ng/dL) (SI: 26.6 nmol/L [4.4-14.9 nmol/L])

On further questioning, the patient admits to taking something else. Which of the following is he most likely taking?

    A. Anastrozole
    B. Clomiphene citrate
    C. Recombinant FSH
    D. Oxandrolone
    E. Stanozolol

35 A 43-year-old woman is referred to you for "treatment-resistant hyperthyroidism." Her primary care physician diagnosed hyperthyroidism 6 months ago and methimazole was prescribed. Despite escalation of her dosage, she remained biochemically hyperthyroid. Ultimately, the patient decided to discontinue her antithyroid medication, as she felt worse while on therapy. Today, the patient feels well and has no symptoms of hyperthyroidism.

On physical examination, her blood pressure is 125/76 mm Hg and pulse rate is 74 beats/min. Her height is 63 in (160 cm), and weight is 124 lb (56.4 kg) (BMI = 22 kg/m^2). Her thyroid gland is of normal size and texture. She has no tremor of her outstretched hands and has normal patellar reflexes.

She does not take any prescribed medications. She does, however, take several over-the-counter supplements and provides you with a list, which includes large doses of the following: ginkgo, biotin, valerian, and bladderwrack.

Serial thyroid function blood test results are shown (*see table*).

Measurement	Time of Assessment			
	6 Months Ago (No Therapy)	3 Months Ago (On Methimazole)	2 Months Ago (Increased Methimazole Dosage)	Today (No Therapy)
TSH	0.01 mIU/L	0.01 mIU/L	0.02 mIU/L	0.01 mIU/L
Free T$_4$	3.4 ng/dL (43.8 pmol/L)	3.7 ng/dL 47.6 pmol/L)	3.3 ng/dL (42.5 pmol/L)	3.5 ng/dL (45.0 pmol/L)
Total T$_3$	500 ng/dL (7.7 nmol/L)	550 ng/dL (8.47 nmol/L)	560 ng/dL (8.6 nmol/L)	510 ng/dL (7.9 nmol/L)

Reference ranges: TSH, 0.5-5.0 mIU/L; free T$_4$, 0.8-1.8 ng/dL (SI: 10.30-23.17 pmol/L); total T$_3$, 70-200 ng/dL (SI: 1.08-3.08 nmol/L).

Which of the following is the best next step to diagnose this patient's condition?

    A. Fecal levothyroxine measurement
    B. Repeated thyroid testing after discontinuation of the patient's supplements
    C. ^{123}I thyroid scan and uptake
    D. Urinary iodine measurement
    E. T$_3$ suppression test

36 A 44-year-old woman with diabetes mellitus is admitted to the hospital with diabetic ketoacidosis. Progress notes from her primary care physician suggest that she has a history of long-term nonadherence to her treatment regimen. Diabetes mellitus was diagnosed 4 years ago, and she was initially treated with metformin and sitagliptin, and then switched to insulin glargine 3 months later. She was given a prescription for premeal rapid-acting insulin, which she has never filled. Her current medications include bupropion; fluoxetine; gabapentin; levothyroxine; phentermine; tapentadol; insulin aspart; and insulin glargine, 15 units every morning. She does not check her glucose levels daily, but when she does, the values are greater than 300 mg/dL (>16.7 mmol/L).

She has been losing weight, but she also notes that she eats infrequently. She is stressed with work and she wonders whether this has contributed to her high blood glucose values. She expresses anger that her boss does not allow her to take breaks to check her blood glucose or to administer insulin injections. The patient states that no one educated her about her diagnosis or the treatment necessary to improve symptoms. However, review of her medical records shows that she has seen a diabetes educator and that she participated in group diabetes education classes. Her hospital record documents that she requested and has been given opioids daily for abdominal pain.

She reports no nausea, vomiting, or abdominal pain at this time. She states that she does not induce vomiting and does not binge eat. She last saw her endocrinologist 6 months ago, and she has no follow-up appointment scheduled. Review of systems is notable for fatigue, insomnia, reduced pleasure in normal activities, and feeling angry about having diabetes. She expresses having muscle pain "all over."

On physical examination, her blood pressure is 109/72 mm Hg and pulse rate is 78 beats/min. Her height is 62 in (157.5 cm), and weight is 116.5 lb (53 kg) (BMI = 21.3 kg/m^2). Examination findings are normal.

Which of the following is the most likely underlying diagnosis?
   A. Depression
   B. Eating disorder
   C. Factitious disorder
   D. Narcotic abuse
   E. Fibromyalgia

37 A 46-year-old man with longstanding type 2 diabetes mellitus presents to discuss his worsening sexual function. Over the past 8 years, his erectile function has gradually declined. Several years ago, he was prescribed tadalafil, 20 mg, as needed for treatment of erectile dysfunction. The medication initially improved his erectile function but this is no longer the case. He has been married for 12 years and has fathered one child. He reports a healthy relationship with his wife and has sexual thoughts daily. He reports no depressive symptoms.

His current medications are atorvastatin, insulin glargine, lisinopril, and metformin.

On physical examination, his blood pressure is 134/88 mm Hg. His height is 69 in (175 cm), and weight is 192 lb (87 kg) (BMI = 28.4 kg/m^2). Physical examination findings are unremarkable. Testes are 20 mL bilaterally without masses.

Laboratory test results:
   Hemoglobin A$_{1c}$ = 7.3% (4.0%-5.6%) (56 mmol/mol [20-38 mmol/mol])
   Total testosterone (8 AM) = 295 ng/dL (300-900 ng/dL) (SI: 10.2 nmol/L [10.4-31.2 nmol/L])

Which of the following would you recommend next for treatment of his erectile dysfunction?
   A. Alprostadil (intracavernosal injection)
   B. Papaverine (intracavernosal injection)
   C. Sildenafil (oral)
   D. Testosterone cypionate (intramuscular injection)
   E. Vacuum constriction device

38 A 24-year-old man is referred to you because of polyuria and polydipsia. He reports drinking 2 to 3 gallons of water daily and urinating a similar amount. He has had this problem for about 10 years, but it has become much worse during the past 6 months. He urinates 2 to 3 times at night. He has a history of depression and currently takes fluoxetine. He is otherwise healthy and has no history of head trauma, weight change, cold intolerance, or erectile dysfunction.

Physical examination findings are normal. His blood pressure is 126/80 mm Hg, and pulse rate is 78 beats/min. His height is 70 in (178 cm), and weight is 215.5 lb (98 kg) (BMI = 30.9 kg/m^2).

Laboratory test results:

Glucose = 112 mg/dL (70-99 mg/dL) (SI: 6.2 mmol/L [3.9-5.5 mmol/L])
Calcium 9.1 mg/dL (8.2-10.2 mg/dL) (SI: 2.3 mmol/L [2.1-2.6 mmol/L])
Sodium = 136 mEq/L (136-142 mEq/L) (SI: 136 mmol/L [136-142 mmol/L])
Uric acid = 3.3 mg/dL (3.5-7.0 mg/dL) (SI: 196.3 μmol/L [208.2-416.4 μmol/L])
Plasma osmolality = 279 mOsm/kg (275-295 mOsm/kg) (SI: 279 mmol/kg [275-295 mmol/kg])
Urine osmolality = 220 mOsm/kg (150-1150 mOsm/kg) (SI: 220 mmol/kg [150-1150 mmol/kg])
Urine glucose, negative

Which of the following is the most likely diagnosis?
A. Nephrogenic diabetes insipidus
B. Primary polydipsia
C. Central diabetes insipidus
D. Syndrome of inappropriate antidiuretic hormone secretion
E. Hyperglycemia

39 A 32-year-old man presents for lipid management. He reports a history of elevated cholesterol detected at age 12 years. He was prescribed colestipol and subsequently lovastatin, which he took until age 18 years. His regimen was then switched to rosuvastatin, and ezetimibe was soon added. He is adopted and therefore family history is unknown. He does not smoke cigarettes or drink alcohol.

On physical examination, his blood pressure is 124/80 mm Hg. His height is 66.5 in (169 cm), and weight is 196 lb (89 kg) (BMI = 31.2 kg/m²). Xanthelasma are present over the left upper and lower eyelids, and you note several tendon xanthomas in both Achilles tendons and dorsum of the hands bilaterally.

Laboratory test results are shown (samples drawn while fasting) (*see table*).

Measurement	No Therapy	On Rosuvastatin, 40 mg Daily	On Rosuvastatin, 40 mg Daily, and Ezetimibe, 10 mg Daily	Reference Ranges
Total cholesterol	473 mg/dL (12.25 mmol/L)	417 mg/dL (10.80 mmol/L)	393 mg/dL (10.18 mmol/L)	<200 mg/dL (optimal) (SI: <5.18 mmol/L)
Triglycerides	133 mg/dL (1.28 mmol/L)	95 mg/dL (1.07 mmol/L)	97 mg/dL 1.10 mmol/L)	<150 mg/dL (optimal) (SI: <3.88 mmol/L)
HDL cholesterol	41 mg/dL (1.06 mmol/L)	38 mg/dL (0.98 mmol/L)	42 mg/dL (1.09 mmol/L)	>60 mg/dL (optimal) (SI: >1.55 mmol/L)
LDL cholesterol	405 mg/dL (10.49 mmol/L)	360 mg/dL (9.32 mmol/L)	332 mg/dL (8.60 mmol/L)	<100 mg/dL (optimal) (SI: <2.59 mmol/L)
Non-HDL cholesterol	432 mg/dL (11.19 mmol/L)	379 mg/dL (9.82 mmol/L)	351 mg/dL (9.09 mmol/L)	<130 mg/dL (optimal) (SI: <3.37 mmol/L)
Apolipoprotein B	...	285 mg/dL (2.85 g/L)	...	50-110 mg/dL (SI: 0.5-1.1 g/L)
Hemoglobin A$_{1c}$	...	5.3% (34 mmol/mol)	...	4.0%-5.6% (20-38 mmol/mol)
TSH	...	1.2 mIU/L	...	0.5-5.0 mIU/L

Which of the following should you add as the best next step in this patient's management?
A. Evolocumab
B. Niacin
C. Colesevelam
D. Fenofibrate
E. Lipoprotein apheresis

40 You are asked to consult on a 68-year-old man with a history of hypertension but no regular medical care who presented to the emergency department with worsening back pain and obstructive urinary symptoms. His only medication is hydrochlorothiazide, 50 mg daily. CT showed a large necrotic prostate mass with metastases to the pelvis and spine. He was admitted to the hospital on the medical oncology service. Laboratory test results at hospital admission were notable for hypercalcemia with a calcium concentration of 15.1 mg/dL (8.2-10.2 mg/dL) (SI: 3.8 mmol/L [2.1-2.6 mmol/L]), and he was given 4 mg of intravenous zoledronic acid. Additionally, high-dosage dexamethasone was initiated for spinal cord compromise, and high-dosage ketoconazole was initiated for rapid medical castration. You are asked to see him, as he has been symptomatically hypocalcemic for 4 days since his admission despite frequent infusions of calcium gluconate, 1 g intravenously.

On physical examination, he is thin and has temporal wasting. His blood pressure is 109/61 mm Hg, pulse rate is 89 beats/min, respiratory rate is 14 breaths/min, and oxygen saturation is 94% on room air. When you tap the skin over his facial nerve, contractions are seen. His reflexes are brisk.

Laboratory test results:
Serum total calcium = 5.6 mg/dL (8.2-10.2 mg/dL) (SI: 1.4 mmol/L [2.1-2.6 mmol/L])
Ionized calcium = 2.9 mg/dL (4.60-5.08 mg/dL) (SI: 0.7 mmol/L [1.2-1.3 mmol/L])
Phosphate = 1.7 mg/dL (2.3-4.7 mg/dL) (SI: 0.5 mmol/L [0.7-1.5 mmol/L])
Serum creatinine = 1.3 mg/dL (0.7-1.3 mg/dL) (SI: 114.9 µmol/L [61.9-114.9 µmol/L])
Alkaline phosphatase = 81 U/L (50-120 U/L) (SI: 1.35 µkat/L [0.84-2.00 µkat/L])
PTH = 245 pg/mL (10-65 pg/mL) (SI: 245 ng/L [10-65 ng/L])
PTHrP = 34.9 pg/mL (14-27 pg/mL) (SI: 34.9 ng/L [14-27 ng/L])
Magnesium = 2.0 mg/dL (1.5-2.3 mg/dL) (SI: 0.8 mmol/L [0.6-0.9 mmol/L])
Albumin = 2.9 g/dL (3.5-5.0 g/dL) (SI: 29 g/L [35-50 g/L])
25-Hydroxyvitamin D = <8 ng/mL ([optimal] 25-80 ng/mL) (SI: <20.0 nmol/L [62.4-199.7 nmol/L])

In addition to this patient's vitamin D deficiency, which other factor had a role in his severe hypocalcemia after bisphosphonate infusion?
  A. Ketoconazole
  B. Osteolytic metastases
  C. Adrenal insufficiency
  D. Hypomagnesemia
  E. Thiazide diuretic use

41 You are asked for advice on a 33-year-old man who has recently moved to your area. His primary care physician documented abnormal thyroid function during a routine health maintenance appointment. The patient reports that he underwent workup for a thyroid problem 5 years ago but that he was never treated. He reports occasional palpitations, but he is otherwise well and asymptomatic. A number of his relatives are treated for thyrotoxicosis.

On physical examination, his height is 73 in (185.4 cm) and weight is 180 lb (81.8 kg) (BMI = 23.7 kg/m²). His blood pressure is 127/96 mm Hg, and pulse rate is 78 beats/min with a regular rhythm. There is no tremor but he has a small, diffuse, palpable goiter. There are no clinical signs of thyroid ophthalmopathy.

Laboratory test results:
TSH = 1.25 mIU/L (0.5-5.0 mIU/L)
Free T$_4$ = 4.2 ng/dL (0.8-1.8 ng/dL) (SI: 54.06 pmol/L [10.30-23.17 pmol/L])
Free T$_3$ = 9.1 pg/mL (2.3-4.2 pg/mL) (SI: 13.98 pmol/L [3.53-6.45 pmol/L]))

Subsequent review of his records at a different hospital confirms the presence of a mutation in the thyroid receptor β gene (*THRB*) (exon 9 [Met310Leu]).

Which of the following is the best next step?
A. Start methimazole
B. Start methimazole and levothyroxine in a block-and-replace regimen
C. Total thyroidectomy
D. Perform ^{131}I radioactive iodine ablation
E. No further treatment

42 A 25-year-old woman with type 1 diabetes mellitus diagnosed at age 5 years wants to discuss her plans for pregnancy. She has had hemoglobin A_{1c} levels ranging from 8.0% to 9.4% (64-79 mmol/mol) over the past 4 years, but she has recently worked on her carbohydrate counting and insulin dosing as she is aware that better glucose control is important for pregnancy. She is sexually active and is not using contraception. Her only medications are insulin glargine and insulin aspart. Her last eye examination was several years ago.

On physical examination, her blood pressure is 130/66 mm Hg and pulse rate is 72 beats/min. Her height is 64 in (162.5 cm), and weight is 124 lb (56.5 kg) (BMI = 21.3 kg/m²). She has no retinopathy on nondilated examination, and findings on heart and lung examination are normal. She has decreased sensation to monofilament testing in her feet.

Laboratory test results:
Hemoglobin A_{1c} = 7.2% (4.0%-5.6%) (55 mmol/mol [20-38 mmol/mol])
Creatinine = 1.2 mg/dL (0.6-1.1 mg/dL) (SI: 106.1 µmol/L [53.0-97.2 µmol/L])
TSH = 2.3 mIU/L (0.5-5.0 mIU/L)
Urinary albumin-to-creatinine ratio = 65 mg/g (<30 mg/g)
Estimated glomerular filtration rate = 65 mL/min per 1.73 m² (>60 mL/min per 1.73 m²)
Pregnancy test, negative

In addition to starting a prenatal vitamin and folic acid supplementation, which of the following is the best next step in this patient's care?
A. Initiate insulin pump therapy
B. Initiate labetalol
C. Initiate levothyroxine
D. Measure proteinuria in a 24-hour collection
E. Recommend a retinal examination

43 A 38-year-old man has had refractory hypertension (blood pressure >190/100 mm Hg) for 3 years despite taking 4 antihypertensive medications. His potassium has always been very low (approximately 2.4 mEq/L [2.4 mmol/L]). Biochemical studies reveal that plasma renin activity and serum aldosterone are both below the limit of assay detection:

Plasma renin activity = <0.6 ng/mL per h (0.6-4.3 ng/mL per h)
Serum aldosterone = <4 ng/dL (4-21 ng/dL) (SI: <111.0 pmol/L [111.0-582.5 pmol/L])

The patient reports drinking approximately 1 L of herbal tea every day that is enriched with glycyrrhizic acid (real licorice root). After discontinuing tea drinking for 3 weeks, his blood pressure is noted to be 138/70 mm Hg on only 1 antihypertensive medication.

Which of the following hormones was most likely contributing to this patient's hypertension and hypokalemia when he was drinking his tea on a daily basis?
- A. 11-Deoxycortisol
- B. Deoxycorticosterone
- C. Angiotensin II
- D. ACTH
- E. Cortisol

44 A 29-year-old woman is referred to you because of hyperprolactinemia. She has been feeling tired for several months, and 3 months ago her menses disappeared and she noted expressible galactorrhea. She has had some scalp hair loss and has gained 4.5 lb (2 kg) over 3 months. On review of systems, she reports reduced frequency of bowel movements.

On physical examination, her blood pressure is 115/90 mm Hg and pulse rate is 54 beats/min. Her height is 65 in (165 cm), and weight is 158.5 lb (72 kg) (BMI = 26.4 kg/m²). There are no features of acromegaly or Cushing syndrome. The thyroid is not enlarged. Findings on cardiac and lung examination are normal.

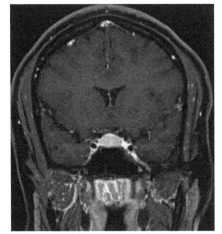

Laboratory test results:
>   Pregnancy test, negative
>   Prolactin = 72 ng/mL (4-30 ng/mL) (SI: 3.1 nmol/L [0.17-1.30 nmol/L])

Pituitary MRI shows an enlarged gland (1.0 × 1.5 cm) with some extension in the suprasellar area, but no chiasmatic compression (*see image*). The radiologist's interpretation is that it is consistent with a pituitary adenoma.

Which of the following is the best next step in this patient's evaluation?
- A. Measure serum IGF-1
- B. Refer to neurosurgery
- C. Perform an ACTH stimulation test to evaluate adrenal reserve
- D. Measure TSH and free T₄
- E. Arrange for a neuro-ophthalmology consultation

45 A 78-year-old woman is a longstanding patient of yours with type 2 diabetes mellitus who returns for routine follow-up. She is concerned that her usual regimen of oral diabetes medications does not appear to be working. Over the last 2 weeks, despite adherence to her treatment regimen, her home glucose values have increased from the usual range of 100-180 mg/dL (5.6-10.0 mmol/L) to 290-300 mg/dL (16.1-16.7 mmol/L). The patient reports that her diet and exercise routine has not changed. She has lost 10 lb (4.5 kg) over the past few months, which she cannot explain.

Her diabetes is complicated by peripheral neuropathy. She also has hypertension, atrial flutter, hypothyroidism, and a history of lung cancer (status post thoracotomy and chemotherapy 7 years ago). Her current diabetes medications are metformin, 500 mg twice daily; glimepiride, 2 mg daily; and pioglitazone, 30 mg daily. She has never used insulin. She has not started any new corticosteroids or steroid-acting medications. The patient lives alone and has several children who check on her regularly.

On physical examination, she is alert and knowledgeable about her diabetes. Her blood pressure is 140/90 mm Hg, and pulse rate is 90 beats/min. Her height is 69 in (175.3 cm), and weight is 130 lb (59.1 kg) (BMI = 19.2 kg/m²). There is mild muscle wasting in her arms and legs.

Laboratory test results:
   Hemoglobin A$_{1c}$ 3 months ago = 8.0% (4.0%-5.6%) (64 mmol/mol [20-38 mmol/mol])
   Hemoglobin A$_{1c}$ today = 11% (4.0%-5.6%) (97 mmol/mol [20-38 mmol/mol])
   TSH = 2.0 mIU/L (0.5-5.0 mIU/L)
   Free T$_4$ = 1.4 ng/dL (0.8-1.8 ng/dL) (SI: 18.0 pmol/L [10.30-23.17 pmol/L])
   Cortisol (8 AM) = 18 µg/dL (5-25 µg/dL) (SI: 496.6 nmol/L [137.9-689.7 nmol/L])

You are concerned that she may have an underlying malignancy that has caused deterioration in her glycemic control. Which of the following tests is most likely to reveal the underlying cause?
   A. Mammography
   B. Whole-body PET/CT
   C. Abdominal CT
   D. Chest CT
   E. Colonoscopy

46 A 61-year-old woman presents to her physician with a 3-week history of weight loss, palpitations, and sweating. She is healthy except for a diagnosis of osteoarthritis and is not taking any medications or supplements. She lives on a farm with her spouse where they raise livestock and grow agricultural produce, which they use for their own consumption. She describes having had 2 previous episodes of similar symptoms over the last 5 years that resolved spontaneously. Her weight has decreased by 8.8 lb (4 kg) over the last 6 months.

On physical examination, she has tachycardia with a pulse rate of 112 beats/min and a tremor of her hands. Her thyroid gland is not enlarged and is nontender; there is no evidence of a bruit. She has no signs of orbitopathy or dermopathy.

Laboratory test results:
   TSH = 0.1 mIU/L (0.5-5.0 mIU/L)
   Free T$_4$ = 2.7 ng/dL (0.8-1.8 ng/dL) (SI: 34.8 pmol/L [10.30-23.17 pmol/L])

A radioactive iodine uptake and scan shows very low uptake. A serum thyroglobulin measurement is low.

At the time of her follow-up visit to her physician 8 weeks later, the patient reports that her symptoms have resolved. Repeated thyroid testing confirms that her serum TSH level is now 0.39 mIU/L and her free T$_4$ level is normal.

Which of the following is the most likely explanation for this patient's thyrotoxicosis?
   A. Iodine contamination of the well water on her farm
   B. Viral thyroiditis
   C. Consumption of pesticide-exposed vegetables
   D. Consumption of bovine thyroid tissue
   E. Consumption of goitrogen-containing vegetables

47 A 76-year-old man is referred to the endocrine clinic for assessment and management of osteoporosis and multiple fractures of bilateral ribs and the right pelvis. He has a 17-year history of hepatitis B virus (treated with tenofovir for more than 10 years), and he developed hepatocellular carcinoma 4 years ago, treated with transarterial chemoembolization at that time. He has not had any evidence of cancer recurrence with normal α-fetoprotein levels.

Six months ago, routine surveillance chest CT identified bilateral rib fractures in varying stages of healing. A bone scan showed focal areas of uptake in bilateral ribs, thoracic spine, and bilateral pelvis. A CT-guided biopsy of a right iliac wing lesion was negative for malignant cells. He had a right forearm fracture after a fall from a ladder 5 years ago. While walking on a beach, he sustained a fracture of his right lateral malleolus and distal tibia 3 years ago. He has no bone pain or loss of height. There is no family history of fracture or osteoporosis.

On physical examination, all vital signs are normal. He is a well-developed man with no bowing of the lower extremities and no pain on palpation of the ribs, spine, or hips. There is no kyphosis.

Laboratory test results:

Mild hyperchloremic metabolic acidosis with progressive renal insufficiency (estimated glomerular filtration rate, 45 mL/min per 1.73 m^2)

Serum urea nitrogen = 25 mg/dL (8-23 mg/dL) (SI: 8.9 mmol/L [2.9-8.2 mmol/L])

Creatinine = 1.79 mg/dL (0.7-1.3 mg/dL) (SI: 158.2 µmol/L [61.9-114.9 µmol/L])

Calcium = 9.0 mg/dL (8.2-10.2 mg/dL) (SI: 2.3 mmol/L [2.1-2.6 mmol/L])

Phosphate = 1.8 mg/dL (2.3-4.7 mg/dL) (SI: 0.6 mmol/L [0.7-1.5 mmol/L])

Albumin = 4.0 g/dL (3.5-5.0 g/dL) (SI: 40 g/L [35-50 g/L])

Alkaline phosphatase = 216 U/L (50-120 U/L) (SI: 3.6 µkat/L [0.84-2.00 µkat/L])

Intact PTH = 27 pg/mL (10-65 pg/mL) (SI: 27 ng/L [10-65 ng/L])

25-Hydroxyvitamin D = 26 ng/mL (25-80 ng/mL [optimal]) (SI: 64.9 nmol/L [62.4-199.7 nmol/L])

1,25-Dihydroxyvitamin D = 24 pg/mL (16-65 pg/mL) (SI: 62.4 pmol/L [41.6-169.0 pmol/L])

Fibroblast growth factor 23 = <50 RU/mL (≤180 RU/mL)

Tubular reabsorption of phosphate = 70% (normal >80%)

TSH, normal

Testosterone, normal

Serum protein electrophoresis, normal

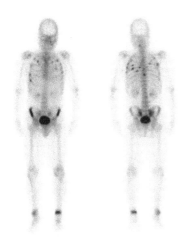

Bone scan.

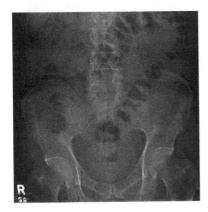

Spine/pelvis x-ray.

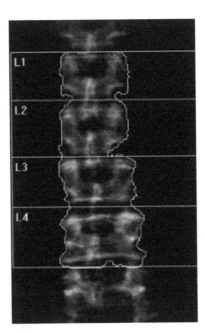

Region	BMD, g/cm²	T Score
L1	0.683	−3.5
L2	0.743	−3.2
L3	0.725	−3.4
L4	0.722	−2.9
Total	0.735	−3.2

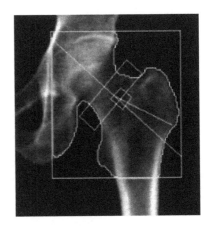

Region	BMD, g/cm²	T Score
Neck	0.410	−3.8
Troch	0.474	−2.4
Inter	0.552	−3.6
Total	0.508	−3.5

Which of the following interventions will most likely improve this patient's overall long-term bone health?
- A. Phosphate replacement
- B. Calcitriol supplementation
- C. Bisphosphonate treatment
- D. Chemotherapy initiation
- E. Switch from tenofovir to entecavir

48 You are asked for advice regarding a 67-year-old man in whom right-sided renal cell carcinoma was recently diagnosed. His preoperative assessment includes a whole-body CT that has identified the presence of a multinodular goiter with a large right-sided nodule measuring 3.8 cm and extending retrosternally. Imaging investigations have not identified any evidence of metastatic disease in the liver, lungs, or skeleton. Surgery is scheduled in 3 days. The patient has been well and asymptomatic. He has no compressive symptoms from the goiter, which was found incidentally during preoperative staging. There is no notable medical history and he is not taking any medications. There is no relevant family history.

On physical examination, his height is 70 in (177.8 cm) and weight is 159 lb (72.3 kg) (BMI = 22.8 kg/m²). His blood pressure is 128/64 mm Hg, and pulse rate is 78 beats/min in a regular rhythm. A small multinodular goiter is palpable in his neck, and there is clinical evidence of retrosternal extension. There is no palpable cervical lymphadenopathy. Findings on systems examination are otherwise unremarkable.

Laboratory test results:
Renal function, normal
Liver function, normal
TSH = 0.28 mIU/L (0.5-5.0 mIU/L)
Free T$_4$ = 1.6 ng/dL (0.8-1.8 ng/dL) (SI: 20.6 pmol/L [10.30-23.17 pmol/L])
Free T$_3$ = 4.0 pg/mL (2.3-4.2 pg/mL) (SI: 6.2 pmol/L [3.53-6.45 pmol/L])
Thyroid-stimulating immunoglobulin = ≤120% of basal activity (≤120% of basal activity)
TPO antibodies = <2.0 IU/mL (<2.0 IU/mL) (<2.0 kIU/L [<2.0 kIU/L])

A technetium ^{99m}Tc pertechnetate scan shows diffuse uptake in both thyroid lobes, which is slightly increased on the right side (*see images*).

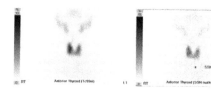

Thyroid ultrasonography shows multiple solid hypoechoic nodules in both lobes with increased internal vascularity (*see images*).

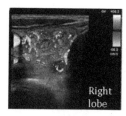 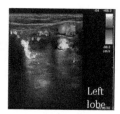

Right lobe / Left lobe

Which of the following is the most likely diagnosis?
- A. Thyroidal metastases from renal cancer
- B. Graves disease
- C. Thyroiditis
- D. Medullary thyroid cancer
- E. Toxic nodular hyperthyroidism

49 A 50-year-old man presents for management of mixed hyperlipidemia and elevated liver enzymes. Cholesteryl ester storage disease was diagnosed at age 18 years, and he is interested in a new enzyme replacement therapy that recently became available. Although he has a prescription for atorvastatin, 40 mg daily, he does not take it regularly. He has no other medical problems. He does not smoke cigarettes, but he does drink 3 to 4 glasses of wine a day. He does not have a regular exercise program and has gained 25 lb (11.4 kg) over the last 2 years.

On physical examination, his blood pressure is 132/78 mm Hg. His height is 70 in (178 cm), and weight is 225 lb (102.3 kg) (BMI = 32.3 kg/m²). Abdominal obesity is present and the liver edge is palpable at the right costal margin. There are no xanthomas. Physical examination findings are otherwise unremarkable.

Laboratory test results (sample drawn while fasting):
   Total cholesterol = 185 mg/dL (<200 mg/dL [optimal]) (SI: 4.79 mmol/L [<5.18 mmol/L])
   Triglycerides = 83 mg/dL (<150 mg/dL [optimal]) (SI: 0.94 mmol/L [<3.88 mmol/L])
   LDL cholesterol = 139 mg/dL (<100 mg/dL [optimal]) (SI: 3.60 mmol/L [<2.59 mmol/L])
   HDL cholesterol = 29 mg/dL (>60 mg/dL [optimal]) (SI: 0.75 mmol/L [>1.55 mmol/L])
   Non-HDL cholesterol = 159 mg/dL (<130 mg/dL) (SI: 4.82 mmol/L [<3.37 mmol/L])
   ALT = 53 U/L (10-40 U/L) (SI: 0.89 µkat/L [0.17-0.67 µkat/L])
   AST = 101 U/L (20-48 U/L) (SI: 1.69 µkat/L [0.33-0.80 µkat/L])
   TSH = 1.39 mIU/L (0.5-5.0 mIU/L)
   Hemoglobin A$_{1c}$ = 5.3% (4.0%-5.6%) (34 mmol/mol [20-38 mmol/mol])

Knowing the risks associated with his underlying disorder, which of the following should be your next management step?
   A. Start ursodeoxycholic acid
   B. Refer to hepatology for possible liver transplant
   C. Restart high-intensity statin therapy
   D. Start ezetimibe
   E. Start sebelipase alfa (enzyme replacement therapy)

50 A 45-year-old man with a 5-year history of type 2 diabetes mellitus presents to the emergency department with worsening fatigue and is found to have acute renal injury. His creatinine concentration on presentation is 3.5 mg/dL (309.4 µmol/L); review of his outpatient records shows his creatinine concentration was 1.8 mg/dL (159.1 µmol/L) 6 months ago. The patient reports having a CT with contrast 1 week ago. He has had no nausea or vomiting.

His current insulin regimen consists of premixed 70/30 insulin, 30 units in the morning and 30 units with his evening meal. He also takes metformin, 1000 mg twice daily. His blood glucose readings at home are 150 to 180 mg/dL (8.3-10.0 mmol/L).

On physical examination, his height is 70 in (177.8 cm) and weight is 200 lb (90.9 kg) (BMI = 28.7 kg/m²).

Recent laboratory test results:
   Hemoglobin A$_{1c}$ = 8.0% (4.0%-5.6%) (64 mmol/mol [20-38 mmol/mol])
   Estimated glomerular filtration rate = 30 mL/min per 1.73 m² (>60 mL/min per 1.72 m²)
   Glucose = 120 mg/dL (70-99 mg/dL) (SI: 6.7 mmol/L [3.9-5.5 mmol/L])

In addition to holding metformin, which of the following scheduled insulin regimens should you recommend?

Answer	Daily Basal Insulin	Prandial Insulin (per meal)	Blood Glucose Target
A.	30 units	10 units	110-140 mg/dL (6.1-7.8 mmol/L)
B.	22 units	5 units	110-140 mg/dL (6.1-7.8 mmol/L)
C.	22 units	7 units	140-180 mg/dL (7.8-10.0 mmol/L)
D.	15 units	5 units	140-180 mg/dL (7.8-10.0 mmol/L)
E.	30 units	10 units	140-180 mg/dL (7.8-10.0 mmol/L)

51 An 18-year-old man presents to endocrine clinic for transition of care from pediatrics. He has had intermittent follow-up care. Osteogenesis imperfecta type 3 was diagnosed when he sustained a femur fracture at birth. He has scoliosis and an extensive fracture history of all extremities including the bilateral femurs and bilateral tibias, which have been complicated by pseudoarthrosis. He is wheelchair-bound and requires assists with transfers. His medical history is also remarkable for iron deficiency anemia. Hearing loss was diagnosed in childhood.

On physical examination, his height is 40 in (101.6 cm) and weight is 52 lb (23.6 kg) (BMI = 22.8 kg/m²). His blood pressure is 120/63 mm Hg, and pulse rate is 94 beats/min. Examination findings are notable for scoliosis and short stature with marked bowing deformities of all extremities. He has frontal bossing and a small jaw. His teeth are misshapen and discolored, and his sclerae are slightly blue. He has diminished breath sounds at the lung bases, joint laxity, and kyphosis.

DXA images are shown (*see images*).

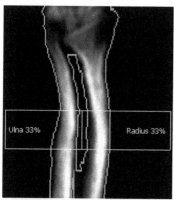

Region	Bone Mineral Density, g/cm²	Age-Matched Z Score
Radius	0.463	–6.0

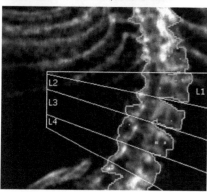

Region	Bone Mineral Density, g/cm²	Age-Matched Z Score
L1	0.447	–6.6
L2	0.544	–6.6
L3	0.476	–7.0
L4	0.551	–6.3
L1-L4	0.504	–6.6

His current medications include calcium, 1000 mg daily, and cholecalciferol, 1000 IU daily, to which he admits intermittent adherence.

Laboratory test results:
Serum total calcium = 9.9 mg/dL (8.2-10.2 mg/dL) (SI: 2.5 mmol/L [2.1-2.6 mmol/L])
Phosphate = 2.7 mg/dL (2.3-4.7 mg/dL) (SI: 0.9 mmol/L [0.7-1.5 mmol/L])
Serum creatinine = 0.59 mg/dL (0.7-1.3 mg/dL) (SI: 52.2 μmol/L [61.9-114.9 μmol/L])
Alkaline phosphatase = 61 U/L (50-120 U/L) (SI: 1.02 μkat/L [0.84-2.00 μkat/L])
PTH = 25 pg/mL (10-65 pg/mL) (SI: 25 ng/L [10-65 ng/L])
Hemoglobin =12.0 g/dL (13.8-17.2 g/dL) (SI: 120 g/L [138-172 g/L])
Hematocrit = 34% (41%-50%) (SI: 0.34 [0.41-0.51])
25-Hydroxyvitamin D = 32 ng/mL (25-80 ng/mL [optimal]) (SI: 79.9 nmol/L [62.4-199.7 nmol/L])

In addition to calcium, vitamin D, and appropriate rehabilitative services, which of the following is the best treatment to reduce this patient's fracture risk?

    A. Alendronate, weekly
    B. Subcutaneous GH therapy, daily
    C. Nasal calcitonin
    D. Intramuscular testosterone cypionate, monthly
    E. Intravenous pamidronate every 3 months

52 Six months ago, you evaluated a 34-year-old woman for medically complicated obesity. At that time, her weight was 222 lb (101 kg) and her BMI was 36 kg/m². She has polycystic ovary syndrome, gastroesophageal reflux disease, hypothyroidism, and chronic back pain. The patient told you that weight had been a concern her entire life and that she had tried multiple diets. She felt as though her life had been characterized by frequent weight loss and weight gain. During your initial evaluation, you learned that she was often eating fast food, her portions were large, and she was eating multiple snacks a day. She was averaging 5000 steps a day. You asked her to meet with a dietitian, and she has been returning for monthly follow-up appointments.

During the first 3 months, she lost 10 lb (4.5 kg). However, the past 3 months her weight has remained unchanged. She is following a meal plan but reports she is hungry all the time. She has been tracking her calories on an app, and she regularly exceeds her calorie limit. Her current medications include levothyroxine and hydrocodone. Her weight is now 211 lb (96 kg). Thyroid function is normal. She is frustrated because despite her efforts to improve her eating habits, hunger continues to be a struggle.

Which of the following is the best next step in her weight-loss management?

    A. Increase activity to 10,000 steps a day and continue the current meal plan
    B. Initiate metformin
    C. Initiate orlistat
    D. Initiate phentermine + topiramate ER
    E. Replace 1 meal each day with a protein bar or shake

53 A man finds his 76-year-old wife unresponsive in the late afternoon. She has had type 2 diabetes mellitus for 9 years. Paramedics are called. Her initial point-of-care glucose measurement is 36 mg/dL (2.0 mmol/L). She is treated with intravenous dextrose, then given glucose gel and transported to the hospital. The initial glucose measurement in the emergency department is 67 mg/dL (3.7 mmol/L). Intravenous 5% dextrose is given and she is admitted to the hospital. Her sensorium gradually clears.

The patient's diabetes treatment regimen has consisted of metformin, 2000 mg daily, and glyburide, 10 mg twice daily, for the last 7 years. Her most recent hemoglobin A_{1c} value was 6.3% (45 mmol/mol) 4.5 weeks ago. She has mild peripheral neuropathy as the only microvascular complication. She has hypertension treated with lisinopril and hydrochlorothiazide. She has stage 3 chronic kidney disease. She is being treated with a statin, but there is no known history of cardiovascular disease. She does not drink alcohol or smoke cigarettes.

The metformin and glyburide were stopped on admission to the hospital. Glucose is measured by fingerstick every 1 to 2 hours. Due to repeated hypoglycemia, the intravenous fluid is changed to 10% dextrose and the rate is increased from 75 to 150 mL/h. She is given several ampules or half ampules of D50 to treat recurrent hypoglycemia. The glucose values are shown (*see table*).

	Time										
	1930	2100	2230	0036	0101	0207	0401	0713	0746	0823	1106
Glucose, mg/dL (mmol/L)	136 (7.5)	*60 (3.3)	89 (4.9)	**45 (2.5)	135 (7.5)	92 (5.1)	83 (4.6)	**48 (2.7)	121 (6.7)	77 (4.3)	*56 (3.1)

* One-half ampule D50; ** 1 ampule D50.

On physical examination, her height is 66 in (168 cm) and weight is 143 lb (65 kg) (BMI = 23.1 kg/m²). Her blood pressure is 136/82 mm Hg, pulse rate is 84 beats/min, and respiratory rate is 12 breaths/min. The patient is alert and oriented. Findings on heart, lung, and abdominal examination are normal. She has mild deficits to monofilament testing in both feet.

Laboratory test results:
   Electrolytes, normal
   Creatinine = 1.4 mg/dL (0.6-1.1 mg/dL) (SI: 123.8 μmol/L [53.0-97.2 μmol/L])
   Estimated glomerular filtration rate = 35 mL/min per 1.73 m² (>60 mL/min per 1.73 m²)
   Serum urea nitrogen = 16 mg/dL (8-23 mg/dL) (SI: 5.7 mmol/L [2.9-8.2 mmol/L])
   Hemoglobin =14.0 g/dL (12.1-15.1 g/dL) (SI: 140 g/L [121-151 g/L])

Electrocardiography demonstrates a normal sinus rhythm without evidence of ischemic changes.

Which of the following is the best next step in the management of this patient's hypoglycemia?
   A. Continue administering ampules of D50 as needed
   B. Give intravenous methylprednisolone
   C. Give everolimus
   D. Give subcutaneous octreotide
   E. Change the infusion to D15 (15% dextrose)

54 You are called to the surgical intensive care unit to evaluate a 21-year-old man admitted 48 hours ago after head trauma caused by a motor vehicle crash. The patient has no notable medical history. Head CT is normal, but he is unresponsive and intubated. The intensive care unit team has had problems maintaining his blood pressure, and the diagnosis of adrenal insufficiency is being considered. He is presently on an epinephrine drip.

   Physical examination findings are normal except for vital signs. His blood pressure is 85/60 mm Hg, and pulse rate is 112 beats/min. Testes are normal size.

Laboratory test results:
   Sodium = 137 mEq/L (136-142 mEq/L) (SI: 137 mmol/L [136-142 mmol/L])
   Potassium = 4.0 mEq/L (3.5-5.0 mEq/L) (SI: 4.0 mmol/L [3.5-5.0 mmol/L])
   Serum urea nitrogen = 21 mg/dL (8-23 mg/dL) (SI: 7.5 mmol/L [2.9-8.2 mmol/L])
   Creatinine = 1.1 mg/dL (0.7-1.3 mg/dL) (SI: 97.2 μmol/L [61.9-114.9 μmol/L])

The intensive care unit team has just performed a 250-mcg ACTH simulation test. The baseline cortisol value was 3.9 μg/dL (107.6 nmol/L). Sixty minutes after administration of 250 mcg of ACTH, it was 24.1 μg/dL (664.9 nmol/L).

Which of the following is the most appropriate next step?
   A. Measure serum aldosterone
   B. Perform another ACTH stimulation test with 1 mcg of ACTH
   C. Administer fludrocortisone
   D. Administer stress-dose steroids
   E. No other testing required

55 A 22-year-old man is referred for management of hypogonadism. He reports that he has been healthy his entire life and underwent normal puberty. He does, however, recall that during a high-school sports physical, the doctor had difficulty locating his testicles. He shaves every 4 days and has regular sexual thoughts. He takes no medications.

   On physical examination, his blood pressure is 115/61 mm Hg. His height is 65 in (165 cm), and weight is 145 lb (66 kg) (BMI = 24.1 kg/m²). He has a normal penis and no gynecomastia. Testes are 3 mL bilaterally without masses.

Laboratory test results:

Total testosterone = 259 ng/dL (300-900 ng/dL) (SI: 9.0 nmol/L [10.4-31.2 nmol/L])

FSH = 29.0 mIU/mL (1.0-13.0 mIU/mL) (SI: 29.0 IU/L [1.0-13.0 IU/L])

LH = 22.0 mIU/mL (1.0-9.0 mIU/mL) (SI: 22.0 IU/L [1.0-9.0 IU/L])

Karyotype = 46,XX

As compared to men with Klinefelter syndrome, what major difference would be expected in men with this syndrome?

A. Higher levels of testosterone

B. Higher body weight

C. Larger testicular volumes

D. Lower rates of gynecomastia

E. Shorter height

56 A 64-year-old man was diagnosed with diabetes mellitus 2 months ago after he presented to his primary care physician with a 3-month history of a 20-lb (9.1-kg) weight loss, polyuria, polydipsia, abdominal pain, and diarrhea. He has no family history of type 2 diabetes. The patient was noted to have a random blood glucose value of 270 mg/dL (15.0 mmol/L) and a hemoglobin A_{1c} value of 8.7% (72 mmol/mol). Metformin and glimepiride were prescribed; however, metformin exacerbated his abdominal symptoms and was discontinued. On glimepiride monotherapy, his blood glucose control improved, and his current average value is 160 mg/dL (8.9 mmol/L). Despite improved glycemic control, he continues to experience abdominal pain and persistent diarrhea. He has regained only 4 to 5 lb (1.8-2.3 kg) of the lost weight. His primary care physician is concerned about unresolved symptoms and sends the patient to you for further evaluation.

On physical examination, his blood pressure is 120/84 mm Hg and pulse rate is 88 beats/min. His height is 71.5 in (181.6 cm), and weight is 180.5 lb (82 kg) (BMI = 24.8 kg/m^2). He looks tired but is otherwise in good health. There is no icterus or jaundice. Findings on head and neck, and heart and lung examinations are normal. His skin is also normal. He has mild discomfort on palpation of the right upper quadrant of the abdomen.

Ultrasonography of the abdomen shows dilation of the common bile duct and evidence of gallstones.

Laboratory test results:

Hemoglobin A_{1c} = 6.7% (4.0%-5.6%) (50 mmol/mol [20-38 mmol/mol])

Comprehensive metabolic panel, normal

Amylase and lipase, normal

In addition to checking antibodies to exclude an autoimmune cause for diabetes, which of the following should be measured next?

A. Fasting somatostatin

B. Fasting glucagon

C. 24-Hour urinary cortisol excretion

D. IGF-1

E. Transferrin saturation and ferritin

57 A 58-year-old postmenopausal woman is referred for evaluation of thigh pain. She has a history of low bone mass (osteopenia) treated with alendronate for 8 years. She now presents with a 2-month history of severe, deep, sharp pain in her right thigh. It is worse when she is walking but remains as a less severe ache when at rest. She has no fatigue, rash, or easy bruising. She has no history of trauma, fracture, or loss of height.

On physical examination, her blood pressure is 143/82 mm Hg and pulse rate is 94 beats/min. Her height is 59 in (150 cm), and weight is 187 lb (85 kg) (BMI = 37.8 kg/m^2). She has no striae and no facial plethora. There is no kyphosis, no bowing of her legs, and no warmth along her legs. Pain is not elicited by rotation of the hips or with flexion/extension at the knees.

Laboratory test results:

Calcium = 8.8 mg/dL (8.2-10.2 mg/dL) (SI: 2.2 mmol/L [2.1-2.6 mmol/L])
Phosphate = 3.0 mg/dL (2.3-4.7 mg/dL) (SI: 1.0 mmol/L [0.7-1.5 mmol/L])
Albumin = 3.8 g/dL (3.5-5.0 g/dL) (SI: 38 g/L [35-50 g/L])
Alkaline phosphatase = 135 U/L (50-120 U/L) (SI: 2.3 µkat/L [0.84-2.00 µkat/L])
25-Hydroxyvitamin D = 19 ng/mL (25-80 ng/mL [optimal])
    (SI: 47.4 nmol/L [62.4-199.7 nmol/L])
1,25-Dihydroxyvitamin D = 30 pg/mL (16-65 pg/mL)
    (SI: 78 pmol/L [41.6-169.0 pmol/L])
Intact PTH = 63 pg/mL (10-65 pg/mL) (SI: 63 ng/L [10-65 ng/L])
Osteocalcin = 21.9 ng/mL (9.0-42.0 ng/mL) (SI: 21.9 µg/L [9.0-42.0 µg/L])
Serum C-telopeptide = 93 pg/mL (104-1008 pg/mL [postmenopausal women])

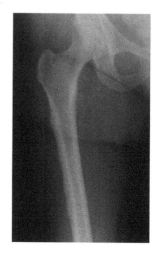

X-ray of the right femur is shown (*see image*).

Which of the following is the most likely cause of her femur pain?

    A. Bone malignancy leading to tumor-induced osteomalacia
    B. Mastocytosis
    C. Paget disease of bone
    D. Prolonged bisphosphonate use
    E. Osteomalacia from vitamin D deficiency

58 A 55-year-old man recently underwent thyroidectomy for a thyroid nodule that had been increasing in size while under observation. He initially underwent FNAB when the nodule was detected 3 years ago, and the cytologic findings were reported to be consistent with a benign nodule. A second FNAB was performed when the nodule increased in size by 20% in 2 of its dimensions, as documented by ultrasonography. On this occasion, the cytologic findings were reported to be atypia of undetermined significance. The patient was advised to have another FNAB with molecular markers. However, the third aspiration sample was deemed by the cytopathologist to clearly show nuclear features of papillary thyroid cancer and the patient was advised to undergo thyroidectomy without the need for molecular markers. The histologic specimen from the patient's thyroid nodule is shown (*see image*). The 3 tumor areas are shown at approximately the same magnification.

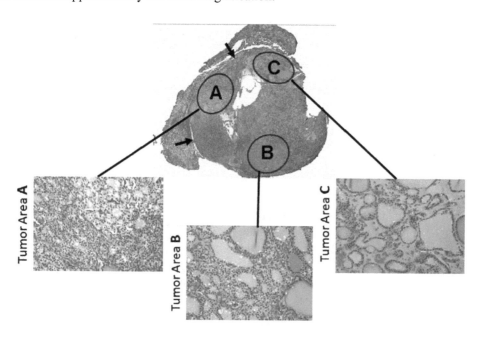

Which of the following describes the histology of the areas of the specimen shown?
- A. All areas of this nodule have benign histology
- B. This nodule shows features of medullary thyroid cancer
- C. This nodule shows features of anaplastic thyroid cancer
- D. The patient's third FNAB likely sampled Area C of the nodule
- E. Area A of the nodule shows nuclear features of papillary thyroid cancer

59 A 72-year-old woman has had type 2 diabetes mellitus since age 44 years, and her clinical course has been complicated by background retinopathy, peripheral neuropathy, and proteinuria. She has hypertension, dyslipidemia, and osteoporosis, but no previous cardiovascular event. Her sister recently had a myocardial infarction, which she was told was due to uncontrolled hypertension. The patient asks whether her blood pressure is adequately controlled. She has no exertional chest or calf claudication pain. She does have some numbness in both feet and periodic orthostatic light-headedness.

Current medications include insulin detemir, sitagliptin, simvastatin, losartan, hydrochlorothiazide, aspirin, alendronate, calcium carbonate, and cholecalciferol.

On physical examination, her height is 66 in (167.6 cm) and weight is 152 lb (69 kg) (BMI = 24.5 kg/m²). Her blood pressure is 136/84 mm Hg, and pulse rate is 66 beats/min. No carotid bruits are detected. Her heart has a regular rate and rhythm with an S_4 and a 2/6 systolic murmur at the right upper sternal border. There is trace lower-leg edema. On neurologic examination, she has decreased sensation to light touch and vibration and reduced proprioception. Her pedal pulses are normal. There are no lesions on her feet.

Laboratory test results:

Hemoglobin A_{1c} = 7.2% (4.0%-5.6%) (55 mmol/mol [20-38 mmol/mol])
Serum urea nitrogen = 14 mg/dL (8-23 mg/dL) (SI: 5.0 mmol/L [2.9-8.2 mmol/L])
Creatinine = 0.8 mg/dL (0.6-1.1 mg/dL) (SI: 70.7 μmol/L [53.0-97.2 μmol/L])
Estimated glomerular filtration rate = 46 mL/min per 1.73 m² (>60 mL/min per 1.73 m²)
Potassium = 4.8 mEq/L (3.5-5.0 mEq/L) (SI: 4.8 mmol/L [3.5-5.0 mmol/L])
Urine albumin = 22 mg/g creat (<30 mg/g creat)
Hematocrit = 34% (35%-45%) (SI: 0.34 [0.35-0.45])

Which of the following blood pressure treatment options would you advise next for this patient?
- A. Add amlodipine
- B. Add lisinopril
- C. Add clonidine
- D. Change hydrochlorothiazide to amlodipine
- E. No change to her current regimen

60 You are asked to evaluate a 62-year-old man who was first noted to have dense bones when he was a teenager. He initially presented with decreased vision from bone impingement on the optic nerve that required surgical intervention. He has an extensive fracture history; his first fracture occurred in high school when he fractured his right humerus throwing a baseball. Since then, he has fractured his upper and lower extremities multiple times, often requiring surgical fixation (*see images*).

He has had multiple complications from his disease, including pancytopenia and portal hypertension from extramedullary hematopoiesis, and he requires periodic blood transfusions. He has developed hearing loss and carpal tunnel syndrome. He has chronic osteomyelitis of the jaw and has required extraction of all of his teeth. His family history is remarkable for his mother and maternal uncle who also have increased bone density and fractures.

On physical examination, his height is 67 in (170 cm) and weight is 165 lb (75 kg) (BMI = 25.8 kg/m²). His blood pressure is 169/59 mm Hg, and pulse rate is 66 beats/min. He has mild frontal bossing with a surgical scar on his skull. He is edentulous, and his sclerae are white. The spleen is firm and very solid in the left upper quadrant and extends 10 cm below the left costal margin.

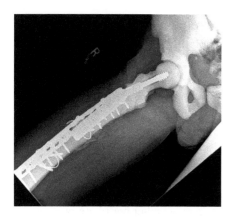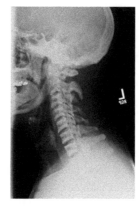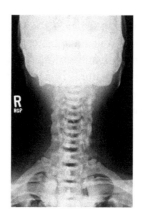

Laboratory test results:
  Serum total calcium = 9.5 mg/dL (8.2-10.2 mg/dL) (SI: 2.4 mmol/L [2.1-2.6 mmol/L])
  Phosphate = 4.5 mg/dL (2.3-4.7 mg/dL) (SI: 1.5 mmol/L [0.7-1.5 mmol/L])
  Serum creatinine = 0.69 mg/dL (0.7-1.3 mg/dL) (SI: 61.0 µmol/L [61.9-114.9 µmol/L])
  Alkaline phosphatase = 162 U/L (50-120 U/L) (SI: 2.7 µkat/L [0.84-2.00 µkat/L])
  PTH = 63 pg/mL (10-65 pg/mL) (SI: 63 ng/L [10-65 ng/L])
  White blood cell count = 1700/µL (4500-11,000/µL) (SI: 1.7×10^9/L [$4.5-11.0 \times 10^9$/L])
  Hemoglobin = 6.1 g/dL g/dL (13.8-17.2 g/dL) (SI: 61 g/L [138-172 g/L])
  Hematocrit = 21% (41%-50%) (SI: 0.21 [0.41-0.51])
  Platelet count = 34×10^3/µL ($150-450 \times 10^3$/µL) (SI: 34×10^9/L [$150-450 \times 10^9$/L])
  Acid phosphatase = 9.8 U/L (0.0-4.3 U/L)
  25-Hydroxyvitamin D = 25 ng/mL (25-80 ng/mL [optimal]) (SI: 62.4 nmol/L [62.4-199.7 nmol/L])
  Lactate dehydrogenase (total) = 356 U/L (105-230 U/L)

Which of the following is the most likely cause of his elevated bone density?
  A. Worth syndrome (gain-of-function mutation in the gene encoding the LDL receptor–related protein 5 [*LRP5*])
  B. Autosomal recessive osteopetrosis (gain-of-function mutation in the gene encoding the osteoclast-specific proton pump [*TCIRG1*])
  C. Albers-Schonberg disease, autosomal dominant osteopetrosis (gain-of-function mutation in the gene encoding a chloride channel [*CLCN7*])
  D. Tumor-induced osteomalacia (fibroblast growth factor 23 abnormality)
  E. Paget disease (mutations in the gene encoding sequestosome 1 [SQSTM1])

61 An 18-year-old woman comes to see you for irregular menses. She underwent menarche at age 12 years and had irregular menstrual cycles, approximately every 3 months, until 3 years ago when they stopped completely. Her weight has been stable. She eats well-balanced meals and has no history of an eating disorder. She has acne but no hirsutism. Her mother had irregular menses her whole life and required clomiphene citrate to achieve pregnancy. The patient is of northern European ethnicity.

On physical examination, her blood pressure is 96/80 mm Hg. Her height is 61.8 in (157 cm), and weight is 120 lb (54.5 kg) (BMI = 22.1 kg/m²). On skin examination, she has acne but no hirsutism. Her thyroid gland is an estimated 20 g and without nodules. She has no galactorrhea on breast examination. Abdominal examination does not reveal striae. Findings on pelvic examination are normal.

Laboratory test results (sample drawn at 8 AM):
  TSH = 1.16 mIU/L (0.5-5.0 mIU/L)
  Prolactin = 6 ng/mL (4-30 ng/mL) (SI: 0.26 nmol/L [0.17-1.30 nmol/L])
  Testosterone = 36 ng/dL (8-60 ng/dL) (SI: 1.25 nmol/L [0.3-2.1 nmol/L])
  17-Hydroxyprogesterone = 50.5 ng/dL (<200 ng/dL) (SI: 1.53 nmol/L [<6.05 nmol/L])
  DHEA-S = 379 µg/dL (44-332 µg/dL) (SI: 10.27 µmol/L [1.19-9.00 µmol/L])
  Sex hormone–binding globulin = 8.43 µg/mL (2.2-14.6 µg/mL) (SI: 75.0 nmol/L [20-130 nmol/L])

LH = 16.0 mIU/mL (1.0-18.0 mIU/mL) (SI: 16.0 IU/L [1.0-18.0 IU/L])
FSH = 7.7 mIU/mL (2.0-12.0 mIU/mL) (SI: 7.7 IU/L [2.0-12.0 IU/L])

Which of the following is the most likely diagnosis?
  A. Nonclassic congenital adrenal hyperplasia
  B. Ovarian tumor
  C. Adrenal adenoma
  D. Polycystic ovary syndrome
  E. Cushing syndrome

62 A 23-year-old woman is referred for management of high triglycerides that were detected during workup for hirsutism. She has a history of irregular menses and is currently on oral contraceptives. She does not smoke cigarettes and drinks alcohol occasionally. She leads an active lifestyle. Her father, a nonsmoker, has treated hypertension and underwent 3-vessel coronary bypass grafting at age 52 years. Her mother is healthy. She has a brother, aged 28 years, who has elevated triglycerides.

On physical examination, her blood pressure is 104/70 mm Hg and pulse rate is 72 beats/min. Her height is 63 in (160 cm), and weight is 175 lb (79.5 kg) (BMI = 31 kg/m^2). There are no xanthomas or hepatosplenomegaly.

Laboratory test results (sample drawn while fasting):
  Total cholesterol = 185 mg/dL (<200 mg/dL [optimal]) (SI: 4.79 mmol/L [<5.18 mmol/L])
  Triglycerides = 703 mg/dL (<150 mg/dL [optimal]) (SI: 7.94 mmol/L [<3.88 mmol/L])
  HDL cholesterol = 29 mg/dL (>60 mg/dL [optimal]) (SI: 0.75 mmol/L [>1.55 mmol/L])
  Non-HDL cholesterol = 156 mg/dL (<130 mg/dL) (SI: 4.04 mmol/L [<3.37 mmol/L])
  ALT = 19 U/L (10-40 U/L) (SI: 0.32 μkat/L [0.17-0.67 μkat/L])
  AST = 16 U/L (20-48 U/L) (SI: 0.27 μkat/L [0.33-0.80 μkat/L])
  TSH = 5.2 mIU/L (0.5-5.0 mIU/L)

Which of the following is the most likely factor contributing to this patient's hypertriglyceridemia?
  A. Polycystic ovary syndrome
  B. Abdominal obesity
  C. Alcohol consumption
  D. Oral contraceptive use
  E. Hypothyroidism

63 A 69-year-old woman has been referred to you for evaluation of osteoporosis. The patient's gynecologist has managed her osteoporosis for the last 11 years with alendronate. According to old clinical records, the patient's baseline DXA documented a T score of –2.9 in the spine. Breast cancer was diagnosed at age 62 years and was treated with surgery and external beam radiation therapy followed by anastrozole, which she tolerated for a total of 14 months. She has no pain in any bones or joints. She has no reflux symptoms and has never had a fracture or loss of height. She has no other medical problems. She has never taken steroids. She drinks 2 to 3 glasses of wine per week and has never smoked cigarettes. There is no family history of vertebral or hip fracture.

On physical examination, her blood pressure is 131/51 mm Hg and pulse rate is 64 beats/min. Her height is 61 in (155 cm), and weight is 121 lb (55 kg) (BMI = 22.9 kg/m^2). Her oropharynx is clear with no exposed bone or gingivitis. She has no kyphosis or scoliosis.

Laboratory test results:
  25-Hydroxyvitamin D = 40 ng/mL (25-80 ng/mL [optimal]) (SI: 99.8 nmol/L [62.4-199.7 nmol/L])
  Serum C-telopeptide = 186 pg/mL (104-1008 pg/mL [postmenopausal women]) (SI: 186 ng/L [104-1008 ng/L])

DXA bone mineral density this year:

    L1-L4 spine T score = –2.4

    Left total hip T score = –2.4

    Femoral neck T score = –2.3

    Right total hip T score = –2.3

    Femoral neck T score = –2.3

There has been no significant change in bone mineral density from studies 2 years ago or 4 years ago.

Which of the following is the best recommendation now?

    A. Stop alendronate and start teriparatide (daily for 2 years)

    B. Stop alendronate and start denosumab (every 6 months for 2 years)

    C. Stop alendronate and start zoledronic acid (every 2 years)

    D. Continue alendronate and reassess DXA and clinical parameters in 2 years

    E. Initiate a bisphosphonate drug holiday and reassess DXA and clinical parameters in 1 to 2 years

64 A 55-year-old man with type 2 diabetes mellitus has had worsening symptoms related to aortic stenosis, and his cardiologist recommends that he have aortic valve replacement. Your records show that his most recent hemoglobin A_{1c} level was 7.0% (53 mmol/mol). He takes metformin, 1000 mg twice daily, and glipizide, 5 mg daily. Additional as-needed medications are salicylates and opioids for back pain. He does not test his blood glucose at home. Review of his chart reveals that his preoperative fasting glucose value the day of surgery was 220 mg/dL (12.2 mmol/L).

    Surgical aortic valve replacement is successful. He is placed on an insulin drip per protocol for 48 hours following surgery. On postoperative day 2, the patient is off all vasopressor medications, is doing well from a cardiac point of view, and is transferred out of the intensive care unit. However, at the end of postoperative day 2, the insulin drip rate remains at 3 units per hour and endocrinology is consulted.

Which of the following is the most likely explanation for the discrepancy between his preoperative hemoglobin A_{1c} value and his postoperative course (requiring insulin)?

    A. Stress hyperglycemia caused by cardiac surgery

    B. False decrease in hemoglobin A_{1c} caused by salicylates and opioids

    C. Nonadherence to his diabetes treatment regimen for several days before surgery

    D. Reduced lifespan of red blood cells due to hemolysis caused by his stenotic aortic valve

    E. β-Cell dysfunction caused by cardiac surgery

65 A 34-year-old man is referred because of weight gain of 30 lb (13.6 kg) over the past 3 years despite eating a healthful diet. He reports no skin changes or muscle weakness. He has a history of hypertension, epilepsy, and a recent diagnosis of impaired glucose tolerance. His medications include lamotrigine, carbamazepine, lisinopril, amlodipine, and atorvastatin.

    On physical examination, he is centrally obese. His height is 72 in (182.9 cm), and weight is 280 lb (127.3 kg) (BMI = 38.0 kg/m²). There are a few pale striae over the abdominal wall but no other skin changes. There is no proximal myopathy. His blood pressure is 151/94 mm Hg.

Laboratory test results:

    Sodium = 138 mEq/L (136-142 mEq/L) (SI: 138 mmol/L [136-142 mmol/L])

    Potassium = 4.9 mEq/L (3.5-5.0 mEq/L) (SI: 4.9 mmol/L [3.5-5.0 mmol/L])

    Serum urea nitrogen = 18 mg/dL (8-23 mg/dL) (SI: 6.4 mmol/L [2.9-8.2 mmol/L])

    Creatinine = 0.9 mg/dL (0.7-1.3 mg/dL) (SI: 79.6 µmol/L [61.9-114.9 µmol/L])

    Glucose = 175 mg/dL (70-99 mg/dL) (SI: 9.7 mmol/L [3.9-5.5 mmol/L])

    TSH = 2.4 mIU/L (0.5-5.0 mIU/L)

    Free T_4 = 1.3 ng/dL (0.8-1.8 ng/dL) (SI: 16.7 pmol/L [10.30-23.17 pmol/L])

    Cortisol (8 AM, after 1-mg overnight dexamethasone suppression test) = 14 µg/dL (SI: 386.2 nmol/L)

In light of these results, which of the following is the most appropriate next investigation?

    A. Perform adrenal CT
    B. Perform pituitary MRI
    C. Measure 24-hour urinary free cortisol
    D. Perform a 2-day low-dose dexamethasone suppression test
    E. Stop lamotrigine and perform another 1-mg overnight dexamethasone suppression test

66 A 28-year-old man presents with a year-long history of poor libido, fatigue, weight gain, and loss of early-morning erections. He has a history of Diamond Blackfan anemia that requires monthly blood transfusions. He has also been treated with regular infusions of subcutaneous desferrioxamine since age 10 years. He reports normal pubertal development and describes no other symptoms. He is married with no children.

On physical examination, he appears pale. His blood pressure is 128/81 mm Hg without significant postural drop, and his resting pulse rate is 52 beats/min. His height is 71 in (180.3 cm), and weight is 198 lb (90 kg) (BMI = 27.6 kg/m^2). He has normal secondary sexual characteristics with 15-mL, smooth testes bilaterally. His skin is dry, and he has a diffuse, nontender goiter.

Laboratory test results:
    Ferritin = 450 ng/mL (15-200 ng/mL) (SI: 1001.2 pmol/L [33.7-449.4 pmol/L])
    Glucose = 165 mg/dL (70-99 mg/dL) (SI: 9.2 mmol/L [3.9-5.5 mmol/L])
    Hematocrit = 65% (41%-50%) (SI: 0.65 [0.41-0.50])
    Hemoglobin =10.2 g/dL (13.8-17.2 g/dL) (SI: 102 g/L [138-172 g/L])
    Mean corpuscular volume = 82 μm^3 (80-100 μm^3) (SI: 82 fL [80-100 fL])
    Platelet count = 210 × 10^3/μL (150-450 × 10^3/μL) (SI: 210 × 10^9/L [150-450 × 10^9/L])
    White blood cell count = 6200/μL (4500-11,000/μL) (SI: 6.2 × 10^9/L [4.5-11.0 × 10^9/L])

Which of the following hormone patterns is most likely to explain this patient's symptoms?

Answer	LH	Testosterone	TSH	Free T$_4$
A.	↓	↓	↓	↓
B.	↑	↓	↓	↓
C.	↓	↓	↑	↓
D.	↔	↔	↓	↓
E.	↑	↓	↔	↔

67 Six months ago, a 26-year-old woman underwent Roux-en-Y gastric bypass surgery for weight management. She has lost 42 lb (19.1 kg) since the operation. Her first pregnancy 4 years ago was complicated by gestational diabetes, and the child's birth weight was 9 lb 5 oz (4200 g). She now presents to discuss plans for a second pregnancy.

On physical examination, her blood pressure is 118/72 mm Hg and pulse rate is 74 beats/min. Her height is 64.5 in (164 cm), and weight is 229 lb (104 kg) (BMI = 38.7 kg/m^2). She is obese but is otherwise healthy appearing. Findings on heart, lung, abdominal, and musculoskeletal examinations are normal.

Her fasting glucose measurement is 90 mg/dL (70-99 mg/dL) (SI: 5.0 mmol/L [3.9-5.5 mmol/L]).

As you counsel her regarding future pregnancy, which of the following would you recommend?

    A. Avoid pregnancy as it is contraindicated following bariatric surgery
    B. Undergo comprehensive nutritional evaluation and continue postbariatric micronutrient replacement with an added prenatal vitamin
    C. Undergo oral glucose tolerance testing before attempting pregnancy
    D. Initiate metformin
    E. Follow usual prenatal care

68 A 19-year-old man presents with severe polyuria and polydipsia (urinates 5 to 6 times per night; 24-hour urine volume of 10 L [hypotonic urine]). Diabetes insipidus is diagnosed. Brain MRI shows enlargement of the pituitary stalk with loss of the posterior bright spot. Anterior pituitary function is normal. Desmopressin therapy is initiated and polyuria resolves. A follow-up MRI 3 months later is unchanged. You decide to continue a watch and wait approach and plan for another MRI in 6 months.

Four months later, a surgeon contacts you regarding the patient to obtain "endocrine clearance" before a planned inguinal hernia repair. You note that the patient has not refilled his desmopressin prescription for 2 months. When you call the patient, he tells you that he ran out of the drug several weeks ago and subsequently discovered that he no longer needed it. Despite stopping the desmopressin, he only wakes once or twice at night to urinate.

Which of the following is the most appropriate next management step?
- A. Measure serum and urinary sodium
- B. Measure vasopressin
- C. Perform an ACTH stimulation test
- D. Perform a formal water deprivation test
- E. Re-start desmopressin

69 A 31-year-old man is referred for management of low libido and infertility. He reports an unremarkable puberty and normal development. He believes that his libido has gradually declined over the past 1 to 2 years from his baseline. The patient married his wife 3 years ago and the couple has been unable to have a child despite unprotected intercourse over the past 15 months. His wife does have a history of a previous pregnancy that was terminated when she was 22 years old. He takes no medications.

On physical examination, his blood pressure is 128/75 mm Hg. His height is 69 in (175 cm), and weight is 168 lb (76 kg) (BMI = 25 kg/m^2). Physical examination findings are unremarkable. He is well virilized without gynecomastia. Testes are 20 mL bilaterally without masses. The vas deferens are palpable.

Laboratory test results:
Total testosterone = 340 ng/dL (300-900 ng/dL) (SI: 11.8 nmol/L [10.4-31.2 nmol/L])
FSH = 6.6 mIU/mL (1.0-13.0 mIU/mL) (SI: 6.6 IU/L [1.0-13.0 IU/L])
LH = 4.7 mIU/mL (1.0-9.0 mIU/mL) (SI: 4.7 IU/L [1.0-9.0 IU/L])
Karyotype = 46,XY
Motile sperm count on semen analysis = 4 million (normal >20 million)

Which of the following tests should you order next?
- A. Chromosome aneuploidy analysis
- B. DNA fragmentation analysis
- C. Semen fructose measurement
- D. Testicular biopsy
- E. Y-chromosome microdeletion testing

70 A 27-year-old man presents to your office with his wife after experiencing severe hypoglycemia with loss of consciousness following a physically active day. Type 1 diabetes mellitus was diagnosed 16 years ago and he has no known diabetes-related end-organ complications. He prides himself on achieving hemoglobin A$_{1c}$ levels below 6.5% (<48 mmol/mol) since his diagnosis. This was his third severe hypoglycemic episode.

His diabetes is managed with insulin degludec, 24 units once daily, and insulin glulisine, 8 units before meals. He tries to keep the carbohydrate content of his meals similar from day to day. He uses an insulin sensitivity factor of 40 to target a glucose concentration of 100 mg/dL (5.6 mmol/L) to treat high glucose levels. Several times per week, he develops vision changes and fatigue when glucose levels fall below 50 mg/dL (<2.8 mmol/L).

A review of his downloaded glucose meter shows that he monitors glucose 4 to 5 times daily with mean concentrations ranging from 120 to 140 mg/dL (6.7-7.8 mmol/L) throughout the day. There is low glucose variability with a standard deviation of glucose values of 41 mg/dL (2.3 mmol/L), but 12% of readings fall below 70 mg/dL (<3.9 mmol/L).

Findings on cardiac and peripheral nerve examinations are normal.

His hemoglobin A$_{1c}$ measurement in your office is 6.4% (46 mmol/mol), and his 11:30 AM fingerstick glucose value is 68 mg/dL (3.8 mmol/L).

Which of the following is the best step to reduce his risk of a severe hypoglycemic reaction in the future?
- A. Change his insulin sensitivity factor from 40 to 20
- B. Switch from set premeal insulin doses to carbohydrate counting
- C. Initiate a continuous glucose monitor
- D. Switch to insulin pump therapy
- E. Switch insulin degludec to insulin detemir

71 A 27-year-old woman with a history of Hodgkin lymphoma and thyroid nodules is referred to you for management of her thyroid nodules. The patient received mantle radiation for Hodgkin lymphoma at age 15 years. Her primary care physician first noted the presence of thyroid nodules at age 24 years. Thyroid ultrasonography at that time showed a left-sided hypoechoic nodule that measured 1.6 × 2.0 × 1.3 cm and 2 isoechoic nodules that measured about 0.9 cm and 0.7 cm in the right lobe. The right lobe was also noted to have heterogeneous echotexture. FNAB of the left-sided nodule showed colloid and follicular cells and was described as an adenomatoid nodule. The cytologic examination from an FNAB of the 0.9-cm nodule revealed lymphoid tangles, and findings were interpreted as being consistent with Hashimoto thyroiditis. The patient was euthyroid at the time, with a TSH value of 2.5 mIU/L and a free T$_4$ value of 1.1 ng/dL (14.2 pmol/L). The patient currently has no symptoms of hypothyroidism and no symptoms referable to her thyroid nodules.

On physical examination, her vital signs are normal, and her BMI is 25 kg/m^2. Her thyroid gland is not enlarged but has an irregular texture. The left-sided thyroid nodule is palpable. It is mobile and nontender. The subcentimeter nodules are nonpalpable.

You perform ultrasonography again and repeat thyroid function tests. The sonographic appearance of the nodules and their size are unchanged.

Thyroid function tests:
  TSH = 1.2 mIU/L (0.5-5.0 mIU/L)
  Free T$_4$ = 1.2 ng/dL (0.8-1.8 ng/dL) (SI: 15.4 pmol/L [10.30-23.17 pmol/L])
  TPO antibodies = 582 IU/mL (<2.0 IU/mL) (SI: 582 kIU/L [<2.0 kIU/L])

Which of the following is the best next step in the management of this patient's thyroid nodules?
- A. Thyroidectomy
- B. Treatment with levothyroxine to achieve a suppressed TSH
- C. Measurement of serum calcitonin
- D. Left lobectomy
- E. Periodic monitoring of the patient's thyroid nodules and serum TSH

72 You are asked to see a 47-year-old man with a 20-year history of Crohn disease for evaluation of recurrent kidney stones. His bowel disease has been difficult to control and it is refractory to multiple therapies. His current regimen includes ustekinumab, 90 mg every 12 weeks, and colestipol, 5 g daily. He has recently undergone resection of the small bowel and ascending colon for strictures and ulcerations.

He has multiple endocrine issues associated with his inflammatory bowel disease including hypogonadism, osteopenia, and adrenal suppression from long-term steroid use. He is taking hydrocortisone replacement. In addition to ustekinumab and colestipol, his current medications include testosterone gel, 1.62% daily, and hydrocortisone, 20 mg daily. He also takes calcium carbonate plus cholecalciferol daily with meals.

Laboratory test results:

Serum total calcium = 9.9 mg/dL (8.2-10.2 mg/dL) (SI: 2.5 mmol/L [2.1-2.6 mmol/L])

Phosphate = 2.7 mg/dL (2.3-4.7 mg/dL) (SI: 0.9 mmol/L [0.7-1.5 mmol/L])

Serum creatinine = 0.97 mg/dL (0.7-1.3 mg/dL) (SI: 85.7 μmol/L [61.9-114.9 μmol/L])

PTH = 47 pg/mL (10-65 pg/mL) (SI: 47 ng/L [10-65 ng/L])

Albumin = 3.0 g/dL (3.5-5.0 g/dL) (SI: 30 g/L [30-50 g/L])

C-reactive protein = 19.9 mg/L (0.8-3.1 mg/L) (SI: 189.5 nmol/L [7.62-29.52 nmol/L])

25-Hydroxyvitamin D = 26 ng/mL (25-80 ng/mL [optimal]) (SI: nmol/L [62.4-199.7 nmol/L])

Urine volume = 2.6 L/24 h

Urinary calcium = 55 mg/24 h (100-300 mg/24 h) (SI: 1.4 mmol/d [2.5-7.5 mmol/d])

Urinary oxalate = 90 mg/24 h (<40 mg/24 h) (SI: 1026 mmol/d [<456 mmol/d])

Urinary uric acid = 300 mg/24 h (342-1191 mg/24 h)

Urinary citrate = 990 mg/24 h (450-1191 mg/24 h)

Urine pH = 6.3

Which of the following is the biggest risk factor for the development of kidney stones in this patient?
  A. Small-bowel resection
  B. Calcium supplementation
  C. Glucocorticoid use
  D. Magnesium supplementation
  E. High urinary citrate excretion

73 A 45-year-old man is referred by his primary care physician for management of longstanding dyslipidemia. He has a history of very high triglycerides detected in his 20s but no history of pancreatitis. Statin therapy was recommended, but he has never wanted to start treatment. He has always struggled with obesity. He leads a sedentary lifestyle, does not smoke cigarettes, and drinks 1 to 2 beers once a month. His dietary habits include regularly eating out and snacking. He has a history of impaired fasting glucose, gout, and newly diagnosed hypertension for which he was prescribed hydrochlorothiazide but has not filled the prescription. His medications include allopurinol, 300 mg daily, and a multivitamin. His 67-year-old father has a history of triglycerides higher than 2000 mg/dL (>22.6 mmol/L) without pancreatitis and recent placement of a coronary stent after presenting with acute dyspnea and chest tightness.

On physical examination, his blood pressure is 142/88 mm Hg. His height is 72 in (183 cm), and weight is 288 lb (131 kg) (BMI = 39.1 kg/m²). There are no xanthomas and no hepatomegaly. Abdominal obesity is present.

Laboratory test results (sample drawn while fasting):

Total cholesterol = 255 mg/dL (<200 mg/dL [optimal]) (SI: 6.60 mmol/L [<5.18 mmol/L])

Triglycerides = 1176 mg/dL (<150 mg/dL [optimal]) (SI: 13.29 mmol/L [<3.88 mmol/L])

HDL cholesterol = 33 mg/dL (>60 mg/dL [optimal]) (SI: 0.85 mmol/L [>1.55 mmol/L])

Non-HDL cholesterol = 222 mg/dL (<130 mg/dL [optimal]) (SI: 5.75 mmol/L [<3.37 mmol/L])

ALT = 43 U/L (10-40 U/L) (SI: 0.72 μkat/L [0.17-0.67 μkat/L])

AST = 39 U/L (20-48 U/L) (SI: 0.65 μkat/L [0.33-0.80 μkat/L])

TSH = 2.1 mIU/L (0.5-5.0 mIU/L)

Hemoglobin A_{1c} = 8.3% (4.0%-5.6%) (67 mmol/mol [20-38 mmol/mol])

In addition to medical nutrition therapy, which of the following should be prescribed?
  A. Metformin and a statin
  B. Metformin and a fibrate
  C. Metformin and fish oil
  D. Basal insulin and a statin
  E. Basal insulin and fish oil

74 A 31-year-old woman first presented 4 years earlier with amenorrhea and galactorrhea. An 11-mm prolactinoma was identified, and she has since been treated with cabergoline. Her current dosage is 0.5 mg twice weekly. She has regular menses and no galactorrhea. She has recently married and wishes to become pregnant as soon as possible; she is using no contraception.

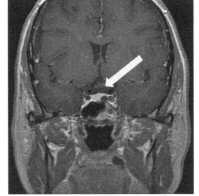

On physical examination, she appears well. Her height is 64 in (162.6 cm), and weight is 140 lb (63.6 kg) (BMI = 24 kg/m²). Her blood pressure is 105/68 mm Hg. No abnormalities are noted.

Laboratory test results:
Prolactin = 26 ng/mL (4-30 ng/mL) (SI: 1.13 nmol/L [0.17-1.30 nmol/L])
β-hCG = 2.1 mIU/mL (<3.0 mIU/mL) (SI: 2.1 mIU/mL [<3.0 IU/L])

Pituitary MRI shows a 5-mm left-sided microadenoma *(see image, arrow)*.

Which of the following is the best advice for this patient?
- A. Stop cabergoline now
- B. Stop cabergoline once pregnant
- C. Switch from cabergoline to bromocriptine once pregnant
- D. Reduce the cabergoline dosage to 0.25 mg once weekly
- E. Continue cabergoline indefinitely

75 A 59-year-old man has type 2 diabetes mellitus that was diagnosed 15 years ago. Five years ago, his therapy was advanced from oral agents to insulin. His treatment regimen consists of insulin detemir, 44 units every 12 hours, plus insulin aspart, 5 to 28 units with meals. The patient's primary symptom is dyspnea when walking 1 block.

His medical history is notable for hypertension, hyperlipidemia, coronary artery disease (status post coronary artery stenting to mid-left anterior descending artery and right coronary artery), New York Heart Association functional class III heart failure, chronic renal insufficiency, obstructive sleep apnea, obesity, and pancreatitis. His cardiologist is adjusting his cardiac medications, including his diuretic dosage, with the goal of removing fluid without adversely affecting his renal function.

On physical examination, his blood pressure is 130/80 mm Hg and pulse rate is 80 beats/min. His height is 69 in (175.3 cm), and weight is 305 lb (138.5 kg) (BMI = 45 kg/m²). Examination findings are remarkable for morbid obesity and 2+ pitting edema below the knees.

Laboratory test results:
Hemoglobin A_{1c} = 8.5% (4.0%-5.6%) (69 mmol/mol [20-38 mmol/mol])
Creatinine = 2.0 mg/dL (0.7-1.3 mg/dL) (SI: 176.8 μmol/L [61.9-114.9 μmol/L])
Estimated glomerular filtration rate = 35 mL/min per 1.73 m² (>60 mL/min per 1.73 m²)

Which of the following interventions do you recommend to reduce his risk for cardiovascular-related death?
- A. Optimize his insulin therapy to achieve a hemoglobin A_{1c} level ≤7.0% (≤53 mmol/mol)
- B. Initiate therapy with pioglitazone
- C. Initiate therapy with empagliflozin
- D. Initiate therapy with liraglutide
- E. No additional therapeutic interventions

76 A 19-year-old woman presents for evaluation after learning that Cowden syndrome (*PTEN* gene mutation) was identified in her sister and mother. She is well and asymptomatic. She was diagnosed with autism spectrum disorder as a child and takes no regular medication. Her older sister and her mother were diagnosed with breast cancer and a maternal aunt has undergone treatment for endometrial cancer.

On physical examination, her height is 65 in (165.1 cm) and weight is 165 lb (75 kg) (BMI = 27.5 kg/m²). Her blood pressure is 132/68 mm Hg, and pulse rate is 72 beats/min. She has a number of small, dome-shaped, skin-colored nodules on her arms and legs. You note that she has a prominent forehead, and her head circumference is 22.8 in (58 cm; >97th percentile). There is no palpable thyroid tissue in her neck. Examination of her breasts does not identify any lumps and there is no axillary lymphadenopathy. Findings on systems examination are otherwise normal.

Laboratory test results:
TSH = 1.3 mIU/L (0.5-5.0 mIU/L)
Free T$_4$ = 1.6 ng/dL (0.8-1.8 ng/dL) (SI: 20.6 pmol/L [10.30-23.17 pmol/L])

Which of the following is the best next step?
A. Total body CT scan
B. Thyroid ultrasonography
C. ¹⁸F-fluorodeoxyglucose PET imaging (FDG-PET)
D. Colonoscopy
E. Transvaginal pelvic ultrasonography

77 An 84-year-old woman with a recent diagnosis of large B-cell lymphoma of the right leg presents to the emergency department with a 3-day history of progressively altered mental status. The patient's daughter, who lives with her, reports that her mother had complaints of nausea and constipation for about a week. There was a diminishment of appetite and oral fluid intake and increased somnolence, leading to today's presentation. According to the daughter, the patient had a nonhealing lesion with an overlying scab on her right leg biopsied 1 week ago, which was identified as large B-cell lymphoma. She has an appointment with the oncologist later this week. The patient takes multiple vitamins including vitamin A and vitamin D. She does not take hydrochlorothiazide or lithium.

On physical examination, she is uncomfortable, moaning, and oriented only to name. Her blood pressure is 98/62 mm Hg, and pulse rate is 106 beats/min. Oxygen saturation is normal on room air. The oropharynx is dry with no lesions. Her chest is clear to auscultation. Cardiac examination is notable only for sinus tachycardia. Her right leg has 2+ edema up to the thigh with a 3 × 2-cm area of skin ulceration over the lateral aspect of the right knee with underlying swelling.

Laboratory test results:
Electrolytes, normal
Serum urea nitrogen = 35 mg/dL (8-23 mg/dL) (SI: 12.5 mmol/L [2.9-8.2 mmol/L])
Creatinine = 1.3 mg/dL (0.6-1.1 mg/dL) (SI: 114.9 μmol/L [53.0-97.2 μmol/L])
Calcium = 14.2 mg/dL (8.2-10.2 mg/dL) (SI: 3.6 mmol/L [2.1-2.6 mmol/L])
Calcium 2 weeks earlier at a routine visit = 10.1 mg/dL (SI: 2.5 mmol/L)
Phosphate = 5.0 mg/dL (2.3-4.7 mg/dL) (SI: 1.6 mmol/L [0.7-1.5 mmol/L])
25-Hydroxyvitamin D = 19 ng/mL (25-80 ng/mL [optimal]) (SI: 47.4 nmol/L [62.4-199.7 nmol/L])
Intact PTH = 3 pg/mL (10-65 pg/mL) (SI: 3 ng/L [10-65 ng/L])

She is admitted to the hospital for intravenous fluid hydration and subcutaneous calcitonin.

Which of the following is the most likely underlying cause of this patient's hypercalcemia?
   A. Ectopic production of 1α-hydroxylase
   B. Ectopic production of authentic PTH by tumoral cells
   C. Prolonged immobilization
   D. Increased production of fibroblast growth factor 23
   E. Increased production of PTHrP

78 A 48-year-old man with a history of nasopharyngeal carcinoma status post surgery and radiation 3 years ago has been feeling unwell, with fatigue and lack of stamina. He was evaluated by another endocrinologist while living in Europe and was told his evaluation was normal and no treatment was indicated. He now presents for a second opinion on whether he has GH deficiency. He brings the following laboratory test results to this visit:

Testosterone (8 AM) = 389 ng/dL (300-900 ng/dL) (SI: 13.5 nmol/L [10.4-31.2 nmol/L])
TSH = 1.6 mIU/L (0.5-5.0 mIU/L)
Free T$_4$ = 1.2 ng/dL (0.8-1.8 ng/dL) (SI: 15.4 pmol/L [10.30-23.17 pmol/L])
Cortisol (8 AM) = 19.7 μg/dL (5-25) (SI: 543.5 nmol/L [137.9-689.7 nmol/L])
Serum IGF-1 = 187 ng/mL (91-246 ng/mL) (SI: 24.5 nmol/L [11.9-32.2 nmol/L])
GHRH plus arginine stimulation test, peak GH = 19.5 ng/mL (SI: 19.5 μg/L)

Physical examination findings are normal. His height is 70 in (177.8 cm), and weight is 167 lb (75.9 kg) (BMI = 24 kg/m^2).

Which of the following is the most appropriate next diagnostic step?
   A. Measure IGFBP3
   B. Measure free IGF-1
   C. Obtain nighttime GH secretion profile
   D. Order a glucagon GH stimulation test
   E. No additional testing is needed; GH deficiency has been ruled out

79 A 46-year-old woman who runs marathons presents to her primary care physician with fatigue and palpitations. She is an endurance athlete who runs several marathons and triathlons per year. She describes constantly feeling tired, unable to run her routine distances, and palpitations when she runs (but also when she is resting).
   On physical examination, the only notable finding is a symmetric goiter.

Laboratory test results:
   TSH = 0.01 mIU/L (0.5-5.0 mIU/L)
   Free T$_4$ = 2.4 ng/dL (0.8-1.8 ng/dL) (SI: 30.9 pmol/L [10.30-23.17 pmol/L])

There is uniform and increased iodine uptake, and Graves disease is diagnosed. She is treated with methimazole and a β-adrenergic blocker for a few weeks and then undergoes successful radioactive iodine ablation. She subsequently becomes hypothyroid (TSH rises to 12 mIU/L), and she is prescribed levothyroxine. Three months after initiating levothyroxine, she reports persistent fatigue and worsening exercise tolerance. In addition, she has unintentionally lost 6.5 lb (3 kg) and describes a lack of appetite. She is concerned she could be depressed.

TSH = 0.8 mIU/L (0.5-5.0 mIU/L)
Free T$_4$ = 1.9 ng/dL (0.8-1.8 ng/dL) (SI: 24.5 pmol/L [10.30-23.17 pmol/L])
Serum cortisol (8 AM) = 17 μg/dL (5-25 μg/dL) (SI: 469.0 nmol/L [137.9-689.7 nmol/L])
Plasma ACTH (8 AM) = 244 pg/mL (10-60 pg/mL) (SI: 53.7 pmol/L [2.2-13.2 pmol/L])

Which of the following is the most likely cause of her current symptoms?
  A. Adrenal insufficiency
  B. Overtreatment with levothyroxine
  C. Recurrent thyrotoxicosis due to residual autonomous thyroid tissue
  D. Celiac disease
  E. ACTH-dependent Cushing syndrome

80 An 18-year-old man is referred by his pediatric endocrinologist to establish care with you. He comes with his mother who tells you that he was diagnosed with Prader-Willi syndrome at age 3 years. As a baby, he had feeding difficulties due to poor muscle tone, but his appetite increased as he got older. His mother must constantly monitor his food intake. She reports that he is hungry all the time and she has resorted to locking kitchen cabinets to ensure he does not have access to food. He takes no medications.

On physical examination, his blood pressure is 120/85 mm Hg, pulse rate is 60 beats/min, and BMI is 41 kg/m². The rest of his examination findings are unremarkable.

During the visit, you discuss the endocrinopathies associated with his medical condition. The patient and his mother are very concerned about his weight and would like to learn about weight-loss options.

Which of the following would you recommend to manage his obesity?
  A. Biliopancreatic diversion
  B. Roux-en-Y gastric bypass
  C. Topiramate
  D. Leptin
  E. Referral to a dietitian for guidance on a supervised and restricted diet

81 A 35-year-old woman is being seen in the endocrinology clinic for follow-up of hypoglycemia. Type 1 diabetes was diagnosed at age 12 years. She was initially treated with multiple daily insulin injections, and her regimen was changed to pump therapy at age 16 years. She has generally had reasonable glycemic control with recent hemoglobin A_{1c} levels in the range of 6.7% to 7.4% (50-57 mmol/mol). She has hypoglycemia unawareness. After experiencing a seizure related to a severe hypoglycemic episode at age 32, she began using a continuous glucose monitor. Two months ago, she was prescribed losartan and atorvastatin. Two weeks ago, streptococcal pharyngitis was diagnosed and she was treated with cefuroxime (she is allergic to penicillin). She also took ibuprofen and acetaminophen for throat pain for 10 days.

At today's appointment, she reports glucose readings on the glucose sensor that are 100 to 150 mg/dL (5.6-8.3 mmol/L) higher than the fingerstick glucose measurements obtained at the same time. On 2 occasions, she administered correctional insulin boluses to treat hyperglycemia without confirming with a fingerstick glucose measurement, and she rapidly developed hypoglycemia. Fortunately, she recognized the hypoglycemic symptoms and was able to self-treat with glucose tablets and carbohydrates. She is now so frustrated with the sensor that she has removed the device.

On physical examination, she appears well. Her height is 66 in (168 cm), and weight is 134 lb (60.9 kg) (BMI = 21.6 kg/m²). Her blood pressure is 107/72 mm Hg, pulse rate is 72 beats/min, and respiratory rate is 12 breaths/min. Findings on funduscopic examination are normal. Her abdomen is without scars or lipohypertrophy. The insulin pump site is on the upper lateral right buttock. No lipohypertrophy is present. The rest of the examination findings are unremarkable.

Laboratory test results:
  Hemoglobin A_{1c} = 7.1% (4.0%-5.6%) (SI: 54 mmol/mol [20-38 mmol/mol])
  Point-of-care glucose = 146 mg/dL (70-99 mg/dL) (SI: 8.1 mmol/L [3.9-5.5 mmol/L])
  Electrolytes, normal
  Creatinine, normal
  Albumin-to-creatinine ratio (4 months ago) = <10 mg/g creat (<30 mg/g creat)

Which of the following is the most likely cause of the spurious glucose readings obtained with this patient's glucose sensor?
- A. Ibuprofen
- B. Cefuroxime
- C. Losartan
- D. Atorvastatin
- E. Acetaminophen

82 A 28-year-old man is seen for follow-up after undergoing pituitary surgery for acromegaly 6 months earlier. There has been marked clinical improvement since surgery, but he still reports arthralgia and night sweats. Three months after surgery, pituitary MRI demonstrated residual tumor in the cavernous sinus, and biochemical evaluation confirmed persistent GH excess. Therefore, octreotide LAR, at an initial dose of 20 mg intramuscular injection every 4 weeks, was prescribed.

On physical examination, he has acromegalic facies with frontal bossing and prognathism. His blood pressure is 152/94 mm Hg. His height is 73 in (185.4 cm), and weight is 225 lb (102.3 kg) (BMI = 29.7 kg/m²).

Laboratory test results:
3 months after surgery:
IGF-1 = 512 ng/mL (117-321 ng/mL) (SI: 67.1 nmol/L [15.3-42.1 nmol/L])
GH = 4.2 ng/mL (0.01-0.97 ng/mL) (SI: 4.2 µg/L [0.01-0.97 µg/L])
6 months after commencing octreotide:
IGF-1 = 385 ng/mL (SI: 50.4 nmol/L)
GH = 2.8 ng/mL (SI: 2.8 µg/L)

Which of the following is the best management step now?
- A. Refer for pituitary radiotherapy
- B. Increase the octreotide dosage to 30 mg every 4 weeks
- C. Stop octreotide and start pegvisomant
- D. Continue octreotide and add pegvisomant
- E. Continue octreotide and add cabergoline

83 A 22-year-old transgender man is referred for management of gender dysphoria. The patient recalls a childhood in which he never felt comfortable in girl's clothing and protested wearing dresses to church. Menarche at age 13 years was distressing. He came out to his friends and family while in college and has been wearing a binder since that time. He established care with a psychologist whom he has being seeing monthly for 1 year. He thinks that he may have depressive symptoms but not major depression or suicidal thoughts. He is interested in starting testosterone therapy and eventually having "top surgery." His only medication is an albuterol inhaler as needed for asthma.

On physical examination, his blood pressure is 124/68 mm Hg. His height is 68 in (173 cm), and weight is 169 lb (77 kg) (BMI = 26 kg/m²). Physical examination findings are unremarkable.

Laboratory test results:
Total testosterone = 28 ng/dL (8-60 ng/dL for women) (SI: 1.0 nmol/L [0.3-2.1 nmol/L])
Estradiol = 95 pg/mL (17-200 pg/mL for women) (SI: 348.7 pmol/L [62.9-739.6 pmol/L])

As you counsel this patient, you explain that which of the following changes are most likely to occur after 1 year of testosterone therapy?

Answer	Depressive Symptoms	Body Weight	Ovaries
A.	Improve	Decrease	Atrophy
B.	Improve	Increase	Hyperplasia
C.	Improve	Increase	Atrophy
D.	No change	Increase	Hyperplasia
E.	No change	Decrease	No change

84 A 62-year-old man presents 3 weeks after being discharged from the hospital with a new diagnosis of diabetes mellitus. He was initially admitted to the hospital with his second myocardial infarction complicated by heart failure (echocardiography showed a left ventricular ejection fraction of 25% to 30% before discharge). He responded well to aggressive medical management, and he was able to ambulate comfortably without dyspnea before discharge. Glucose levels were elevated during his hospitalization and were treated with a high-dose supplemental insulin aspart scale. His hemoglobin A_{1c} measurement (sample drawn during admission) was 8.0% (64 mmol/mol). Since hospital discharge, his glucose levels have been between 160 and 200 mg/dL before breakfast and before his evening meal. He walks for 30 minutes daily. His medications include isosorbide, furosemide, hydralazine, metoprolol, and pravastatin.

On physical examination, his blood pressure is 116/74 mm Hg and pulse rate is 58 beats/min. His height is 72.5 in (184.2 cm), and weight is 217 lb (98.6 kg) (BMI = 29 kg/m²). There is no jugular venous distention. On cardiac examination, there are no murmurs, rubs, or gallops. His lungs are clear. There is 2+ ankle edema.

Laboratory test results:
Glucose = 187 mg/dL (70-99 mg/dL) (SI: 10.4 mmol/L [3.9-5.5 mmol/L])
Creatinine = 2.4 mg/dL (0.7-1.3 mg/dL) (SI: 212.2 µmol/L [61.9-114.9 µmol/L])
Estimated glomerular filtration rate = 28 mL/min per 1.73 m² (>60 mL/min per 1.73 m²)

Which of the following agents would be the best therapeutic option to lower his hemoglobin A_{1c} level?
A. Sitagliptin
B. Glyburide
C. Canagliflozin
D. Pioglitazone
E. Metformin

85 A 32-year-old woman recently saw a primary care physician because of frequent urinary tract infections over the last 10 years. Laboratory testing noted a slightly elevated serum calcium level (10.6 mg/dL [2.7 mmol/L]), and urinalysis results were consistent with a bacterial infection. An antibiotic was prescribed, and she was referred to you for further evaluation of hypercalcemia.

She was first told she had an elevated calcium level 8 years ago. She recalls that the value was approximately 10 mg/dL (2.5 mmol/L). Last year, she was noted to have a serum calcium level of 11.3 mg/dL (2.8 mmol/L) at a routine check-up (albumin not measured). She does not believe she has ever had a calcium measurement higher than 11.3 mg/dL (>2.8 mmol/L).

She has excessive thirst with polyuria and nocturia 2 times a night. She feels fatigued and has insomnia. She has no history of renal stones, acid reflux symptoms, fractures, loss of height, arthralgias, or myalgias. She is not known to have persistent hypertension and takes no medications or supplements. Her family history is notable for her mother having hypercalcemia and taking lithium for bipolar disorder.

Laboratory test results:

Creatinine = 0.59 mg/dL (0.6-1.1 mg/dL) (SI: 52.2 μmol/L [53.0-97.2 μmol/L])

Calcium = 10.4 mg/dL (8.2-10.2 mg/dL) (SI: 2.6 mmol/L [2.1-2.6 mmol/L])

Phosphate = 3.0 mg/dL (2.3-4.7 mg/dL) (SI: 10.0 mmol/L [0.7-1.5 mmol/L])

Albumin = 3.9 g/dL (3.5-5.0 g/dL) (SI: 39 g/L [35-50 g/L])

Intact PTH = 38 pg/mL (10-65 pg/mL) (SI: 38 ng/L [10-65 ng/L])

25-Hydroxyvitamin D = 32 ng/mL (25-80 ng/mL [optimal]) (SI: 79.9 nmol/L [62.4-199.7 nmol/L])

Analyte	24-Hour Value	Concentration
Urinary calcium	91 mg/24 h (2.3 mmol/d)	6.5 mg/dL
Urinary creatinine	1.2 g/24 h (10.6 mmol/d)	85.5 mg/dL

Reference ranges: urinary calcium, 100-300 mg/24 h (2.5-7.5 mmol/d); urinary creatinine, 1.0-2.0 g/24 h (8.8-17.7 mmol/d).

Thyroid ultrasonography (*see image*) demonstrates 2 subcentimeter hypoechoic nodules (0.5 × 0.8 cm and 0.4 × 0.5 cm) just inferior to the right thyroid lobe that are of indeterminate etiology. No nodules are observed in the thyroid gland.

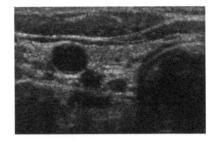

Sestamibi scan does not demonstrate any identifiable parathyroid adenomas.

DXA findings include a Z score of –1.4 in the left total hip and a Z score of 1.5 in the distal one-third forearm.

Which of the following is the most appropriate recommendation for this patient?

A. Reassure her that no further treatment is needed

B. Refer for exploratory neck surgery for parathyroidectomy

C. Measure PTHrP

D. Order urine protein electrophoresis

E. Perform FNAB of the largest nodule inferior to the right thyroid

86 You are consulted regarding the management of a thyroid nodule in a 38-year-old man. The patient is a newscaster, and the nodule was first noted 2 years ago when a television viewer called into the network to advise him to see an endocrinologist. The patient subsequently underwent thyroid ultrasonography, which showed a 4.9 × 3 × 4.2-cm right-sided nodule. The nodule was described as solid with a central hypoechoic region. A 0.7-cm isoechoic nodule without intranodular calcifications was also documented on the left side. FNAB of the 4.9-cm nodule was performed, and cytologic examination documented a Hurthle-cell nodule, with a differential diagnosis including a Hurthle-cell neoplasm. The patient has no other medical conditions. He has no compressive symptoms related to his larger thyroid nodule.

On physical examination, he is a euthyroid-appearing individual. His blood pressure is 128/78 mm Hg. His height is 70 in (177.8 cm), and weight is 156 lb (70.9 kg) (BMI = 22.4 kg/m²). His right thyroid lobe is clearly visible. The right-sided nodule is firm, nontender, and not associated with any other palpable nodules or lymphadenopathy. There is no apparent tracheal deviation. The rest of his physical examination findings are unremarkable. The sonographic appearance of the 4.9-cm nodule is shown (*see image*).

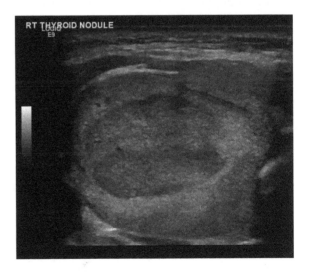

Which of the following courses of action would you recommend to this patient and his primary care physician?
- A. Repeated thyroid ultrasonography in 1 year
- B. Repeated FNAB of the 4.9-cm nodule with Gene Expression Classifier testing
- C. Percutaneous ethanol injection into the 4.9-cm nodule
- D. Right lobectomy
- E. FNAB of the left thyroid nodule

87 A 54-year-old postmenopausal woman with a 15-year history of rheumatoid arthritis presents for management of lipids. She was found to have an abnormal lipid panel 2 years ago and was prescribed atorvastatin, 40 mg daily, but she developed myalgias and stopped the medication after 2 months. Her rheumatoid arthritis is quiescent and is treated with low-dosage prednisone and methotrexate. She has treated hypothyroidism, but is otherwise healthy. She does not smoke cigarettes and drinks 1 glass of wine 3 times a week. There is no family history of premature or early cardiovascular disease.

On physical examination, her blood pressure is 120/64 mm Hg. Her height is 65 in (165 cm), and weight is 164 lb (74.5 kg) (BMI = 27.3 kg/m²). She has some abdominal obesity and chronic arthritic deformities of the metacarpophalangeal joints of both hands.

Laboratory test results (sample drawn while fasting):

Total cholesterol = 228 mg/dL (<200 mg/dL [optimal]) (SI: 2.91 mmol/L [<5.18 mmol/L])
Triglycerides = 143 mg/dL (<150 mg/dL [optimal]) (SI: 1.62 mmol/L [<3.88 mmol/L])
LDL cholesterol = 161 mg/dL (<100 mg/dL [optimal]) (SI: 4.17 mmol/L [<2.59 mmol/L])
HDL cholesterol = 38 mg/dL (>60 mg/dL [optimal]) (SI: 0.98 mmol/L [>1.55 mmol/L])
TSH = 1.53 mIU/mL (0.5-5.0 mIU/L)
Hemoglobin A_{1c} = 6.1% (4.0%-5.6%) (43 mmol/mol [20-38 mmol/mol])

On the basis of the above lipid panel and using the American College of Cardiology/American Heart Association 2013 risk calculator, her 10-year risk for atherosclerotic cardiovascular disease is 3.9%.

Which of the following should you recommend in the management of this patient's lipids?
- A. No therapy now
- B. Colesevelam
- C. Ezetimibe
- D. Trial of a statin at a lower dosage
- E. A proprotein convertase subtilisin/kexin type 9 (PCSK9) inhibitor

88 A 38-year-old nulliparous woman with type 2 diabetes mellitus is contemplating pregnancy in the next 6 months, and she is seeking advice regarding her diabetes control. Diabetes was diagnosed at age 35 years, and her treatment regimen consists of metformin and glyburide. Her most recent hemoglobin A_{1c} measurement was 6.8% (51 mmol/mol).

On physical examination, her blood pressure is 135/75 mm Hg. Her height is 64 in (162.6 cm), and weight is 175 lb (79.5 kg) (BMI = 30 kg/m²). Her most recent eye examination documented evidence of retinopathy with hard exudates and microaneurysms.

Laboratory test results (sample drawn while fasting):

Hemoglobin A_{1c} = 6.8% (4.0%-5.6%) (51 mmol/mol [20-38 mmol/mol])
Total cholesterol = 192 mg/dL (<200 mg/dL [optimal]) (SI: 4.97 mmol/L [<5.18 mmol/L])
LDL cholesterol = 110 mg/dL (<100 mg/dL [optimal]) (SI: 2.85 mmol/L [<2.59 mmol/L])
HDL cholesterol = 28 mg/dL (>60 mg/dL [optimal]) (SI: 0.73 mmol/L [>1.55 mmol/L])
Triglycerides = 270 mg/dL (<150 mg/dL [optimal]) (SI: 3.05 mmol/L [<3.88 mmol/L])
Estimated glomerular filtration rate = 88 mL/min per 1.73 m² (>60 mL/min per 1.73 m²)

She asks what she must do to reduce her pregnancy-related risks.

Which of the following is the best next step before conception?
  A. Target hemoglobin A_{1c} value 6.0%-6.5% (42-48 mmol/mol)
  A. Target weight loss of 10%
  B. Target blood pressure <120/80 mm Hg
  C. Undergo retinal laser therapy
  D. Target triglycerides <150 mg/dL [<1.70 mmol/L])

89 You are asked to evaluate a 39-year-old woman who is in the emergency department. She describes a 3-day history of frontal headache, vomiting, and fatigue. She has a history of stage IV melanoma and type 2 diabetes mellitus. She is currently treated with ipilimumab immunotherapy (for the past 3 months), premixed insulin twice daily, ramipril, simvastatin, and pancrelipase. She reports noticing more hypoglycemia recently.

On physical examination, she is drowsy but arousable. She appears dehydrated. Her temperature is 99.5°F (37.5°C), blood pressure is 105/68 mm Hg, and pulse rate is 110 beats/min. There are no focal neurologic findings, and visual fields are normal.

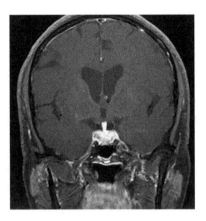

Laboratory test results:
  White blood cell count = 13,500/μL (4500-11,000/μL)
    (SI: 13.5×10^9/L [4.5-11.0×10^9/L])
  C-reactive protein = 5.0 mg/L (0.8-3.1 mg/L) (SI: 48 nmol/L [7.62-29.52 nmol/L])
  Sodium = 129 mEq/L (136-142 mEq/L) (SI: 129 mmol/L [136-142 mmol/L])
  Potassium = 4.5 mEq/L (3.5-5.0 mEq/L) (SI: 4.5 mmol/L [3.5-5.0 mmol/L])
  Serum urea nitrogen = 28 mg/dL (8-23 mg/dL) (SI: 10.0 mmol/L [2.9-8.2 mmol/L])
  Creatinine = 1.8 mg/dL (0.6-1.1 mg/dL) (SI: 159.1 μmol/L [53.0-97.2 μmol/L])
  Cortisol = 4.8 μg/dL (5-25 μg/dL) (SI: 132.4 nmol/L [137.9-689.7 nmol/L])
  TSH = 0.8 mIU/L (0.5-5.0 mIU/L)
  Free T_4 = 0.65 ng/dL (0.8-1.8 ng/dL) (SI: 8.4 pmol/L [10.30-23.17 pmol/L])

Contrast-enhanced pituitary MRI is shown (*see image*).

Which of the following is the most likely cause of this patient's pituitary abnormality?
  A. Hypophysitis
  B. Hemorrhage
  C. Abscess
  D. Metastasis
  E. Adenoma

90 A 22-year-old woman with polycystic ovary syndrome comes to you for treatment advice. She underwent menarche at age 13 years and has always had irregular menstrual cycles, every 4 to 6 months. She weighed 140 to 150 lb (63.6-68.2 kg) in high school, but she gained weight in college and has been unable to lose it. She also developed hirsutism on her chin, and she shaves daily.

On physical examination, her blood pressure is 118/76 mm Hg. Her height is 68 in (172.7 cm), and weight is 167 lb (76.0 kg) (BMI = 25.5 kg/m²). Skin examination reveals acanthosis on the neck and hirsutism over the chin and on the lower abdomen and upper thighs. Her Ferriman-Gallwey score is 20. Her thyroid is an estimated 20 g and without nodules. On breast examination, there are no masses or galactorrhea.

Laboratory test results:

Testosterone = 69 ng/dL (8-60 ng/dL) (SI: 2.4 nmol/L [0.3-2.1 nmol/L])

DHEA-S = 122 µg/dL (44-332 µg/dL) (SI: 3.3 µmol/L [1.19-9.00 µmol/L])

Insulin = 34 µIU/mL (1.4-14.0 µIU/mL) (SI: 236.1 pmol/L [9.7-97.2 pmol/L])

Total cholesterol = 259 mg/dL (<200 mg/dL [optimal]) (SI: 6.71 mmol/L [<5.18 mmol/L])

Triglycerides = 118 mg/dL (<150 mg/dL [optimal]) (SI: 1.33 mmol/L [<3.88 mmol/L])

LDL cholesterol = 197 mg/dL (<100 mg/dL [optimal]) (SI: 5.10 mmol/L [<2.59 mmol/L])

HDL cholesterol = 62 mg/dL (>60 mg/dL [optimal]) (SI: 1.61 mmol/L [>1.55 mmol/L])

Hemoglobin A_{1c} = 5.4% (4.0%-5.6%) (36 mmol/mol [20-38 mmol/mol])

Which of the following is the best treatment option for this patient?
A. Combination hormonal contraception
B. Levonorgestrel-coated intrauterine device
C. Spironolactone
D. Dexamethasone
E. Metformin

91 A 37-year-old woman with no notable medical history except for hysterectomy 5 years ago (after the birth of her second child) started developing headaches about 4 months ago. Initial head CT was normal. Over the following 2 months, her headaches became worse, and she developed panhypopituitarism and diabetes insipidus. Brain MRI showed diffuse enlargement of the pituitary gland and stalk thickening (4 mm). Lymphocytic hypophysitis was presumptively diagnosed, and she was treated with high-dosage dexamethasone, 4 mg twice daily. Now, 2 months later, her headaches have not improved. Her vision remains subjectively normal. She has no fever or chills. She has gained 20 lb (9.1 kg) since starting dexamethasone. Her pituitary mass has further enlarged. In addition to dexamethasone, she takes levothyroxine, 100 mcg daily, and desmopressin, 0.2 mg twice daily orally, with good control of polyuria.

On physical examination, her height is 65 in (165 cm) and weight is 196 lb (89 kg) (BMI = 32.6 kg/m²). Her blood pressure is 124/78 mm Hg, and pulse rate is 89 beats/min. She is afebrile. She has normally pigmented skin, normal findings on neurologic examination, and no tremors.

Chest x-ray is normal.

Which of the following is the most appropriate next step?
A. Perform a pituitary biopsy
B. Perform a tuberculin skin test
C. Measure transferrin saturation and ferritin
D. Measure serum angiotensin-converting enzyme levels
E. Measure pituitary antibodies

92 A 26-year-old man returns to your clinic for management of his cystic fibrosis–related diabetes mellitus. He is followed by a multidisciplinary team of providers, including a pulmonologist and endocrinologist. His diabetes was diagnosed at age 19 years with a 2-hour oral glucose tolerance test. You have been following him since he graduated from college at age 22 years. His current hemoglobin A_{1c} value is 7.8% (62 mmol/mol). The patient has been married for 2 years and the couple is now interested in having a child. At the end of the visit, he inquires about his fertility potential. Neither the patient nor his wife has attempted to have a child in the past. His wife has asthma that is well controlled with inhalers. She reports having regular menses.

The patient's current medications are insulin glargine once daily, insulin aspart before meals, pancreatic enzyme supplements, multivitamins, a mucolytic agent, and oral antibiotics.

On physical examination, his blood pressure is 116/62 mm Hg. His height is 72 in (183 cm), and weight is 143 lb (65 kg) (BMI = 19.4 kg/m²). Physical examination findings are unremarkable. His testes are 15 mL bilaterally without any masses.

Regarding his fertility, which of the following referrals is the best next step?
   A. Adoption agency
   B. Genetic counseling and genetic testing
   C. Andrology laboratory for a complete semen analysis
   D. Urology for percutaneous epididymal sperm aspiration
   E. Urology for testicular excisional biopsy with sperm extraction

93 A 48-year-old woman presents with a 12-month history of weight gain (30 lb [13.6 kg]), skin thinning, and bruising. Type 2 diabetes mellitus and hypertension have also been recently diagnosed. She has a history of degenerative lumbar spine disease causing chronic back pain. She is currently treated with candesartan, metformin, amitriptyline, and acetaminophen.

On physical examination, she has central obesity and a dorsocervical fat pad. Examination of the skin reveals some bruising over the forearms and pale striae over the abdominal wall. There are multiple freckles on her shoulders, but none over the mucous membranes. Her blood pressure is 162/99 mm Hg. She is obese (BMI = 36 kg/m²).

Laboratory test results:
   ACTH = 4.0 pg/mL (10-60 pg/mL) (SI: 0.88 pmol/L
      [2.2-13.2 pmol/L])
   Cortisol (8 AM after 1-mg overnight dexamethasone suppression
      test) = 7.5 μg/dL (SI: 207 nmol/L)
   24-Hour urinary free cortisol = 85 μg/24 h (4-50 μg/24 h)
      (SI: 235 nmol/d [11-138 nmol/d])
   17α-Hydroxyprogesterone = 78 ng/dL (<80 ng/dL [follicular
      phase]) (SI: 2.36 nmol/L [<2.42 nmol/L])
   Plasma metanephrine = 56 pg/mL (<57 pg/mL)
      (SI: 283.9 pmol/L [<289 pmol/L])
   Plasma normetanephrine = 280 pg/mL (<148 pg/mL)
      (SI: 1528.8 pmol/L [<808 pmol/L])

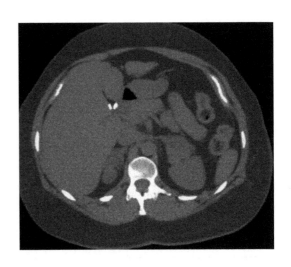

CT of the adrenal glands is shown (*see image*).

Which of the following diagnoses is most likely responsible for this patient's condition?
   A. Carney complex
   B. Primary pigmented nodular adrenal hyperplasia
   C. Bilateral pheochromocytoma
   D. Bilateral macronodular adrenal hyperplasia
   E. Nonclassic congenital adrenal hyperplasia

94 A 22-year-old woman has questions about the treatment of her diabetes mellitus. In childhood, she was told that she had elevated glucose levels, but diabetes was not diagnosed until she was 21. She has been taking metformin, 750 mg twice daily, for the last year and has intermittent bloating and loose stools. She saw a nutritionist 2 months ago to review a diet plan. Her 2-week average glucose value is 124 mg/dL (6.9 mmol/L). She has no hypoglycemia. She does not have hypertension and is not on lipid-lowering medication. She has regular menses and has an intrauterine device in place. She exercises regularly. She does not smoke cigarettes.

Her mother was diagnosed with diabetes in her mid-teens, as was the patient's older brother. Her maternal grandfather also had diabetes. The patient's brother was found to have a mutation in the glucokinase gene (*GCK*).

On physical examination, her height is 66 in (168 cm) and weight is 136 lb (61.8 kg) (BMI = 21.9 kg/m²). Her blood pressure is 106/72 mm Hg, and pulse rate is 62 beats/min. Examination findings are normal.

Laboratory test results:

Hemoglobin A$_{1c}$ = 5.9% (4.0%-5.6%) (41 mmol/mol [20-38 mmol/mol])

Creatinine = 0.7 mg/dL (0.6-1.1 mg/dL) (SI: 61.9 μmol/L [53.0-97.2 μmol/L])

Estimated glomerular filtration rate = >90 mL/min per 1.73 m^2 (>60 mL/min per 1.73 m^2)

Electrolytes, normal

TSH, normal

C-peptide = 1.8 ng/mL (0.9-4.3 ng/mL) (SI: 0.6 nmol/L [0.30-1.42 nmol/L])

Glucose = 136 mg/dL (70-99 mg/dL) (SI: 7.5 mmol/L [3.9-5.5 mmol/L])

Glutamic acid decarboxylase antibodies, undetectable

Which of the following is the best next step in the treatment of diabetes in this patient?
A. Continue metformin
B. Stop metformin and continue with diet treatment
C. Stop metformin and start a sulfonylurea
D. Stop metformin and start a sodium-glucose cotransporter 2 inhibitor
E. Stop metformin and start a glucagonlike peptide 1 analogue

95 A 61-year-old woman is referred to you with a 3-year history of increasing fatigue and weight gain of 5 lb (2.3 kg), but no other concerns. She takes ramipril to treat hypertension, but does not take any other regular medication. Her mother has rheumatoid arthritis.

On physical examination, her height is 68 in (172.7 cm) and weight is 210 lb (95.5 kg) (BMI = 31.9 kg/m^2). Her blood pressure is 146/85 mm Hg, and pulse rate is 68 beats/min. There is no palpable thyroid enlargement in her neck. She has normal knee and ankle reflexes on neurologic evaluation. Findings on systems examination are otherwise unremarkable.

She has had her thyroid function tested on several occasions in the last 5 years (*see table*).

Date	Serum TSH	Serum Free T$_4$	TPO Antibodies
5 years ago	5.7 mIU/L	1.1 ng/dL (14.2 pmol/L)	320 IU/mL (320 kIU/L)
18 months ago	5.3 mIU/L	1.2 ng/dL (15.4 pmol/L)	...
6 months ago	5.8 mIU/L	1.1 ng/dL (14.2 pmol/L)	...
Today	5.5 mIU/L	1.2 ng/dL (15.4 pmol/L)	120 IU/mL (<2.0 kIU/L)

Reference ranges: TSH, 0.5-5.0 mIU/L; free T$_4$, 0.8-1.8 ng/dL (SI: 10.30-23.17 pmol/L); TPO antibodies, <2.0 IU/mL (SI: <2.0 kIU/L).

Which of the following would result in you recommending levothyroxine replacement therapy?
A. Reduced serum free T$_3$ concentration
B. Her blood pressure of 146/85 mm Hg
C. Total cholesterol concentration greater than 220 mg/dL (>5.70 mmol/L)
D. Evidence of thyroiditis on thyroid ultrasonography
E. Levothyroxine therapy is not indicated

96 A 40-year-old man presents to the emergency department with a 1-week history of progressive weakness of his arms and legs, intermittent cramps in his fingers and feet, and pain in "all of his bones." These symptoms have limited his activity level. He reports having sharp and dull pain in the bilateral ribs and feet for the past 2 years. Over the course of the last year, he has had progressive pain involving his shoulders, arms, and legs, as well as joint pain in his wrists, knees, and ankles. He has no trauma or fracture history or fever. He has no known medical problems, no history of renal stones, and no loss of height.

On physical examination, his vitals signs are stable. He is afebrile and normotensive with a pulse rate of 96 beats/min. His height is 71 in (177.8 cm). He appears weak and in distress from pain. On musculoskeletal examination, he has full range of motion against gravity but not to slight resistance in the bilateral upper and lower extimities. There is no muscle atrophy in the hands or feet. Pain is elicited on palpation of muscles in the upper arms, lower arms, thighs, and calves. There is no joint swelling or effusions.

Laboratory test results:

Basic chemistry panel, normal

Complete blood cell count, normal

Calcium = 8.9 mg/dL (8.2-10.2 mg/dL) (SI: 2.2 mmol/L [2.1-2.6 mmol/L])

Phosphate = 1.1 mg/dL (2.3-4.7 mg/dL) (SI: 0.4 mmol/L [0.7-1.5 mmol/L])

Albumin = 4.2 g/dL (3.5-5.0 g/dL) (SI: 42 g/L [35-50 g/L])

Alkaline phosphatase = 150 U/L (50-120 U/L) (SI: 2.5 μkat/L [0.84-2.00 μkat/L])

Intact PTH = 104 pg/mL (10-65 pg/mL) (SI: 104 g/L [10-65 ng/L])

25-Hydroxyvitamin D = 20 ng/mL (25-80 ng/mL [optimal]) (SI: 49.9 nmol/L [62.4-199.7 nmol/L])

1,25-Dihydroxyvitamin D = <8 pg/mL (16-65 pg/mL) (SI: 20.8 pmol/L [41.6-169.0 pmol/L])

Chest x-ray shows bilateral rib fractures in various stages of healing but no abnormal masses in the bones or lungs. The patient is admitted to the hospital for medical treatment and further testing.

Which of the following is the best next test to evaluate for the underlying etiology of this patient's condition?

    A. Serum protein electrophoresis

    B. Fibroblast growth factor 23 measurement

    C. Bone-specific alkaline phosphatase measurement

    D. Bone mineral density assessment

    E. Serum C-telopeptide measurement

97 A 36-year-old woman has a 10-year history of anxiety and depression. She has been treated with venlafaxine for 5 years with substantial improvements in her anxiety, but over the last year she has developed more frequent anxiety episodes and occasional palpitations. Alprazolam was prescribed several weeks ago, but it has not relieved her symptoms. During a routine primary care appointment, her blood pressure was 162/90 mm Hg, her pulse rate was 102 beats/min, and she was noted to be anxious. Her primary care physician ordered thyroid function tests, which were normal, and then ordered measurement of plasma metanephrines to evaluate whether she could have a catecholamine-producing tumor contributing to her anxiety.

Plasma normetanephrine = 222 pg/mL (<148 pg/mL) (SI: 1212.1 pmol/L [<808 pmol/L])

Plasma metanephrine = 80 pg/mL (<57 pg/mL) (SI: 405.6 pmol/L [<289 pmol/L])

Which of the following is the most likely interpretation of these results?

    A. Anxiety

    B. "False-positive" results related to venlafaxine use

    C. "False-positive" results related to alprazolam use

    D. Paraganglioma

    E. Pheochromocytoma

98 An 18-year-old man presents for an initial consultation after his primary care physician received positive results of *RET* proto-oncogene genetic testing. The testing was ordered because a disease-causing mutation (Leu790Phe [L790F]) had been identified in the patient's mother. The same mutation was identified in the patient. He is asymptomatic and has not yet had any evaluation. The patient's relevant family history includes 3 family members with medullary thyroid cancer. His 38-year-old mother recently underwent a thyroidectomy and central compartment lymph node dissection. She had 2 foci of medullary thyroid cancer in her thyroid gland and lymph node metastases, but she has had no evidence of residual disease on follow-up testing. His 35-year-old maternal uncle also recently underwent thyroidectomy and was found to have medullary thyroid cancer metastatic to the cervical lymph nodes. His surgery was complicated by a hypertensive crisis resulting in an aborted surgery, so the planned lymph node dissection was not completed. His serum calcitonin level has remained elevated after the operation. The patient's maternal grandmother died at age 57 years of metastatic medullary cancer involving the liver. There is no known family history of hyperparathyroidism or pheochromocytoma.

On physical examination, the patient's vital signs are normal. His height is 72 in (182.9 cm), and weight is 170 lb (77.1 kg) (BMI = 23.1 kg/m²). His blood pressure is 138/90 mm Hg. The patient has a normal-sized thyroid gland with no palpable nodules. There is no palpable cervical adenopathy.

You research the Leu790Phe mutation and find that although is it associated with less aggressive disease than many other *RET* mutations, medullary thyroid cancer has been documented in mutation carriers as young as 12 years. The typical age of progression to medullary thyroid cancer is 30 to 47 years.

In addition to screening the patient for pheochromocytoma, which of the following is the best next step in his care?
  A. Measure serum gastrin
  B. Measure serum prolactin
  C. Measure serum calcitonin and perform neck ultrasonography
  D. Recommend immediate thyroidectomy
  E. Nothing additional now; routine annual physical examinations until he is 30 years old

99 A 64-year-old woman is being seen in clinic for yearly follow-up of hypertension and dyslipidemia. She had laboratory tests done for an insurance physical 6 weeks ago. At that time, her fasting glucose concentration was 116 mg/dL (6.4 mmol/L) and her hemoglobin A₁c level was 6.1% (45 mmol/mol). Six months ago, her fasting glucose level was 109 mg/dL (6.0 mmol/L). She is being treated with valsartan/hydrochlorothiazide, 160 mg/12.5 mg daily, and carvedilol, 12.5 mg twice daily. She takes atorvastatin, 80 mg daily. She underwent stenting of a right coronary artery lesion 3 years ago. She has gained 12 lb (5.5 kg) in the last 3 years and would like to lose weight. She does not smoke cigarettes. She has a glass of wine 3 to 4 times per week. She is sedentary most of the day.

On physical examination, her height is 65 in (165 cm) and weight is 163 lb (74.1 kg) (BMI = 27.1 kg/m²). Her blood pressure is 132/83 mm Hg, and pulse rate is 66 beats/min. Findings on heart, lung, abdominal, and neurologic examinations are normal.

Laboratory test results:
    Creatinine = 1.0 mg/dL (0.6-1.1 mg/dL) (SI: 88.4 µmol/L [53.0-97.2 µmol/L])
    Estimated glomerular filtration rate = >60 mL/min per 1.73 m² (>60 mL/min per 1.73 m²)
    Electrolytes, normal
    TSH, normal
    Urine albumin, normal
    Total cholesterol = 156 mg/dL (<200 mg/dL [optimal]) (SI: 4.04 mmol/L [<5.18 mmol/L (optimal)])
    HDL cholesterol = 48 mg/dL (>60 mg/dL [optimal]) (SI: 1.24 mmol/L [>1.55 mmol/L (optimal)])
    LDL cholesterol = 76 mg/dL (<100 mg/dL [optimal]) (SI: 1.97 mmol/L [<2.59 mmol/L (optimal)])
    Triglycerides = 156 mg/dL (<150 mg/dL [optimal]) (SI: 1.76 mmol/L [<3.88 mmol/L (optimal)])

Which of the following is the best next step in this patient's treatment?
  A. Decrease the atorvastatin dosage to 40 mg daily
  B. Stop the atorvastatin
  C. Start metformin
  D. Start sitagliptin
  E. Recommend intensive lifestyle modifications

100 A 37-year-old man comes to your clinic for advice regarding weight management. He is currently at his heaviest weight of 242 lb (110 kg) (BMI = 37 kg/m^2). His lowest adult weight was 169.5 lb (77 kg). He has a history of hypertension (well controlled), chronic kidney disease (glomerular filtration rate, 45 mL/min per 1.73 m^2), nephrolithiasis, cholelithiasis, and chronic back pain. When reviewing his weight history, he tells you that his weight problem started after college and his weight has slowly increased over the years. The 2 main factors for his weight gain seem to be poor eating choices and lack of physical activity. His medications include lisinopril and methadone. He would like to make lifestyle changes to help with weight loss.

Over the next 4 months, he is able to lose 15 lb (6.8 kg) by adhering to an 1800-calorie per day diet and participating in aerobic exercise 5 times a week. However, now, 8 months after his initial visit, he has been unable to lose any additional weight. He has a friend who is taking naltrexone sustained release/bupropion sustained release and has successfully lost weight. The patient is interested in learning more about this medication and is wondering whether it would be appropriate for him.

Which of the following aspects of his clinical picture is a contraindication to naltrexone/bupropion?
- A. Cholelithiasis
- B. Hypertension
- C. Methadone use
- D. Glomerular filtration rate
- E. Nephrolithiasis

101 A 57-year-old woman is referred to you by her orthopedic surgeon for medical management of a bone lesion before surgical fixation. She was just evaluated for new-onset right wrist pain and deformity that occurred after an injury at work. The pain has worsened and is now refractory to anti-inflammatory medication. This has made it difficult for her to work because she is right-handed. She received a recommendation to proceed with surgery to decrease the deformity of her bow and to stabilize the bone with plate, screw, and cement fixation. A whole-body bone scan shows markedly increased activity involving the entire right radius (*see image*).

An x-ray shows enlargement of her right forearm with cortical thickening, trabecular coarsening, and bowing (*see image*).

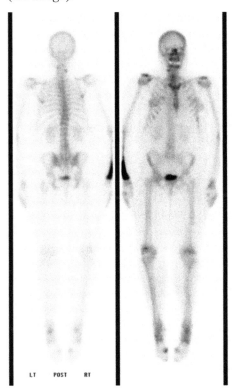

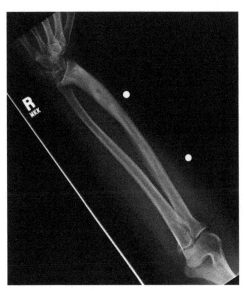

She now describes paresthesias in her right fingers, as well as pain that extends up to her right shoulder.

On physical examination, her height is 68 in (173 cm) and weight is 185 lb (84.1 kg) (BMI = 28.1 kg/m^2). Her blood pressure is 165/67 mm Hg, and pulse rate is 76 beats/min. She has no axillary lymphadenopathy. Her right upper extremity has an obvious distal radial deformity with an apex dorsal bow. She has a neurovascularly intact hand and no sensory deficits. There is tenderness to palpation along her radius.

Laboratory test results:
    Serum total calcium = 9.4 mg/dL (8.2-10.2 mg/dL) (SI: 2.4 mmol/L [2.1-2.6 mmol/L])
    Phosphate = 3.7 mg/dL (2.3-4.7 mg/dL) (SI: 1.2 mg/dL [0.7-1.5 mmol/L])
    Serum creatinine = 0.7 mg/dL (0.6-1.1 mg/dL) (SI: 61.9 μmol/L [53.0-97.2 μmol/L])
    Alkaline phosphatase = 381 U/L (50-120 U/L) (SI: 6.4 μkat/L [0.84-2.00 μkat/L])
    PTH = 47 pg/mL (10-65 pg/mL) (SI: 47 ng/L [10-65 ng/L])
    Urinary N-telopeptide = 189 nmol BCE/mmol creat (24-124 nmol BCE/mmol creat)

Which of the following is the best management plan?
   A. Denosumab
   B. Palliative radiation therapy
   C. Surgical correction of the radius
   D. Intravenous zoledronic acid
   E. Teriparatide

102 A 55-year-old woman presents with episodic palpitations, sweats, and headaches. Biochemical testing reveals that her plasma normetanephrine level is 5-fold greater than the upper limit of the reference range. Abdominal CT identifies a 3-cm left adrenal mass with a lipid-poor density of 34 Hounsfield units and a malignant-appearing, 2.5-cm right renal mass suggestive of renal cell carcinoma. Relevant family history includes a gastrointestinal stromal tumor in her 48-year-old brother and metastatic pheochromocytoma in her 58-year-old sister.

Which of the following genes is most likely to harbor a pathogenic mutation in this patient?
   A. *SDHB*
   B. *RET*
   C. *SDHAF2*
   D. MEN1
   E. NF1

103 A 41-year-old woman comes to you for advice regarding hormone therapy. She underwent menarche at age 15 years and has always had regular menstrual cycles. For the last year, she has had hot flashes at the time of her menstrual cycles. Her second child was born 3 years ago and she does not want any further pregnancies. She does not smoke cigarettes.

On physical examination, her blood pressure is 108/68 mm Hg. Her height is 59 in (149.9 cm), and weight is 118 lb (53.6 kg) (BMI = 23.9 kg/m^2). She has no breast masses or discharge. Pelvic examination reveals no masses.

Laboratory test results on day 3 of the menstrual cycle:
    FSH = 11.3 mIU/mL (2-12 mIU/mL) (SI: 11.3 IU/L [2-12 IU/L])
    Estradiol = 43 pg/mL (10-180 pg/mL) (SI: 157.9 pmol/L [36.7-660.8 pmol/L])
    Prolactin = 5.7 ng/mL (4-30 ng/mL) (SI: 0.25 nmol/L [0.17-1.30 nmol/L])
    TSH = 1.22 mIU/L (0.5-5.0 mIU/L)
    β-hCG = <6 mIU/mL (<3.0 mIU/mL) (SI: <6 IU/L [<3.0 IU/L])

Which of the following would be the best therapy for this patient?
  A. Ethinyl estradiol, 35 mcg daily, and norethindrone, 1 mg daily
  B. Estradiol, 0.025 mg transdermal daily, and micronized progesterone, 100 mg daily
  C. Ethinyl estradiol, 20 mcg daily, and norethindrone acetate, 1 mg daily
  D. Estradiol, 0.5 mg daily, and medroxyprogesterone, 2.5 mg daily
  E. Estradiol, 0.62 mg daily, and norethindrone acetate, 2.7 mg transdermal daily

104 An 11-year-old girl with type 1 diabetes mellitus is seen for follow-up. Diabetes was diagnosed 3 years ago. Her hemoglobin A_{1c} has been maintained in the mid-7% range (53 mmol/mol). Her pediatrician has noted decreased growth velocity over the past 2 years. Her height has decreased from the 50th percentile to the 25th percentile, with weight remaining unchanged around the 25th percentile. The patient does not have any specific concerns such as fatigue and has no gastrointestinal symptoms such as nausea, loose stool, or constipation. She does experience occasional abdominal bloating. She has had no change in skin pigmentation and has had no dizziness. The only worry her mother notes is increased frequency of hypoglycemia that is not explained by change in diet or activity level.

On physical examination, her blood pressure is 102/60 mm Hg and pulse rate is 94 beats/min. No mucosal hyperpigmentation is noted. She has grade 1 enamel defects on dental evaluation (some areas are yellow/brown). The thyroid is normal in size and texture, and no nodularity is noted. Findings on examination of the heart, lungs, abdomen, and extremities are normal. Reflexes are normal.

Laboratory test results:
  Hemoglobin A_{1c} = 7.2% (4.0%-5.6%) (55 mmol/mol [20-38 mmol/mol])
  Complete metabolic panel, normal
  25-Hydroxyvitamin D = 16 ng/mL (25-80 ng/mL) (SI: 39.9 nmol/L [62.4-199.7 nmol/L])

Which of the following is the most likely cause of her short stature?
  A. GH deficiency
  B. Gastroparesis
  C. Adrenal insufficiency
  D. Celiac disease
  E. Hypothyroidism

105 A 23-year-old woman with hyperthyroidism whom you managed during her pregnancy returns for a postpartum follow-up visit. She had been treated with propylthiouracil during the first trimester and then methimazole subsequently. During the latter part of pregnancy, she required 40 mg of methimazole daily to maintain her thyroid hormone levels slightly above the upper limit of the normal range. Her baby has done well and has not had problems with abnormal thyroid function.

The patient remains on a methimazole dosage of 40 mg daily and is taking a daily multivitamin containing 150 mcg of iodine. She has no symptoms that are unexpected in the postpartum period. She is tired and not sleeping through the night because of nursing and caring for her infant. She is breastfeeding but notes some limitation in the quantity of her milk production and she is concerned about this.

On physical examination, her vital signs are normal and she is currently 13.2 lb (6 kg) above her prepregnancy weight. She appears euthyroid.

Thyroid function test results (sample drawn in preparation for today's visit):
  TSH = 2.5 mIU/L (0.5-5.0 mIU/L)
  Free T_4 = 1.1 ng/dL (0.8-1.8 ng/dL) (SI: 14.2 pmol/L [10.30-23.17 pmol/L])

Considering this patient's concerns, which of the following is the best next step in her management?

A. Decrease her methimazole dosage
B. Maintain her methimazole dosage
C. Maintain her methimazole dosage and add iodine, 400 mcg daily
D. Maintain her methimazole dosage and add a dopamine antagonist
E. Switch from methimazole to an equivalent dosage of propylthiouracil

106 A 57-year-old obese man has been followed in your clinic for evaluation of possible hypogonadism. He reports a normal puberty and has fathered 3 children. He has longstanding erectile dysfunction. Five years ago, sarcoidosis was diagnosed. At that time, he recalls that he had a low testosterone level, and he was prescribed testosterone replacement therapy for several years with either a topical gel or intramuscular testosterone undecanoate. Nonetheless, he has not been on testosterone replacement therapy for the past 12 months. Since his last clinic visit 2 months ago, the patient has unintentionally lost 16 lb (7.3 kg) and reports sweating, tremors, and palpitations. He is not exercising but has a gym membership. His current medications are celecoxib and avanafil as needed.

On physical examination, his blood pressure is 132/83 mm Hg and pulse rate is 94 beats/min. His height is 70 in (178 cm), and weight is 231 lb (105 kg) (BMI = 33.1 kg/m^2). He has a normal-sized thyroid gland with no palpable nodules. The rest of the examination findings are normal.

Laboratory test results:
   TSH = 0.005 mIU/L (0.5-5.0 mIU/L)
   Free T$_4$ = 3.7 ng/dL (0.8-1.8 ng/dL) (SI: 47.6 pmol/L [10.30-23.17 pmol/L])

Compared with his baseline values, which of the following hormonal profiles is he most likely to have?

Answer	Total Testosterone	Bioavailable Testosterone	Sex Hormone–Binding Globulin
A.	↓	↓	↓
B.	↓	No change	No change
C.	↓	No change	↓
D.	↑	↑	↑
E.	↑	↓	↑

107 A 58-year-old man with a history of polycystic kidney disease and hemodialysis for the last 13 years is referred by his nephrologist for excessive soft-tissue calcifications. He has severe coronary artery disease with a history of 3-vessel coronary artery bypass graft surgery and placement of 2 coronary stents. His arteriovenous fistula has undergone revision 3 times over the last 8 years because of vascular disease.

The patient reports the presence of firm nodules on his lower legs, arms, and elbows for the last several years. The nodules grow until they rupture the skin and a "chalky" substance "bursts out." This leads to prolonged nonhealing wounds. He is taking sevelamer, 3200 mg 3 times daily. He could not tolerate low-dosage cinacalcet because of nausea and hypocalcemia. Conversely, calcitriol and paricalcitol were stopped due to development of hypercalcemia and worsening hyperphosphatemia.

On physical examination, he appears older than his stated age and is sitting in a wheelchair. His blood pressure is 102/64 mm Hg, pulse rate is 90 beats/min, and respiratory rate is 16 breaths/min. His height is 66 in (167.6 cm), and weight is 188 lb (85.5 kg) (BMI = 30.3 kg/m^2). His examination findings are notable only for multiple areas along his leg and thigh with shallow-based ulcers, although there is no evidence of a white, chalky substance or discharge. There is firm nodularity in the left elbow. No kyphosis or scoliosis is noted.

Laboratory test results:

Estimated glomerular filtration rate = 8 mL/min
per 1.73 m² (>60 mL/min per 1.73 m²)

Calcium = 9.5 mg/dL (8.2-10.2 mg/dL)
(SI: 2.4 mmol/L [2.1-2.6 mmol/L])

Phosphate = 9.7 mg/dL (2.3-4.7 mg/dL)
(SI: 3.1 mmol/L [0.7-1.5 mmol/L])

Intact PTH = 685 pg/mL (10-65 pg/mL)
(SI: 685 ng/L [10-65 ng/L])

25-Hydroxyvitamin D = 10 ng/mL
(25-80 ng/mL [optimal])
(SI: 25.0 nmol/L [62.4-199.7 nmol/L])

1,25-Dihydroxyvitamin D = 53 pg/mL
(16-65 pg/mL) (SI: 137.8 pmol/L
[41.6-169.0 pmol/L])

Serum C-telopeptide = >6000 pg/mL (35-836 pg/mL)

Osteocalcin = 282 ng/mL (9.0-42.0 ng/mL)
(SI: 282 µg/L [9.0-42 µg/L])

Bone-specific alkaline phosphatase = 118 µg/L (≤20 µg/L)

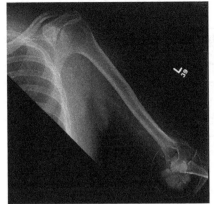
Left elbow x-ray.

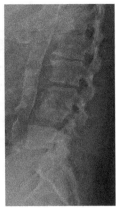
Lateral spine x-ray.

Radiologic studies are shown (*see images*).

Which of the following is the best treatment step for this patient now?

A. Increase the dosage of sevelamer
B. Restart cinacalcet
C. Restart calcitriol
D. Initiate ergocalciferol
E. Perform subtotal parathyroidectomy

108 A 65-year-old man with hypertension was diagnosed with diabetes mellitus on routine blood work 3 months ago. At that time, his hemoglobin A$_{1c}$ level was 8.7% (72 mmol/mol) and his fasting blood glucose concentration was 218 mg/dL (12.1 mmol/L). Since his diagnosis, he has followed recommended lifestyle measures including caloric restriction, moderation of carbohydrate intake, and walking for 30 minutes most days of the week. At his follow-up visit today, he reports feeling more energetic. He has lost 3 lb (1.4 kg), and his fasting glucose levels at home have ranged between 165 and 190 mg/dL (9.2-10.5 mmol/L). Current medications include lisinopril, hydrochlorothiazide, atenolol, and simvastatin.

On physical examination, his blood pressure is 138/84 mm Hg and pulse rate is 84 beats/min. His height is 70.5 in (179.1 cm), and weight is 227 lb (103 kg) (BMI = 31.1 kg/m²). Findings on cardiovascular examination are normal except for reduced pedal pulses. Findings on peripheral nerve examination are normal.

Fasting laboratory test results:

Hemoglobin A$_{1c}$ = 8.1% (4.0%-5.6%) (65 mmol/mol [20-38 mmol/mol])

Glucose = 168 mg/dL (70-99 mg/dL) (SI: 9.3 mmol/L [3.9-5.5 mmol/L])

Serum urea nitrogen = 32 mg/dL (8-23 mg/dL) (SI: 11.4 mmol/L) [2.9-8.2 mmol/L])

Creatinine = 1.6 mg/dL (0.7-1.3 mg/dL) (SI: 141.4 µmol/L [61.9-114.9 µmol/L])

Estimated glomerular filtration rate = 48 mL/min per 1.73 m² (>60 mL/min per 1.73 m²)

Cholesterol = 168 mg/dL (<200 mg/dL [optimal]) (SI: 4.35 mmol/L [<5.18 mmol/L])

Triglycerides = 235 mg/dL (<150 mg/dL [optimal]) (SI: 2.66 mmol/L [<3.88 mmol/L])

HDL cholesterol = 34 mg/dL (>60 mg/dL [optimal]) (SI: 0.88 mmol/L [>1.55 mmol/L])

LDL cholesterol = 78 mg/dL (<100 mg/dL [optimal]) (SI: 2.02 mmol/L [<2.59 mmol/L])

You plan to start metformin for persistently uncontrolled diabetes. In addition to a lower hemoglobin A_{1c} level, which of the following patterns would you expect to find in 6 months?

Answer	Weight	Triglycerides	Hypoglycemia	Creatinine	Vitamin B_{12}
A.	↔/↓	↓	↔	↔	↔/↓
B.	↔/↓	↑	↔	↑	↔/↓
C.	↔	↓	↑	↔	↔
D.	↔	↔	↔	↑	↔/↑
E.	↔/↑	↓	↑	↔	↔/↑

109 A 32-year-old woman with hypothyroidism after thyroidectomy for Graves disease presents for adjustment of her levothyroxine dosage during her second pregnancy. She is currently 18 weeks' gestation and will also be seeing her obstetrician today. Her levothyroxine dosage before pregnancy was 100 mcg daily and she is currently taking 125 mcg levothyroxine daily. Her last serum TSH value was 1.1 mIU/L. Her first pregnancy resulted in a low–birth weight baby who initially failed to thrive but reached normal growth milestones thereafter.

Her physical examination findings are normal, with her pregnancy-associated weight gain being at the lower end of the normal range. She has no palpable thyroid tissue in the thyroid bed. Her abdomen is gravid. Her deep tendon reflexes are normal. You have repeated her thyroid function tests and her TSH value is 2.1 mIU/L. You ask her to continue her current levothyroxine dosage and plan to reevaluate her in 4 weeks.

Later that day, you receive a call from her obstetrician saying that fetal ultrasonography was performed and the patient's fetus had a heart rate of 190 beats/min. The obstetrician expresses concern about this tachycardia.

Which of the following findings would you predict?
A. Elevated titers of TSH receptor antibodies (TRAb) in the mother
B. High T_3 levels in the mother
C. High free T_4 levels in the mother
D. Evidence of delayed bone maturation in the fetus
E. Normal TSH in umbilical cord blood

110 A 31-year-old woman comes to you for advice regarding primary ovarian insufficiency. She had a birth control implant removed 1 year ago to become pregnant, but has remained amenorrheic. She notes new hot flashes. Her medical history is otherwise unremarkable.

On physical examination, her blood pressure is 118/78 mm Hg. Her height is 68 in (172.7 cm), and weight is 142 lb (64.4 kg) (BMI = 21.6 kg/m²). She has no hyperpigmentation. Her thyroid is estimated to be 20 g and no nodules are detected. Pelvic examination reveals no masses.

Laboratory test results:
  FSH = 96.4 mIU/mL (2-12 mIU/mL) (SI: 96.4 IU/L [2-12 IU/L])
  Estradiol = <10 pg/mL (10-180 pg/mL) (SI: <36.7 pmol/L [36.7-660.8 pmol/L])
  TSH = 3.5 mIU/L (0.5-5.0 mIU/L)
  Karyotype = 46,XX
  FMR1 repeat number = 20 and 32 (normal)
  21-Hydroxylase antibodies = 13.0 U/mL (<1.0 U/mL)

You prescribe an estradiol patch and oral progesterone.

Which of the following is the most important test to order next?
- A. Ovarian antibody measurement
- B. ACTH stimulation test
- C. Antimullerian hormone measurement
- D. TPO antibody measurement
- E. Hemoglobin A_{1c} measurement

111 A 58-year-old man is admitted to the hospital for pneumonia with hypoxia. Intravenous antibiotics and oxygen therapy have been initiated, and admission is anticipated to last 3 to 4 days. He has a 20-year history of type 2 diabetes mellitus complicated by peripheral neuropathy and impaired renal function. His diabetes has been relatively poorly controlled with hemoglobin A_{1c} values ranging from 8.2% to 9.8% (66-84 mmol/mol) over the past few years. One year ago, his regimen was transitioned to U500 insulin and his current dose is 340 units before breakfast and 280 units before his evening meal (total daily dose 620 units). Other medications include losartan, atorvastatin, aspirin, and gabapentin. He admits that he does not follow a diabetes diet, but instead grazes continuously throughout the day. His most recent hemoglobin A_{1c} value 5 weeks ago was 8.4% (68 mmol/mol).

On physical examination, he is febrile with a temperature of 101.2°F (38.4°C), but he is alert and cheerful. His blood pressure is 133/95 mm Hg, pulse rate is 96 beats/min, and respiratory rate is 18 breaths/min. His height is 69 in (175.3 cm), and weight is 265 lb (120.5 kg) (BMI = 39.1 kg/m²). He has general obesity with no features of lipodystrophy. A carbohydrate-consistent diabetes diet has been ordered.

Which of the following is the best management plan?
- A. Continue U500 insulin twice daily before meals—total daily dose 620 units
- B. Continue U500 insulin twice daily before meals at 90% of home doses—total daily dose 560 units
- C. Change to insulin glargine, 300 units once daily, and insulin aspart, 100 units with meals + correction dosing—total daily dose 600 units
- D. Change to insulin glargine, 150 units, and insulin aspart, 50 units, with meals + correction dosing—total daily dose 300 units
- E. Change to intravenous insulin at 15 units/h—total daily dose 360 units

112 A 72-year-old man is referred to you by his primary care physician because of abnormal thyroid function test results and a right-sided neck swelling. The patient reports no symptoms of thyroid dysfunction and was not aware of the neck swelling until his physician noted it. He takes lisinopril to treat hypertension.

On physical examination, his height is 68 in (172.7 cm) and weight is 161 lb (73.2 kg) (BMI = 24.5 kg/m²). His blood pressure is 134/76 mm Hg, and pulse rate is 76 beats/min. Examination of his neck confirms a right-sided neck swelling (2 cm in maximal diameter) that moves with swallowing. There is no palpable cervical lymphadenopathy. There is no tremor and no obvious signs of thyroid-related ophthalmopathy.

Laboratory test results:
TSH = 0.06 mIU/L (0.5-5.0 mIU/L)
Free T_4 = 1.6 ng/dL (0.8-1.8 ng/dL) (SI: 20.6 pmol/L [10.30-23.17 pmol/L])
Free T_3 = 4.0 pg/mL (2.3-4.2 pg/mL) (SI: 6.1 pmol/L [3.53-6.45 pmol/L])

In view of the low TSH level, a technetium ^{99m}Tc pertechnetate scan is performed (*see images*).

Thyroid ultrasonography confirms multinodular thyroid enlargement with a dominant mixed cystic/solid right-sided nodule (16 × 20 × 23 mm) with internal colloid. On the left side, there is a solid, isoechoic nodule (14 × 15 × 12 mm) with no microcalcifications and no internal blood flow (*see images*).

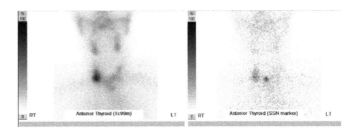

Which of the following is the best next step in this patient's management?
- A. Ultrasound-guided FNAB of both right- and left-sided thyroid nodules
- B. Ultrasound-guided FNAB of the right-sided thyroid nodule
- C. Ultrasound-guided FNAB of the left-sided thyroid nodule
- D. Measurement of serum thyroglobulin
- E. Measurement of serum thyroid-stimulating immunoglobulin

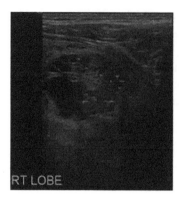 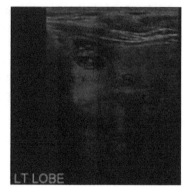

RT LOBE   LT LOBE

113 A 63-year-old man is evaluated in the diabetes clinic. His chief concern is muscle pain in the thighs and legs. The pain started in the right thigh but has progressed to both lower extremities over the last 3 months. He has had aching, burning pain, predominantly in the thighs. He has trouble getting out of bed and walking up stairs. His appetite is poor and he has lost 23 lb (10.5 kg) since symptoms began.

Diabetes mellitus was diagnosed at age 56 years, and he takes metformin, 850 mg twice daily. He has a history of microalbuminuria and peripheral neuropathy, but he has never had a foot ulcer. He has hypertension and dyslipidemia for which he takes enalapril, 10 mg twice daily, and pravastatin, 40 mg daily. Depression was recently diagnosed, and duloxetine, 60 mg daily, was initiated 1 week ago. He does not exercise. He has 3 servings of alcohol per week and does not smoke cigarettes.

On physical examination, his height is 70 in (178 cm) and weight is 178 lb (80.9 kg) (BMI = 25.5 k/m^2). His blood pressure is 142/84 mm Hg, pulse rate is 86 beats/min, and respiratory rate is 12 breaths/min. Findings on examination of the heart, lungs, and abdomen are normal. There is wasting of the right quadriceps and decreased muscle strength with hip and knee flexion and extension and to a lesser degree in the ankles. Neurologic examination reveals absent ankle reflexes, diminished vibrational sense, and diminished response to monofilament testing in both feet.

Laboratory test results:
Hemoglobin A$_{1c}$ = 8.0% (4.0%-5.6%) (64 mmol/mol [20-38 mmol/mol])
Creatinine = 1.3 mg/dL (0.7-1.3 mg/dL) (SI: 114.9 μmol/L [61.9-114.9 μmol/L])
Estimated glomerular filtration rate = 60 mL/min per 1.73 m^2 (>60 mL/min per 1.73 m^2)
Electrolytes, normal
TSH, normal
Vitamin B$_{12}$ and folic acid, normal
Creatine kinase, normal
Serum electrophoresis, no monoclonal protein
Erythrocyte sedimentation rate = 24 mm/h (0-20 mm/h)

Which of the following is the best next step in this patient's management?
- A. Add insulin
- B. Add gabapentin
- C. Add prednisone
- D. Add pregabalin
- E. Stop metformin and start insulin

114 A 43-year-old man presents with hypertension and symptoms of Cushing syndrome. A 12-cm left adrenal mass and numerous liver metastases are identified. Radical left adrenalectomy is performed and pathology reveals high-grade adrenocortical carcinoma. Stage 4 adrenocortical carcinoma is diagnosed, and adjuvant mitotane therapy is initiated. His mitotane dosage is escalated to 4 g daily and he achieves a therapeutic mitotane level of 18 ng/mL (suggested therapeutic level >14 ng/mL). He now reports fatigue, nausea, vomiting, and dizziness.

Laboratory test results:
  Sodium = 134 mEq/L (136-142 mEq/L) (SI: 134 mmol/L [136-142 mmol/L])
  Potassium = 5.6 mEq/L (3.5-5.0 mEq/L) (SI: 5.6 mmol/L [3.5-5.0 mmol/L])
  Morning cortisol = 14 µg/dL (5-25 µg/dL) (SI: 386.2 nmol/L [137.9-689.7 nmol/L])
  ACTH = 274 pg/mL (10-60 pg/mL) (SI: 60.3 pmol/L [2.2-13.2 pmol/L])

Which of the following is the most appropriate next step?
  A. Stop mitotane
  B. Administer sodium chloride tablets
  C. Administer ondansetron
  D. Administer hydrocortisone
  E. Administer metyrapone

115 A 19-year-old woman with a history of polycystic ovary syndrome, prediabetes, and obesity (BMI = 33 kg/m^2) comes for a follow-up appointment. She tells you that since her last clinic visit 6 months ago she was diagnosed with a seizure disorder. An anticonvulsant drug was prescribed, which caused a 10% weight gain. The patient admits she stopped taking the medication because she was dismayed by the weight gain. She is very hesitant to start a different agent, as she read on the Internet that all anticonvulsant drugs have this adverse effect. You have a long discussion regarding the importance of restarting an agent to control her seizures. You recommend that she contact her neurologist and discuss the possibility of switching to topiramate, as this medication would not cause weight gain and it could actually help with weight loss.

Which of the following anticonvulsant drugs was most likely responsible for her initial weight gain?
  A. Valproic acid
  B. Levetiracetam
  C. Phenytoin
  D. Lamotrigine
  E. Zonisamide

116 A 52-year-old man is referred by his oncologist. A malignant melanoma on his back was diagnosed 2 years ago, and he developed multiple liver metastases over the last 4 months. Immune checkpoint inhibitor treatment has been initiated, consisting of ipilimumab (a cytotoxic T-lymphocyte antigen-4 [CTLA-4] blocker) and nivolumab (an antiprogrammed cell death 1 [PD1] receptor antibody). The patient reports increasing fatigue and lethargy over the last 4 weeks. He has no symptoms of cold intolerance or constipation, and he has lost 5 lb (2.3 kg) over the last 2 months. He has a 5-year history of bipolar disorder that has been successfully treated with lithium. His mother and sister take levothyroxine to treat hypothyroidism.

On physical examination, his height is 70 in (177.8 cm) and weight is 150 lb (68.2 kg) (BMI = 21.5 kg/m^2). His blood pressure is 128/72 mm Hg, and pulse rate is 72 beats/min in a seated position. There is no postural drop in blood pressure. Examination of his neck does not identify any thyroid enlargement and there is no palpable cervical lymphadenopathy. Abdominal examination reveals a palpable liver with an irregular hard edge. There is mild pedal edema. No other abnormalities are found on systems examination.

Laboratory test results:

TSH = 6.2 mIU/L (0.5-5.0 mIU/L)

Free T_4 = 0.65 ng/dL (0.8-1.8 ng/dL) (SI: 8.4 pmol/L [10.30-23.17 pmol/L])

Free T_3 = 2.1 pg/mL (2.3-4.2 pg/mL) (SI: 3.2 pmol/L [3.53-6.45 pmol/L])

TPO antibodies = 5.0 IU/L (<2.0 IU/mL) (SI: 5.0 kIU/L [<2.0 kIU/L])

Sodium = 138 mEq/L (136-142 mEq/L) (SI: 138 mmol/L [136-142 mmol/L])

Potassium = 4.1 mEq/L (3.5-5.0 mEq/L) (SI: 4.1. mmol/L [3.5-5.0 mmol/L])

Creatinine = 1.0 mg/dL (0.7-1.3 mg/dL) (SI: 88.4 µmol/L [61.9-114.9 µmol/L])

Cortisol (8 AM) = 28 µg/dL (5-25 µg/dL) (SI: 772.5 nmol/L [137.9-689.7 nmol/L])

Which of the following is the most likely explanation for the observed thyroid function test results?

A. Lithium-induced hypothyroidism

B. Euthyroid sick syndrome

C. Ipilimumab-induced hypophysitis

D. Ipilimumab/nivolumab–induced hypothyroidism

E. Hashimoto thyroiditis

117 A 52-year-old woman with type 1 diabetes mellitus since age 8 years has panmicrovascular complications, including proliferative retinopathy, painful neuropathy, and renal insufficiency that has progressed to stage 5 chronic kidney disease. She also has coronary artery disease previously requiring 4-vessel bypass surgery. Her appetite is reduced but she has no nausea, early satiety, diarrhea, constipation, or orthostatic light-headedness.

Her diabetes is treated with insulin glargine, 14 units each morning, and insulin aspart, 5 units before meals. She uses an insulin sensitivity factor of 1:60 to target a glucose value of 120 mg/dL (6.7 mmol/L). Other medications include metoprolol, 50 mg daily; nifedipine extended release, 90 mg daily; furosemide, 40 mg daily; and gabapentin, 300 mg 3 times daily.

On physical examination, her blood pressure is 128/60 mm Hg and pulse rate is 78 beats/min. Her height is 67 in (170.2 cm), and weight is 137 lb (62 kg) (BMI = 21.5 kg/m²). Her eyes have bilateral panretinal laser scars. On neurologic examination, she has markedly decreased vibration sense in both first toes and absent monofilament light-touch sensation in both feet. Pedal pulses are 2+.

Laboratory test results:

Hemoglobin A_{1c} = 8.4% (4.0%-5.6%) (68 mmol/mol [20-38 mmol/mol])

Fasting glucose = 221 mg/dL (70-99 mg/dL) (SI: 12.3 mmol/L [3.9-5.5 mmol/L])

Serum urea nitrogen = 62 mg/dL (8-23 mg/dL) (SI: 22.1 mmol/L [2.9-8.2 mmol/L])

Creatinine = 4.6 mg/dL (0.6-1.1 mg/dL) (SI: 406.6 µmol/L [53.0-97.2 µmol/L])

Estimated glomerular filtration rate = 12 mL/min per 1.73 m² (>60 mL/min per 1.73 m²)

Hematocrit = 32.1 (35%-45%) (SI: 0.321 [0.35-0.45])

Urine protein = 3+

She is being evaluated for combined kidney and pancreas transplants but is concerned about the potential risks of having both organs transplanted during the same surgical procedure.

You counsel this patient that she could expect which of the following outcomes if she were to receive a simultaneous kidney-pancreas transplant vs a pancreas after kidney transplant?

A. Increased risk of cardiovascular events

B. Increased risk that the transplanted kidney will be rejected

C. Improvement in retinopathy

D. Greater longevity of the transplanted pancreas

E. Increased risk of long-term mortality

118

A 38-year-old woman with a microprolactinoma comes to you 6 weeks after delivering a healthy baby girl. She presented with irregular menstrual cycles and galactorrhea 2 years ago. MRI revealed a 0.8-cm hypointense lesion in the pituitary gland, and a prolactin level of 56 ng/mL (2.4 nmol/L) was documented. She was treated with bromocriptine until she became pregnant, at which time the medication was stopped. Visual field testing throughout pregnancy was normal. She is breastfeeding and does not want more children.

On physical examination, her blood pressure is 120/70 mm Hg. Her height is 56.5 in (143.5 cm), and weight is 149 lb (67.7 kg) (BMI = 32.8 kg/m²). Visual fields are full to confrontation. Breast examination reveals galactorrhea.

Laboratory test results:
    Prolactin = 71 ng/mL (4-30 ng/mL) (SI: 3.1 nmol/L [0.17-1.30 nmol/L])
    Free T$_4$ = 1.3 ng/dL (0.8-1.8 ng/dL) (SI: 16.7 pmol/L [10.30-23.17 pmol/L])

Which of the following medications would be most appropriate for this patient?
A. Bromocriptine
B. Norethindrone
C. Ethinyl estradiol/norethindrone
D. Cabergoline
E. Metoclopramide

119

A 26-year-old woman with cystic fibrosis is referred for evaluation and treatment of diabetes mellitus. Diabetes was diagnosed on the basis of an abnormal 2-hour glucose tolerance test at age 24 years. She is being treated with glyburide, 10 mg twice daily, and sitagliptin, 100 mg daily. Recently, she has experienced more hyperglycemia. Nine months ago, her hemoglobin A$_{1c}$ level was 6.8% (51 mmol/mol). Three weeks ago, it was 8.3% (67 mmol/mol). She measures her glucose level twice daily, and her 2-week average glucose value is 183 mg/dL (10.2 mmol/L). Fasting glucose measurements range from 106 to 184 mg/dL (5.9-10.2 mmol/L). She has not had any hypoglycemia recently. She has no microvascular complications. She has lost 11 lb (5 kg) in the last 9 months. She met with the dietician 4 months ago.

Cystic fibrosis was diagnosed at age 6 years. She uses inhalers and was treated for atypical community-acquired pneumonia 3 months ago. She has not been treated with glucocorticoids for 18 months. She has regular menses and is not sexually active. She walks 1 mile, 3 days per week. She does not smoke cigarettes. Her younger brother also has cystic fibrosis and was diagnosed with impaired glucose tolerance 9 months ago. He is being treated with diet.

On physical examination, her height is 67.5 in (171cm) and weight is 146 lb (66.4 kg) (BMI = 22.5 kg/m²). Her blood pressure is 114/68 mm Hg, pulse rate is 83 beats/min, and respiratory rate is 12 breaths/min. Examination findings are normal.

Laboratory test results:
    Creatinine = 0.9 mg/dL (0.6-1.1 mg/dL) (SI: 79.6 μmol/L [53.0-97.2 μmol/L])
    Estimated glomerular filtration rate = >90 mL/min per 1.73 m² (>60 mL/min per 1.73 m²)
    Electrolytes, normal
    C-peptide = 1.5 ng/mL (0.9-4.3 ng/mL) (SI: 0.50 nmol/L [0.30-1.42 nmol/L])
    Glucose = 148 mg/dL (70-99 mg/dL) (SI: 8.2 mmol/L [3.9-5.5 mmol/L])

Which of the following is the best treatment for this patient's diabetes?
A. Continue the 2 antihyperglycemic medications and start basal insulin in the evening
B. Stop the 2 antihyperglycemic medications and start basal plus bolus insulin
C. Stop the 2 antihyperglycemic medications and start basal insulin in the evening
D. Continue the 2 antihyperglycemic medications and start a glucagonlike peptide 1 analogue
E. Double the dosage of glyburide and continue the sitagliptin

120 A 57-year-old woman has a 3-year history of hypertension. She is treated with lisinopril, amlodipine, and atenolol, but despite these medications her blood pressure has remained greater than 150/90 mm Hg and her potassium concentration has been noted to be between 3.0 and 3.5 mEq/L (3.0-3.5 mmol/L) on multiple occasions.

Her primary care physician screened her for primary aldosteronism:
Serum aldosterone = 16.4 ng/dL (4.0-21.0 ng/dL) (SI: 454.9 pmol/L [111.0-582.5 pmol/L])
Plasma renin activity = 0.4 ng/mL per h (0.6-4.3 ng/mL per h)
Aldosterone-to-renin ratio = 41

A confirmatory salt-suppression test reveals nonsuppressible aldosterone, and primary aldosteronism is diagnosed. Abdominal CT identifies (1) a 1.6-cm left adrenal mass that is described as round with a lipid-rich density of 4 Hounsfield units and (2) a 1.2-cm right adrenal mass that is described as round with a lipid-rich density of –2 Hounsfield units.

The patient expresses a strong interest in surgical resection to achieve cure if it is feasible. Therefore, adrenal venous sampling is performed to localize the source of aldosterone. Sampling is obtained simultaneously from the inferior vena cava and each adrenal vein at baseline and 5 minutes after administration of 250 mcg of ACTH. Cortisol and aldosterone values are sampled twice, simultaneously, from each adrenal vein.

Measurement	Inferior Vena Cava (baseline)	Inferior Vena Cave (5 min after ACTH)
Cortisol	14.4 µg/dL (397.3 nmol/L)	28.6 µg/dL (789.0 nmol/L)
Aldosterone	25 ng/dL (693.5 pmol/L)	39 ng/dL (1081.9 pmol/L)

Measurement	Left Adrenal Vein		Right Adrenal Vein	
	Baseline Sample	5 min After ACTH Sample	Baseline Sample	5 min After ACTH Sample
Cortisol	155.2 µg/dL (4281.7 nmol/L)	516 µg/dL (14,235.4 nmol/L)	34.4 µg/dL (949.0 nmol/L)	1580 µg/dL (43,589.0 nmol/L)
Aldosterone	39 ng/dL (1081.9 pmol/L)	227 ng/dL (6297.0 pmol/L)	161.0 ng/dL (4464.1 pmol/L)	10,585 ng/dL (293,627.9 pmol/L)
Aldosterone-to-Cortisol Ratio	0.25	0.44	4.7	6.7

Lateralization ratio (ratio of the right aldosterone-to-cortisol ratio to left aldosterone-to-cortisol ratio): 18.8

Which of the following is the most appropriate recommendation?
A. Surgical resection of the left adrenal gland
B. Surgical resection of the right adrenal gland
C. No surgery; treatment with a mineralocorticoid receptor antagonist
D. Repeated adrenal venous sampling due to inadequate catheterization of the left adrenal vein
E. Repeated adrenal venous sampling due to inadequate catheterization of the right adrenal vein

ENDOCRINE SELF-ASSESSMENT PROGRAM 2018

Part II

1 ANSWER: E) Liraglutide

All of the listed choices would lower this patient's hemoglobin A_{1c}. Factors that should weigh into decision-making when adding an antihyperglycemic medication to the regimen of patients with type 2 diabetes include effectiveness, weight effects, hypoglycemia risk, other potential adverse effects, and cost. Because patients with type 2 diabetes have a high risk of cardiovascular disease, which is the leading cause of death in this population, the effect of diabetes medications on cardiovascular outcomes is an additional factor that should be considered.

In 2008, the US FDA introduced guidelines for studies of new diabetes medications to track longer-term cardiovascular outcomes to document safety. Large clinical trials have now demonstrated that several diabetes medications have longer-term beneficial cardiovascular effects. In the United Kingdom Prospective Diabetes Study, metformin therapy for 10 years, when compared with conventional nutritional therapy in overweight patients with type 2 diabetes, significantly reduced the risk of myocardial infraction by 39% and all-cause mortality by 36%. Premeal rapid-acting insulin (Answer A), sulfonylureas (Answer B), and acarbose (Answer C) have not been shown to reduce cardiovascular events. When compared with placebo, 3 years of sitagliptin treatment (Answer D) in the TECOS study (Trial Evaluating Cardiovascular Outcomes with Sitagliptin) was not associated with lower rates of major cardiovascular events.

In addition to glucose-lowering actions, glucagonlike peptide 1 receptor agonists have been associated with favorable cardiometabolic effects, including weight loss and lower systolic blood pressure, triglycerides, and C-reactive protein. The LEADER trial (Liraglutide Effect and Action in Diabetes: Evaluation of Cardiovascular Outcome Results) showed a 13% lower rate of major cardiovascular events after 3.8 years in patients with type 2 diabetes at high risk for a cardiovascular event who were randomly assigned to liraglutide (Answer E) vs placebo. Thus, liraglutide is the best recommendation for this patient.

Although not listed as an option here, the sodium-glucose cotransporter 2 inhibitor empagliflozin has also been shown to have cardiovascular benefits. A median treatment duration of 2.6 years with empagliflozin in the EMPA-REG OUTCOME trial led to a relative risk reduction of 38% in death of cardiovascular causes among patients with type 2 diabetes at increased cardiovascular risk. However, empagliflozin use is controversial in patients with an impaired glomerular filtration rate, as in this case.

Educational Objective
Recommend antihyperglycemic agents associated with improved cardiovascular outcomes.

UpToDate Topic Review(s)
Glucagon-like peptide-1 receptor agonist for the treatment of type 2 diabetes mellitus

Reference(s)

UK Prospective Diabetes Study (UKPDS) Group. Effect of intensive blood-glucose control with metformin on complications in overweight patients with type 2 diabetes (UKPDS 34).Referred to by *Lancet.* 1998;352(9131):854-865. PMID: 9742977

Varanasi A, Patel P, Makdissi A, Dhindsa S, Chaudhuri A, Dandona P. Clinical use of liraglutide in type 2 diabetes and its effects on cardiovascular risk factors. *Endocr Pract.* 2012;18(2):140-145. PMID: 21856595

Marso SP, Daniels GH, Brown-Frandsen K, et al; LEADER Trial Investigators. Liraglutide and cardiovascular outcomes in type 2 diabetes. *N Engl J Med.* 2016;375(4):311-322. PMID: 27295427

Zinman B, Wanner C, Lachin JM, et al; EMPA-REG OUTCOME Investigators. Empagliflozin, cardiovascular outcomes, and mortality in type 2 diabetes. *N Engl J Med.* 2015;373(22):2117-2128. PMID: 26378978

2 ANSWER: E) Serum IGF-2 to IGF-1 ratio

All aspects of the Whipple triad have been fulfilled in this vignette (symptoms of hypoglycemia, biochemical confirmation, and improvement of symptoms with carbohydrates), making this a case of genuine, intractable hypoglycemia. The patient was previously well and is taking no prescribed medications that could lower blood glucose. In these circumstances, a number of diagnoses should be considered, including adrenal insufficiency, factitious hypoglycemia, endogenous hyperinsulinism (insulinoma/or a functional disorder of the pancreatic β cells), or non–islet-cell–mediated hypoglycemia.

This patient has some clinical features of cortisol excess (overweight, striae, hypertensive) and has an early-morning plasma cortisol value at the high end of the reference range. While the diagnostic criteria for relative adrenal insufficiency in acute illness are unclear, the clinical presentation and high-normal early-morning cortisol level make it unlikely in this case. Thus, further examination of the hypothalamic-pituitary-adrenal axis with an ACTH stimulation test (Answer A) is unnecessary.

This patient's plasma insulin and C-peptide levels are appropriately low, which excludes endogenous hyperinsulinism as a possible etiology. Plasma insulin and C-peptide levels can sometimes be suppressed by 10% dextrose infusion (as a consequence of hyperglycemia), but this is not a concern here as this patient is simply euglycemic on this regimen. Selective arterial calcium stimulation (Answer B) with hepatic venous sampling is a complex test performed in cases of hyperinsulinism and unremarkable imaging studies. It is useful in distinguishing (and localizing) a small insulinoma from diffuse pancreatic pathology (eg, islet-cell hypertrophy/nesidioblastosis), but it is unnecessary in this patient with an obvious tumor.

Amphetamine toxicity can present with clinical features similar to those of hypoglycemia (confusion, tachycardia, diaphoresis, and seizures), but low blood glucose is not common. Alcohol can lead to hypoglycemia, as can many other drugs. However, hypoglycemia in such circumstances should be short-lived and responsive to treatment, which is not the case in this vignette. Therefore, a urine toxicology screen (Answer C) is not the best next step.

Factitious or accidental hypoglycemia should always be considered when the cause is not immediately obvious. This patient could, in theory, have access to glucose-lowering medications, as his mother has type 2 diabetes mellitus. However, such cases are unusual and, most importantly, plasma insulin and C-peptide are easily detectable in the setting of sulfonylurea misuse because these drugs are insulin secretagogues. Therefore, a sulfonylurea screen (Answer D) is not required.

The most obvious clinical abnormalities outlined in this vignette are profound hypoglycemia despite continuous 10% dextrose infusion and a large (16-cm) right adrenal mass compressing the right lobe of the liver, which is evident on CT. These findings, along with undetectable plasma insulin, make non–islet-cell hypoglycemia the most likely diagnosis. This is a rare complication of malignancy. It has most often been reported with epithelial tumors (hepatocellular carcinoma most commonly) or mesenchymal tumours (eg, fibrosarcoma). There have been reports of adrenocortical carcinoma and non–islet-cell hypoglycemia, although this is very rare. The main cause of non–islet-cell hypoglycemia is increased glucose use and inhibition of hepatic glucose release due to secretion of incompletely processed IGF-2 (also termed "big" IGF-2) by the tumor. Therefore, affected persons have low serum insulin and C-peptide concentrations but low β-hydroxybutyrate, which is consistent with insulinlike activity. Although not always available in routine laboratories, measurement of "big" IGF-2 or the IGF-2 to IGF-1 ratio (Answer E) can be diagnostic.

This patient had a large adrenocortical carcinoma producing IGF-2 and demonstrated a grossly elevated IGF-2 to IGF-1 ratio. After debulking surgery, he achieved temporary respite from his hypoglycemia although it returned after several months. Hypoglycemia due to such an etiology is usually unresponsive to somatostatin analogues and diazoxide. This patient required continuous 10% dextrose infusion, glucagon infusion, oral glucocorticoid, and nasogastric feeding and still remained hypoglycemic. Eventually, he was given supraphysiologic doses of human GH, which rendered him euglycemic for a short while. GH can increase IGF-binding protein and acid-labile subunit, which can bind IGF-2 and prevent interaction with the insulin receptor.

Educational Objective
Identify the biochemistry associated with hypoglycemia mediated by a non–islet-cell tumor and describe the mechanism underlying this phenomenon.

UpToDate Topic Review(s)
Nonislet cell tumor hypoglycemia

Reference(s)

Bodnar TW, Acevedo MJ, Pietropaolo M. Management of non-islet-cell tumor hypoglycemia: a clinical review. *J Clin Endocrinol Metab*. 2014;99(3):713-722. PMID: 24423303

Dynkevich Y, Rother KI, Whitford I, et al. Tumors, IGF-2, and hypoglycemia: insights from the clinic, the laboratory, and the historical archive. *Endocr Rev*. 2013;34(6):798-826. PMID: 23671155

Drake WM, Miraki F, Siddiqi A, et al. Dose-related effects of growth hormone on IGF-I and IGF-binding protein-3 levels in non-islet cell tumour hypoglycaemia. *Eur J Endocrinol*. 1998;139(5):532-536. PMID: 9849819

3 ANSWER: B) Abnormal parathyroid development

HDR syndrome (hypoparathyroidism, sensorineural deafness, and renal disease) is a rare genetic disorder inherited in an autosomal dominant manner with variable penetrance. This syndrome was first described by Barakat et al in 1977 and is also referred to as Barakat syndrome. Deletions or mutations in the *GATA3* gene affect the embryonic development of the parathyroid glands, auditory system, and kidneys. This patient has Barakat syndrome as evidenced by her hypoparathyroidism, deafness, ovarian cysts, and renal anomalies. Thus, her hypocalcemia has resulted from abnormal parathyroid development (Answer B). Another cause of the absence or dysfunction of the parathyroid glands leading to hypocalcemia is 22q11.2 deletion syndrome (previously known as DiGeorge syndrome), which is not listed as an option.

Patients with HDR syndrome can present with symptoms of hypocalcemia at any age. Hearing loss is usually bilateral and ranges from mild to profound impairment. Kidney abnormalities include nephrotic syndrome, chronic kidney disease, hematuria, proteinuria, congenital kidney anomalies (eg, cystic kidney; renal dysplasia, hypoplasia, or agenesis), and urologic abnormalities (eg, pelvicalyceal deformity, vesicoureteral reflux). Other abnormalities associated with the syndrome include female genital malformations, Hirschsprung disease, ocular abnormalities (eg, retinitis pigmentosa, nystagmus, pseudopapilledema, ptosis), psychomotor delay, and growth failure.

Autosomal dominant hypocalcemia is caused by an activating mutation in the *CASR* gene, which shifts the set point of the calcium-sensing receptor so that PTH is not released at serum calcium concentrations that normally trigger PTH release. This leads to low serum calcium levels. Additionally, renal calcium reabsorption in these patients is lower than anticipated because of the absence of PTH secretion leading to elevated urinary calcium excretion. Patients with this disorder are usually asymptomatic (thus, Answer A is incorrect).

Pseudohypoparathyroidism is caused by a group of disorders characterized by low calcium, high phosphate, and elevated PTH levels due to organ resistance to PTH. Given the inappropriately normal PTH level in this patient, PTH resistance (Answer C) is incorrect. Several subtypes of pseudohypoparathyroidism are caused by mutations in the *GNAS* gene, which lead to G protein's inability to activate adenylyl cyclase upon the binding of PTH to its receptor and eventual end-organ response to PTH. *GNAS* is imprinted in humans, such that expression of the allele in a specific tissue is dependent on whether the allele is maternally or paternally inherited.

Hypocalcemia due to hypoparathyroidism is also associated with the autoimmune polyglandular syndrome type 1 (or APS type 1) also referred to as autoimmune polyendocrinopathy-candidiasis-ectodermal dystrophy (APECED) syndrome. Autoimmune destruction of the parathyroid gland occurs with destruction of other endocrine glands, and the loss of parathyroid function usually occurs in childhood along with mucocutaneous candidiasis. The APS type 1 syndrome is caused by mutations in the *AIRE* gene, which is expressed in the parathyroid glands, thymus, pancreas, adrenal cortex, and fetal liver. This patient has no evidence of primary adrenal insufficiency, chronic mucocutaneous candidiasis, or other autoimmune disorders, making the scenario of autoimmune destruction of the parathyroid glands (Answer D) unlikely.

Wilson disease (Answer E) is caused by a defect in cellular copper transport, which results in the accumulation of copper in the liver, brain, and other tissues, including the parathyroid glands. Damage to organs occurs from the accumulation of copper and results in hepatic, neurologic, and psychiatric manifestations, as well as hypoparathyroidism. Wilson disease is an autosomal recessive disorder and is the result of mutations in *ATP7B*, a gene encoding a hepatic copper transport protein. The earliest lesions in Wilson disease are seen in the liver, the site of initial copper accumulation. The absence of a history of liver disease, neurologic deficits, and Kayser-Fleischer rings in this patient make Wilson disease an unlikely diagnosis.

Educational Objective
Diagnose HDR syndrome (Barakat syndrome) as a cause of hypoparathyroidism and review the differential diagnosis of hypocalcemia in the setting of low parathyroid hormone.

UpToDate Topic Review(s)
Hypoparathyroidism

Reference(s)

Shoback D. Clinical practice. Hypoparathyroidism. *N Engl J Med.* 2008;359(4):391-403. PMID: 18650515

Shim YS, Choi W, Hwang IT, Yang S. Hypoparathyroidism, sensorineural deafness, and renal dysgenesis syndrome with a GATA3 mutation. *Ann Pediatr Endocrinol Metab.* 2015;20(1):59-63. PMID: 25883929

4 ANSWER: B) Upper gastrointestinal series

Sleeve gastrectomy is one of the most frequently performed bariatric operations. It reduces the gastric capacity to 25%, which restricts oral intake. Loss of excess weight of 67.1% has been reported 12 months after surgery. Postoperative complications after sleeve gastrectomy include leaks, fistulas, bleeding, stenosis, and gastroesophageal reflux disease. When a patient who has a history of sleeve gastrectomy presents with abdominal symptoms, the clinician should determine whether they are secondary to a surgical complication.

The patient in this vignette presents with dysphagia, nausea, and an episode of emesis, all of which are symptoms associated with gastric stenosis after sleeve gastrectomy. This complication can occur in the early postoperative period or in the months following the operation. When it presents later, the symptoms may be gradual in onset. In most cases, resolution of the stenosis is achieved by endoscopic dilatation.

Some of the patient's symptoms could be explained by severe gastroesophageal reflux disease. The diagnostic test that will help determine the etiology of her symptoms is an upper gastrointestinal series (Answer B), which will show stenosis if present. If the upper gastrointestinal series is negative, esophageal pH testing (Answer A) would be an appropriate next step. This test is especially useful in patients with atypical gastroesophageal reflux disease symptoms, as it helps determine whether reflux is the etiology.

Abdominal CT or ultrasonography (Answers C and D) would be useful if the patient presented with symptoms due to an abscess secondary to a leak. This complication usually occurs days to weeks after surgery. Additional symptoms from an abdominal abscess would be abdominal pain and fever.

A gastric emptying study (Answer E) is used to evaluate gastric motor function and is usually performed after a mechanical obstruction has been ruled out.

Educational Objective
Evaluate for complications associated with sleeve gastrectomy.

UpToDate Topic Review(s)
Late complications of bariatric surgical operations

Reference(s)

Irizarry KA, Miller M, Freemark M, Haqq AM. Prader Willi syndrome: genetics, metabolomics, hormonal function, and new approaches to therapy. *Adv Pediatr.* 2016;63(1):47-77. PMID: 27426895

Goldstone AP, Holland AJ, Hauffa BP, Hokken-Koelega AC, Tauber M;, speakers contributors at the Second Expert Meeting of the Comprehensive Care of Patients with PWS. Recommendations for the diagnosis and management of Prader-Willi syndrome [published correction appears in *J Clin Endocrinol Metab.* 2008;93(11):4183-4197]. *J Clin Endocrinol Metab.* 2008;93(11):4183-4197. PMID: 18697869

Irizarry KA, Bain J, Butler MG, et al. Metabolic profiling in Prader-Willi syndrome and nonsyndromic obesity: sex differences and the role of growth hormone. *Clin Endocrinol (Oxf).* 2015;83(6):797-805. PMID: 25736874

Scheimann AO, Butler MG, Gourash L, Cuffari C, Klish W. Critical analysis of bariatric procedures in Prader-Willi syndrome. *J Pediatr Gastroenterol Nutr.* 2008;46(1):80-83. PMID: 18162838

5 ANSWER: A) Abdominal ultrasonography

Androgen insensitivity syndrome results from mutations in the gene encoding the androgen receptor and can be complete or partial. In complete androgen insensitivity syndrome, as in this vignette, there is no androgen-mediated genital development in the fetus. Therefore, there is an absence of male external genitalia. There is also absence of androgen-mediated hair growth from adrenal androgens (pubic and axillary hair) and testicular androgens (male-hair pattern). The testes are present and may be found in the inguinal canal, presenting as hernias, or as masses in the labioscrotal folds, but they are most commonly found intraabdominally (78%). The testes make antimullerian hormone. Therefore, there is regression of the mullerian structures: the uterus, tubes, and upper two-thirds of the vagina. Testosterone is also produced and aromatized to estradiol, resulting in breast development. Patients with complete androgen insensitivity have female features, primary amenorrhea, and absence of sexual hair in the presence of an XY karyotype. Partial androgen insensitivity syndrome is caused by a less deleterious mutation in the androgen receptor gene that results in partial activity. Development of male external genitalia can be partial and incomplete.

Studies examining the fate of the testes in patients with complete androgen insensitivity syndrome have been small. The current data suggest that the risk for testicular cancer is 0.8% before puberty and 2% to 3.6% in adults. The tumors that develop in adults with complete androgen insensitivity are seminomas and gonadoblastomas. Gonadoblastomas are noninvasive in situ lesions that precede seminomas and are the most common lesion. One theory suggests that they arise from failed gonocytes (germ cells before differentiation), but little is understood about their pathophysiology. They contain germ cells, stroma, and Sertoli cells. When the germ-cell material invades the stroma, it is diagnosed as a seminoma. It is recommended that individuals with androgen insensitivity syndrome undergo gonadectomy after puberty is complete because of the increased risk of invasive tumors in adults. However, some families choose to leave gonads intact so that the patient can make an informed decision about gonadectomy in adulthood. Few data are available to suggest appropriate monitoring strategies or to provide outcome information to patients who elect to keep gonads intact. Testes can be moved to a location that is easier to view if they are intraabdominal and ultrasonography can then be used to improve detection in follow-up. Existing protocols recommend that ultrasonography or MRI be performed every 6 to 12 months to look for changes in testicular size or morphology (Answer A). Ultrasonography can also be combined with biopsy to look for in situ lesions, which are the most common initial presentation.

With intact gonads, testosterone levels are in the male range and testosterone is converted to estradiol. Bone density is normal when gonads are intact, but can be low after gonadectomy if estrogen replacement is delayed. Therefore, a bone density scan (Answer E) should be performed for screening purposes only in a patient who has undergone gonadectomy. Testosterone levels will remain elevated, produced by the testes, but it is not necessary to measure levels (Answer D). Measurement of hCG (Answer C) will detect some seminomas, but it is not secreted in most cases and is therefore not a good screening tool by itself. Rather, yearly measurement should be combined with MRI or ultrasonography. α-Fetoprotein is not secreted by seminomas (the invasive tumor), so its measurement (Answer B) is not useful to detect potentially invasive disease.

Educational Objective
Recommend the best monitoring strategy for malignancy in a patient with complete androgen insensitivity syndrome.

UpToDate Topic Review(s)
Diagnosis and treatment of disorders of the androgen receptor

Reference(s)

Ulbright TM, Young RH. Gonadoblastoma and selected other aspects of gonadal pathology in young patients with disorders of sex development. *Sem Diag Pathol.* 2014;31(5):427-440. PMID: 25129544

Gomez-Lobo V, Amies Oelschlager AM; North American Society for Pediatric and Adolescent Gynecology. Disorders of sexual development in adult women. *Obstet Gynecol.* 2016;128(5):1162-1173. PMID: 27741188

Patel V, Kastl RK, Gomez-Lobo V. Timing of gonadectomy in patients with complete androgen insensitivity syndrome-current recommendations and future directions. *J Pediatr Adolesc Gynecol.* 2016;29(4):320-325. PMID: 26428189

6 **ANSWER: B) Start high-dosage glucocorticoid treatment**
There is ongoing controversy regarding the diagnosis of steroid-responsive encephalopathy associated with autoimmune thyroiditis (SREAT), also known as Hashimoto encephalopathy. While many clinicians do not believe this is a real disease entity, endocrinologists are often asked to provide advice on patients in whom the condition is suspected. A comprehensive literature review published in 2015 identified 251 reported cases. The clinical picture of SREAT is variable. The hallmark presenting feature is a nonspecific encephalopathy that is characterized by alteration of mental state and consciousness ranging from confusion to coma and impaired cognitive function. Additional manifestations include stroke-like episodes, seizures, aphasia, extrapyramidal signs, myoclonus, gait disorder, and neuropsychiatric symptoms. The onset of symptoms is usually acute or subacute. Diagnostic criteria of SREAT consist of (1) the presence of neurologic and/or psychiatric dysfunction, (2) elevated serum thyroid antibodies, (3) absence of other identifiable causes of encephalopathy by laboratory and neuroimaging investigations, and (4) good corticosteroid responsiveness.

The diagnosis is usually one of exclusion of other causes of acute or subacute encephalopathy with or without seizures such as systemic, infectious, toxic, metabolic, structural, neoplastic, and psychiatric causes;

seizure-related disorders; and trauma. Serum TPO antibodies are usually quite elevated and are almost essential for confirming the diagnosis. TPO antibodies can also be found in the cerebrospinal fluid of affected patients although this finding is not required to make the diagnosis. Findings of elevated serum thyroglobulin antibodies and TSH-receptor antibodies have been described. There is no clear evidence of correlation between the severity of the clinical picture and the type or level of antibodies. The pathogenic role of these antibodies, however, has not been demonstrated unambiguously. Several mechanisms have been proposed, including the induction of CNS inflammation, vasculitis, vasculopathy, and vasogenic brain edema and cerebral hypoperfusion, as well as direct toxic effects of the antibodies. Most patients are euthyroid at the time of neurologic presentation and it therefore seems unlikely that the condition is caused by a dysthyroid state. Measurement of thyroid hormone levels and ultrasonography of the thyroid gland usually are not helpful in the diagnosis of SREAT. Cerebrospinal fluid analysis in adult and pediatric patients with SREAT most consistently shows elevated protein levels without pleocytosis, and electroencephalography usually demonstrates mild to severe generalized slowing, confirming the encephalopathic state. Neuroimaging via CT or MRI is typically performed to exclude other causes of encephalopathy, although there are no specific radiologic findings to confirm a diagnosis of SREAT.

The treatment of SREAT consists of a combination of supportive measures such as maintaining fluid balance and avoiding hypoxia, especially if significant seizure activity is present. The specific treatment combines immunosuppressive agents, thyroid-acting drugs, anticonvulsant agents, and sometimes antipsychotic and sedative drugs. The term SREAT indicates the disorder's responsiveness to steroid treatment. While the pathophysiologic link with thyroid autoimmunity remains unclear, there is good evidence that certain forms of encephalopathy are steroid responsive, similar to a number of other disease states that appear to improve with glucocorticoids without a clear pathophysiologic explanation. The administration of high-dosage glucocorticoids (Answer B) therefore seems appropriate for this patient. There are no randomized controlled trials demonstrating benefits of this therapy. High-dosage steroids was the first-line treatment in 193 of the 251 cases reported in the literature. The duration before improvement is observed is variable and has been reported from as soon as one day to several weeks.

The successful use of other immunosuppressive agents, including rituximab and azathioprine, has been reported, as has plasmapheresis (Answer C) and administration of immunoglobulins (Answer D), although these are usually used as second-line strategies when response to high-dosage steroids is poor. It is imperative that euthyroidism is maintained, and because thyroid function in this patient is normal, increasing the levothyroxine dosage (Answer A) seems unnecessary. Furthermore, there is no indication to administer liothyronine (Answer E) either in addition to levothyroxine or as monotherapy. Since the presentation of SREAT is rather nonspecific in many patients, empirical treatment with antibiotics and antiviral agents is usually administered and these should be continued in this patient. However, since there has been no response to the current therapies and the patient's condition has remained unchanged after 72 hours, the administration of glucocorticoids seems appropriate.

Educational Objective
Recommend the best therapy for a patient with steroid-responsive encephalopathy associated with autoimmune thyroiditis (SREAT).

UpToDate Topic Review(s)
Hashimoto encephalopathy

Reference(s)

Laurent C, Capron J, Quillerou B, et al. Steroid-responsive encephalopathy associated with autoimmune thyroiditis (SREAT): characteristics, treatment and outcome in 251 cases from the literature. *Autoimmun Rev.* 2016;15(12):1129-1133. PMID: 27639840

Montagna G, Imperiali M, Agazzi P, et al. Hashimoto's encephalopathy: a rare proteiform disorder. *Autoimmun Rev.* 2016;15(5):466-476. PMID: 26849953

7 **ANSWER: E) Ask the patient how the insulin was initially stored after picking it up from the pharmacy**
Identifying the underlying cause of diabetic ketoacidosis is very important, since failure to find an etiology will most likely result in recurrence. This patient's blood glucose was recently well controlled and taking additional insulin doses only transiently reduced his glucose level. These clues suggest that his insulin has lost potency.

The proper storage of insulin is often overlooked in young adults, as the patient's parents may have been in control of the insulin when the patient lived with them. In such scenarios, it is critical to ask the patient how the insulin is stored after picking it up from the pharmacy, how the insulin is handled on trips, and whether the insulin has ever been kept out of the refrigerator or in a car (Answer E). In this particular case, the patient picked up his insulin from the pharmacy and placed it in the glove compartment of a car. Later that evening, he retrieved the insulin and placed it in the refrigerator, not realizing that the insulin had already lost potency due to heat exposure.

Patients should be counseled on the handling of insulin, with tips such as those provided by consumermedsafety.org:

- Do not keep insulin in hot places (such as a car)
- Do not keep insulin in freezing places (such as a freezer)
- Do not leave insulin in sunlight
- Never use expired insulin
- Write the date on the insulin vial on the day it is opened or the day it is removed from the fridge
- Inspect the insulin before each use
- Be aware of unusual or weird smells

Guidelines by the major insulin companies state that unused insulin should be stored in refrigerator. Once insulin is opened and used, the insulin vial or pen should be kept at room temperature, below 86°F (<30°C). Any unused insulin in the pen or vial should be discarded after 28 days.

This patient did not make the transition from his pediatric endocrinologist to an adult endocrinologist, and young adulthood is a time of life when diabetes control often deteriorates. Referral to an endocrinologist now (Answer A) is clearly a priority, but it would not identify the immediate cause of his diabetic ketoacidosis. Initiating new technologies such as insulin pump therapy (Answer B) or continuous glucose monitoring (Answer C) may be useful for this patient in the future, but they would not diagnose or adequately address the current problem. Changing from insulin glargine to insulin detemir (Answer D) also does not address the problem of insulin storage, as all insulins are vulnerable to heat.

Educational Objective
Identify improper storage of insulin and subsequent loss of potency as a potential cause of diabetic ketoacidosis.

UpToDate Topic Review(s)
General principles of insulin therapy in diabetes mellitus

Reference(s)
Brange J, Langkjoer L. Insulin structure and stability. In: Brange J, Langkjoer L, eds. *Pharmaceutical Biotechnology*. Vol 5. New York, NY: Springer US; 1993:315-350.

Brange J, Havelund S, Hougaard P. Chemical stability of insulin. 2. Formation of higher molecular weight transformation products during storage of pharmadeutical preparations. *Pharm Res*. 1992;9(6):727-734. PMID: 1409352

8 ANSWER: B) Initiate denosumab
In patients with prostate cancer, androgen-deprivation therapy with bilateral orchiectomy or GnRH analogues (leuprolide, goserelin, triptorelin, histrelin), either alone or in combination with an antiandrogen (flutamide, bicalutamide, nilutamide), causes profound hypogonadism characterized by loss of libido, muscle mass, and bone density. Abiraterone is a CYP17 inhibitor that prevents adrenal biosynthesis of androgen. Significant bone loss can be seen in men within 6 to 12 months of castration or initiation of a GnRH analogue. Fractures occur within 2 years of beginning androgen-deprivation treatment and increase in frequency with longer duration therapy. Importantly, skeletal fractures in patients with prostate cancer may be associated with shorter survival, independent of the pathologic stage of the cancer. The National Comprehensive Cancer Network guidelines recommend treatment with denosumab subcutaneously every 6 months, as it is the only agent approved by the US FDA to increase bone mass and prevent fracture in men at high risk who are receiving androgen-deprivation therapy for prostate cancer. However, these guidelines also consider the use of zoledronic acid intravenously every year or alendronate orally every week. In this case, it is important to ensure that vitamin D deficiency is corrected before initiating any antiresorptive therapy.

In this patient with osteoporosis who is taking abiraterone, initiating denosumab (Answer B) is the best recommendation now. Given the presence of chronic kidney disease, a bisphosphonate (either alendronate [Answer D] or zoledronic acid [Answer E]) is not the best choice. Teriparatide (Answer C) is not recommended because of the potential risk for occult bone metastases in the setting of active prostate cancer and the possible adverse development of osteosarcoma. This patient's prednisone dosage is not supraphysiologic and should not be contributing to bone loss. Additionally, discontinuing glucocorticoid replacement therapy (Answer A) in a patient taking abiraterone, which leads to adrenal insufficiency, is not recommended.

Educational Objective
Explain why men treated with androgen-deprivation therapy are at risk for developing low bone mass and osteoporosis and recommend appropriate treatment.

UpToDate Topic Review(s)
Side effects of androgen deprivation therapy

Reference(s)

Bienz M, Saad F. Androgen-deprivation therapy and bone loss in prostate cancer patients: a clinical review. *Bonekey Rep.* 2015;4:716. PMID: 26131363

Gralow JR, Biermann JS, Farooki A, et al. NCCN Task Force Report: bone health in cancer care. *J Natl Compr Canc Netw.* 2013;11(Suppl 3):S1-S50. PMID: 23997241

Kaufman JM, Lapauw B, Goemaere S. Current and future treatments of osteoporosis in men. *Best Pract Res Clin Endocrinol Metab.* 2014;28(6):871-874. PMID: 25432358

9 ANSWER: C) Stop all insulin and start metformin

Ketosis-prone diabetes mellitus is a heterogeneous disorder that is intermediate in features between type 1 and type 2 diabetes. Affected patients usually present with diabetic ketoacidosis but do not have the typical phenotype of patients with type 1 diabetes. These patients are almost always obese and usually have a family history of type 2 diabetes. Most often the syndrome occurs in ethnic minority groups. After recovery from the episode of ketoacidosis and resolution of glucose toxicity, β-cell function improves in most but not all patients.

Patients with ketosis-prone diabetes mellitus do not fit well into the diabetes classification scheme promulgated by the American Diabetes Association. An attempt to use the presence or absence of autoimmune markers and β-cell reserve (by measuring C-peptide) has led to the development of the Aβ system of classification of patients with ketosis-prone diabetes. Four subgroups have been defined, and categorizing patients into one of these groups can help guide appropriate treatment.

The Aβ categories are as follows:

- A+β-   Autoantibodies are present, β-cell function is absent
- A+β+   Autoantibodies are present, β-cell function is present
- A-β-   Autoantibodies are absent, β-cell function is absent
- A-β+   Autoantibodies are absent, β-cell function is present

Types A+β- and A-β- are distinct immunologically, but these patients are considered to have type 1 diabetes by the American Diabetes Association classification scheme. Types A+β+ and A-β+ are also distinct but have characteristics typical of patients with type 2 diabetes. Most patients with ketosis-prone diabetes present with the A-β+ subtype. The patient in the vignette would fit into this subgroup.

Patients with ketosis-prone diabetes should be treated in the usual manner for diabetic ketoacidosis, including intravenous fluids, continuous intravenous insulin infusion, and correction of electrolyte abnormalities. Once the diabetic ketoacidosis has resolved, patients should be discharged on intensive insulin therapy. Assessment of β-cell reserve should be done once glucose toxicity has resolved (weeks to months later). This can be accomplished with a fasting or glucagon-stimulated C-peptide measurement. Most clinicians use the presence or absence of glutamic acid decarboxylase antibodies as a marker of autoimmune status, although the insulin-associated protein 2 (IA-2) antibody can also be measured.

Management of ketosis-prone diabetes can be guided on the basis of the Aβ subtype. Patients with autoantibodies (A+β+ and A+β-) are at higher risk for recurrent ketoacidosis and require long-term insulin therapy. Patients with the β+ subtypes have reversible β-cell function and can be treated with oral antihyperglycemic agents. Metformin (Answer C) is the preferred medication for patients with the subtype A-β+. A randomized, placebo-controlled trial of obese African American patients who had originally presented with diabetic ketoacidosis or hyperglycemic crisis demonstrated that after resolution of severe hyperglycemia, metformin (1000 mg daily) and sitagliptin (100 mg daily) were both effective in preventing hyperglycemic relapse over a 4-year follow-up period. Patients with prolonged remission had improved β-cell function. This patient has intact β-cell function and the insulin doses are quite small given his BMI. Therefore, the insulin can be stopped.

No clinical data are available regarding the use of sodium-glucose cotransporter 2 inhibitors, such as empagliflozin (Answer A), in the treatment of patients with ketosis-prone diabetes, so this is not the best step. Because this patient is obese and should be treated with an insulin sensitizer, glimepiride (Answer B) is not the drug of choice. According to the American Diabetes Association treatment guidelines, all patients with type 2 diabetes should be treated with metformin as initial treatment, so diet therapy alone (Answer D) is insufficient. Continuing the same low-dosage insulin regimen (Answer E) is a treatment option, but not the best one. This patient currently has excellent glycemic control. Insulin is not needed and the patient should do well on metformin alone.

Educational Objective
Diagnose and manage ketosis-prone diabetes mellitus.

UpToDate Topic Review(s)
Syndromes of ketosis-prone diabetes mellitus

Reference(s)
Banerji MA, Chaiken RL, Huey H, et al. GAD antibody negative NIDDM in adult black subjects with diabetic ketoacidosis and increased frequency of human leucocyte antigen DR3 and DR4. Flatbush diabetes. *Diabetes*. 1994;43(6):741-745. PMID: 8194658

Umpierrez GE, Smiley D, Kitabchi AE. Narrative review: Ketosis-prone type 2 diabetes mellitus. *Ann Intern Med*. 2006;144(5):350-357. PMID: 16520476

Balasubramanyan A, Nalini R, Hampe CS, Maldonado M. Syndromes of ketosis-prone diabetes mellitus. *Endocr Rev*. 2008;29(3):292-302. PMID: 18292467

American Diabetes Association. 2. Classification and Diagnosis of Diabetes. *Diabetes Care*. 2016;39(Suppl 1):S13-S22. PMID: 26696675

Vellanki P, Smiley DD, Stefanovski D, et al. Randomized controlled study of metformin and sitagliptin on long-term normoglycemia remission in African American patients with hyperglycemic crises. *Diabetes Care*. 2016;39(11):1948-1955. PMID: 27573938

10 ANSWER: D) Prednisone

This patient has sarcoidosis with respiratory symptoms and abdominal lymphadenopathy. It is important to pursue a diagnosis, and this is often done by bronchoscopy if hilar lymph nodes are amenable or biopsy of other lymph nodes. Biopsy of this patient's abdominal lymph nodes confirmed the diagnosis of sarcoidosis. Hypercalcemia has been described in most granulomatous disorders and is most often associated with sarcoidosis. Dysregulation of calcium metabolism is a common complication of this disease. Hypercalcemia results from increased intestinal calcium absorption induced by extrarenal calcitriol production and possibly calcitriol-induced bone resorption. Under normal circumstances, calcitriol synthesis occurs primarily in the kidneys and renal 1α-hydroxylation of vitamin D is tightly regulated by PTH, fibroblast growth factor 23, and calcitonin. High levels of calcitriol down-regulate 1α-hydroxylase and up-regulate 24,25α-hydroxylase, converting substrate favorably to the inactive metabolite 24,25-dihydroxyvitamin D. In sarcoidosis, there is loss of this negative feedback system. The activated mononuclear cells, primarily the macrophage, in the lung and lymph nodes containing the 1α-hydroxylase enzyme are resistant to down-regulation of the enzyme in response to high levels of calcitriol. PTH is typically suppressed because of high levels of calcium and calcitriol.

This patient has marked hypercalcemia that merits therapy. The mainstay of therapy is to enhance renal clearance of calcium with the use of intravenous fluid resuscitation and, if needed, loop diuretics to prevent fluid overload. Loop diuretics, such as furosemide, have not been studied in a prospective fashion in this setting, but they have little direct effect on calcium excretion and hence are considered inappropriate. In contrast, thiazide diuretics act to inhibit the sodium–calcium exchange in the collecting system to enhance sodium excretion and retain calcium in the circulation.

After initial management with intravenous fluid resuscitation and loop diuretics, glucocorticoids (Answer D) are indicated to diminish intestinal absorption of calcium and to inhibit the 1α-hydroxylase enzyme in granulomas. Steroids have no effect on renal tubular 1α-hydroxylase activity, but they are postulated to suppress granuloma enzyme activity via effects on interleukin 2 and interferon gamma. Steroid therapy may initially worsen hypercalciuria, so a follow-up 24-hour urine collection to measure calcium excretion may be indicated.

Because of PTH suppression, bone remodeling in patients with sarcoidosis and hypercalcemia is low. In that light, antiresorptive agents such as bisphosphonates (Answer C), denosumab (Answer B), and selective estrogen receptor modulators (Answer E) have little or no effect on calcium levels. In addition, bisphosphonates are contraindicated in patients with a markedly reduced glomerular filtration rate, as is the case in this patient.

Cinacalcet (Answer A) is a calcium-sensing receptor–sensitizing agent. It can lower calcium levels in patients with PTH-dependent hypercalcemia because the calcium-sensing receptor is expressed on the parathyroid cells. However, as noted in the preceding text, this patient has PTH-independent hypercalcemia and cinacalcet would be unlikely to alter calcium levels.

Educational Objective
Diagnose sarcoidosis as a cause of non–PTH-mediated hypercalcemia and recommend appropriate treatment.

UpToDate Topic Review(s)
Sarcoid: Muscle, bone, and vascular disease manifestations

Reference(s)
Conron M, Young C, Beynon HL. Calcium metabolism in sarcoidosis and its clinical implications. *Rheumatology (Oxford)*. 2000;39(7):707-713. PMID: 10908687

11 **ANSWER: C) Blood pressure → hypertension; potassium → hypokalemia; uterine endometrium → thick**
Hypercortisolism can result in the clinical manifestations of Cushing syndrome, which include hypertension and hypokalemia. Although many aspects of Cushing syndrome are induced by excessive activation of the glucocorticoid receptor, the major mechanism by which hypercortisolism induces hypertension and hypokalemia is via excessive activation of the mineralocorticoid receptor. Cortisol is a potent mineralocorticoid receptor agonist that typically circulates in the blood at concentrations that are 100- to 1000-fold higher than that of aldosterone. However, the action of the 11β-hydroxysteroid dehydrogenase 2 enzyme inactivates cortisol to cortisone, which thereby minimizes the influence of cortisol on the mineralocorticoid receptor to permit a high-affinity interaction between aldosterone and the mineralocorticoid receptor. In hypercortisolism, 11β-hydroxysteroid dehydrogenase 2 can be overwhelmed by a high cortisol substrate resulting in mineralocorticoid receptor activation and a state of pseudohyperaldosteronism: a clinical syndrome of mineralocorticoid receptor excess (hypertension and hypokalemia) in which renin and aldosterone are appropriately suppressed.

Mifepristone is a progesterone receptor antagonist and glucocorticoid receptor antagonist. It is generally very effective at blocking the glucocorticoid receptor and reducing the symptoms of Cushing syndrome. However, blocking the glucocorticoid receptor when cortisol levels are very high essentially provides more cortisol substrate for 11β-hydroxysteroid dehydrogenase 2 and the mineralocorticoid receptor. Thus, one known effect of mifepristone is increased mineralocorticoid receptor activation that can increase blood pressure and urinary potassium excretion. For this reason, patients taking mifepristone should be carefully monitored for elevations in blood pressure and decreases in potassium. Potassium concentrations should be corrected before starting mifepristone and carefully monitored during treatment. Hypokalemia can be treated with potassium supplements and mineralocorticoid receptor antagonists, which will improve potassium homeostasis and blood pressure. Lastly, the progesterone receptor antagonism induced by mifepristone can induce endometrial hypertrophy in women, which may manifest as unexpected spotting or bleeding. Thus, the effects most likely to result from mifepristone therapy in this patient are hypertension, hypokalemia, and thickened uterine endometrium (Answer C). Excessive glucocorticoid receptor antagonism with mifepristone can induce a syndrome of adrenal insufficiency. Close monitoring for the clinical signs and symptoms of adrenal insufficiency is paramount during mifepristone treatment since cortisol levels remain high and are therefore nondiagnostic. Symptoms that may suggest adrenal insufficiency are subtle and nonspecific, and can include unexplained fatigue, nausea, vomiting, weight loss, and low blood pressure.

Educational Objective

Explain the mechanism of action and adverse effects of mifepristone.

UpToDate Topic Review(s)

Pharmacology and toxicity of adrenal enzyme inhibitors and adrenolytic agents

Reference(s)

Nieman LK, Biller BM, Findling JW, et al; Endocrine Society. Treatment of Cushing's syndrome: an Endocrine Society Clinical Practice Guideline. *J Clin Endocrinol Metab.* 2015;100(8):2807-2831. PMID: 26222757

Fleseriu M, Molitch ME, Gross C, Schteingart DE, Vaughan TB 3rd, Biller BM. A new therapeutic approach in the medical treatment of Cushing's syndrome: glucocorticoid receptor blockade with mifepristone. *Endocr Pract.* 2013;19(2):313-326. PMID: 23337135

12 ANSWER: B) Gestational fasting blood glucose level

Gestational diabetes mellitus is a well-recognized risk factor for future development of type 2 diabetes. Estimates of risk vary, but in studies with longer-term follow-up, up to half of women with gestational diabetes progress to type 2 diabetes. In women with gestational diabetes, there is a marked increase in the incidence of type 2 diabetes in the first 5 years postpartum. Recognizing other clinical risk factors leads to improved risk stratification and interventions.

Potential risk factors in pregnancy are shown (*see table*).

Prepregnancy maternal characteristics	Higher prepregnancy weight
	Older age
	Ethnicity (eg, South Asian, Pacific islander)
	Parity (>5 pregnancies)
	Family history of type 2 diabetes
Pregnancy-specific maternal factors	High fasting glucose levels
	Elevated glucose levels on postglucose challenge
	Increased pregnancy weight gain
	Elevated blood pressure
Delivery and postpartum factors	Preterm delivery
	Macrosomia
	Not breastfeeding

Systematic reviews reveal that gestational glycemic control (fasting blood glucose levels during pregnancy) (Answer B) is the strongest predictor of both early postpartum and long-term development of type 2 diabetes in the mother.

When the glycemic parameters are controlled in multivariate analysis, maternal BMI (Answer D) is still associated with increased risk of type 2 diabetes, but it is not as strongly predictive as glycemic parameters. Although the other factors such as parity (>5 pregnancies) (Answer A), ethnicity (Answer C), and family history of type 2 diabetes (Answer E) are associated with increased risk in univariate analysis, when glycemic parameters are accounted for in multivariate analysis, none of these factors is independently associated with development of diabetes.

The limitation of such analyses is the variability in the studies with respect to definition of gestational diabetes and type 2 diabetes, testing frequency, length of follow-up, and definition of ethnic subgroup. Ethnic subgroups may be as broadly defined as "nonwhite." Further studies focusing on specific subgroups are required to elucidate the role of ethnicity in clinical outcomes for the mother. Women of certain ethnic backgrounds, including South Asian ancestry, are at risk for type 2 diabetes at much lower BMIs than white women.

Educational Objective

Counsel women with gestational diabetes mellitus on the likelihood of developing type 2 diabetes in the future.

Reference(s)

Kim C, Newton KM, Knopp RH. Gestational diabetes and the incidence of type 2 diabetes: a systematic review. *Diabetes Care.* 2002;25(10):1862-1868. PMID: 12351492

Ratner RE. Prevention of type 2 diabetes in women with previous gestational diabetes [published correction appears in *Diabetes Care.* 2007;30(12):3154]. *Diabetes Care.* 2007;30(Suppl 2):S242-S245. PMID: 17596479

Rayanagoudar G, Hashi AA, Zamora J, Khan KS, Hitman GA, Thangaratinam S. Quantification of the type 2 diabetes risk in women with gestational diabetes: a systematic review and meta-analysis of 95,750 women. *Diabetologia.* 2016;59(7):1403-1411. PMID: 27073002

13 ANSWER: D) A statin

This patient is seeking advice regarding primary prevention of cardiovascular disease. Several available guidelines for cardiovascular risk assessment use traditional variables such as age, sex, smoking status, waist circumference, and presence of hypertension or diabetes.

The American College of Cardiology/American Heart Association guidelines for cholesterol lowering released in 2013 have now been adopted widely in the United States and focus on global cardiovascular risk assessment. These guidelines recommend high-intensity statin therapy for adults with clinical atherosclerotic cardiovascular disease, adults with an LDL-cholesterol concentration greater than 190 mg/dL (>4.92 mmol/L), and adults with type 1 or type 2 diabetes between 40 and 79 years of age. For primary prevention of atherosclerotic cardiovascular disease in adults without diabetes, risk assessment is performed using the cardiovascular risk calculator available as part of the guidelines. Moderate- to high-intensity statin therapy is recommended if the 10-year risk of a cardiovascular event is greater than 7.5%. The variables used to calculate an individual's 10-year atherosclerotic cardiovascular disease risk are age, sex, race, systolic blood pressure, diabetes status, total cholesterol level, and HDL-cholesterol level.

Thus, on the basis of these categories, this patient's calculated risk is less than 5% and she does not necessarily need to be treated. However, her LDL-cholesterol level is greater than 160 mg/dL (>4.14 mmol/L) and she has a very strong family history of premature atherosclerotic cardiovascular disease (onset <55 years in a first-degree male relative or <65 years in a first-degree female relative). Family history is not considered in the risk calculator, which is a major drawback to its use for this patient. This situation requires that the clinician have a discussion with the patient about risk and engage in shared decision-making. Statins, the first-line therapy for atherosclerotic cardiovascular disease prevention, should be recommended in view of her genetic risk (Answer D). While at least a moderate-intensity statin should be offered in her case, it is reasonable to start a lower-dosage statin and escalate the dosage as tolerated.

It should be noted that in the absence of active liver disease (as evidenced by stable liver function tests), there is no contraindication to statin therapy. Patients with severe cholestasis due to primary biliary cirrhosis can present with severe hyperlipidemia due to formation of large lipoprotein particles called lipoprotein X. These are abnormal lipoproteins composed of phospholipid and unesterified cholesterol. Management of the liver disease, usually by liver transplant, resolves the marked hypercholesterolemia.

Dietary modification is a mainstay of cardiovascular disease risk reduction. Clear evidence demonstrates the benefit of decreasing saturated fat intake and replacing saturated fat with other macronutrients in lowering LDL cholesterol. The 2013 American College of Cardiology/American Heart Association guidelines on lifestyle management to reduce cardiovascular risk recommend that adults who would benefit from LDL-cholesterol lowering should aim for a diet that consists of 5% to 6% of calories from saturated fat. Low-fat diets can decrease LDL cholesterol by 10% to 15%. While a low-fat diet (Answer A) should be part of her treatment plan, it alone is not sufficient in view of her genetic risks.

Ezetimibe (Answer C) prevents intestinal cholesterol reabsorption and can reduce LDL-cholesterol by 10% to 15%. It is seldom used as monotherapy and has more benefit when added to statin therapy. Additionally, there are no randomized controlled trials evaluating the role of ezetimibe in primary prevention of cardiovascular disease. However, in patients who truly cannot take a statin, use of ezetimibe monotherapy is a reasonable alternative.

Colesevelam (Answer B), a bile acid sequestrant, could be considered. These agents result in a 10% to 20% reduction in LDL cholesterol. Gastrointestinal adverse effects are a major limiting factor. In the setting of this patient's underlying liver disease, colesevelam is not the best therapeutic option.

Metformin (Answer E) is the first-line therapy for type 2 diabetes and it can beneficially influence body weight, lipid profile, and liver fat. The United Kingdom Prospective Diabetes Study reported that use of metformin monotherapy in obese patients with type 2 diabetes decreased cardiovascular disease–related end points such as myocardial infarction and stroke. Nevertheless, evidence that metformin is beneficial for overall cardiovascular primary risk reduction is very limited. Additionally, the patient in this vignette does not have diabetes, so the addition of metformin is not the best choice.

Educational Objective
Assess the risk for atherosclerotic cardiovascular disease in a patient with moderate LDL-cholesterol elevations and recommend appropriate management.

UpToDate Topic Review(s)
Treatment of lipids (including hypercholesterolemia) in primary prevention

Reference(s)

Stone NJ, Robinson JG, Lichtenstein AH, et al; American College of Cardiology/American Heart Association Task Force on Practice Guidelines. 2013 ACC/AHA guideline on the treatment of blood cholesterol to reduce atherosclerotic cardiovascular risk in adults: a report of the American College of Cardiology/American Heart Association Task Force on Practice Guidelines. *J Am Coll Cardiol*. 2014;63(25 Pt B):2889-2934. PMID: 24239923

Eckel RH, Jakicic JM, Ard JD, de Jesus JM, et al; American College of Cardiology/American Heart Association Task Force on Practice Guidelines. 2013 AHA/ACC guideline on lifestyle management to reduce cardiovascular risk: a report of the American College of Cardiology/American Heart Association Task Force on Practice Guidelines [published corrections appear in *J Am Coll Cardiol*. 2014;63(25 Pt B):3024-3025 and *J Am Coll Cardiol*. 2015;66(24):2812]. *J Am Coll Cardiol*. 2014;63(25 Pt B):2960-2984. PMID: 24239922

Martin SS, Sperling LS, Blaha MJ, et al. Clinician-patient risk discussion for atherosclerotic cardiovascular disease prevention: importance to implementation of the 2013 ACC/AHA Guidelines. *J Am Coll Cardiol*. 2015;65(13):1361-1368. PMID: 25835448

14 ANSWER: C) Refer to neurosurgery

When evaluating a sellar mass, one must determine whether it is secreting an excessive amount of any hormone, causing hypopituitarism, or damaging the surrounding structures (mainly optic nerves and chiasm). This patient has a large sellar mass causing central hypogonadism, but no evidence of Cushing disease or acromegaly. His morning cortisol level rules out adrenal insufficiency. The chiasmatic compression and abnormal visual field test make surgery necessary to address the mass effect (thus, Answer C is correct).

The patient's prolactin is elevated, but if he had a prolactinoma, the value would be much higher (>100 ng/mL [>4.3 nmol/L]). The moderate increase in prolactin is most likely due to stalk compression. Therefore, dopaminergic therapy (Answer B), although likely to reduce the prolactin level, would not cause tumor shrinkage and would place the patient at risk of further vision damage. Conversely, if prolactin were markedly elevated, a trial of dopaminergic drug therapy with repeated imaging in 3 months would be reasonable. Macroprolactinemia occurs when prolactin is elevated due to accumulation of biologically inactive prolactin that is bound to immunoglobulins. About 15% of cases of hyperprolactinemia are due to macroprolactinemia. However, diagnosing macroprolactinemia (Answer A) would not help in this case because the presence of macroprolactinemia would only indicate that real (monomeric) prolactin is normal, and it would not change the surgical indication.

Starting testosterone therapy (Answer D), although reasonable, would not address the main issue (mass effect). Furthermore, there is a good possibility that testosterone may normalize after decompressive surgery. Hypogonadism does not increase surgical risk.

Finally, α subunit measurement (Answer E) (often increased in nonfunctioning macroadenomas) would not independently change the surgical indication regardless of whether it is normal or elevated.

Educational Objective
Distinguish prolactinoma from hyperprolactinemia due to stalk compression.

Reference(s)

Karavitaki N, Thanabalasingham G, Shore HC, et al. Do the limits of serum prolactin in disconnection hyperprolactinaemia need re-definition? A study of 226 patients with histologically verified non-functioning pituitary macroadenoma. *Clin Endocrinol (Oxf)*. 2006;65(4):524-529. PMID: 16984247

Molitch ME. Disorders of prolactin secretion. *Endocrinol Metab Clin North Am*. 2001;30(3):585-610. PMID: 11571932

15 ANSWER: D) Inactivating mutation in the *CYP24A1* gene

Hypercalcemia is a common clinical problem, with primary hyperparathyroidism and malignancy accounting for most cases. The initial goal of evaluating the cause of hypercalcemia is to distinguish PTH-mediated hypercalcemia from non–PTH-mediated hypercalcemia, which primarily includes malignancy, vitamin D intoxication, and granulomatous disease.

Several case reports describe mutations in the *CYP24A1* gene (Answer D), which are a rare cause of non–PTH-mediated hypercalcemia and are indeed the etiology of this patient's hypercalcemia. Given that this is a disorder that often goes undiagnosed, the actual prevalence is not known. The *CYP24A1* gene encodes the vitamin D 24-hydroxylase enzyme, which catalyses the hydroxylation of the biologically active form of vitamin D, $1,25$-dihydroxyvitamin D_3, and its precursor, 25-hydroxyvitamin D_3, to the inactive form, $24,25$-dihydroxyvitamin D, for excretion. Mutations in *CYP24A1* inhibit these functions, resulting in increased levels of active vitamin D, low metabolites, and subsequent persistent hypercalcemia. This disorder is known to cause a range of clinical phenotypes and presentations, including idiopathic infantile hypercalcemia and adult-onset nephrocalcinosis and nephrolithiasis. The mainstay of treatment for these patients is avoidance of calcium and vitamin D supplementation. In the context of raised or borderline-high serum calcium levels, suppressed PTH, and persistently elevated $1,25$-dihydroxyvitamin D levels, this rare condition should be considered after other causes are excluded by measuring $24,25$-dihydroxyvitamin D, which is now available at some institutions.

Hypercalcemia can be associated with ingestion of excessive vitamin D (Answer A). Daily intake of more than 10,000 IU should raise suspicion of vitamin D intoxication, especially in the setting of hypercalcemia and hypercalciuria. This patient admits to sporadically taking supplements. The symptoms associated with vitamin D toxicity are similar to other causes of both PTH-mediated hypercalcemia and non–PTH-mediated hypercalcemia. Laboratory findings in patients with vitamin D intoxication include hypercalcemia, hyperphosphatemia due to increased intestinal in renal phosphate absorption, and suppressed PTH concentrations. The normal phosphate levels in this patient make vitamin D intoxication unlikely.

Another cause of non–PTH-mediated hypercalcemia is the abnormal calcium metabolism seen in granulomatous diseases, including sarcoidosis (Answer B). In sarcoidosis and other granulomatous diseases, activated macrophages in the lung and lymph nodes produce calcitriol independent of PTH. In comparison, monocytes in patients with granulomatous disease both produce more calcitriol and lack the normal feedback control of calcitriol production, which would normally prevent excess production. Additionally, PTHrP may also contribute to the hypercalcemia in some patients with sarcoidosis. Hypercalcemia is caused by excess substrate of $1,25$-dihydroxyvitamin D and one would expect all metabolites, including $24,25$-dihydroxyvitamin D, to be elevated and not suppressed.

Similarly, hypercalcemia is caused by PTH-independent extrarenal production of calcitriol from calcidiol by activated mononuclear cells in patients with lymphoma (Answer C). Hypercalcemia has also been well described in Hodgkin lymphoma, nonHodgkin lymphoma, and adult T-cell leukemia/lymphoma. Increasing levels of $1,25$-dihydroxyvitamin D have been implicated in the pathogenesis in all cases of lymphoma and in about 30% of cases of nonHodgkin lymphoma.

Inactivating mutations in the *CASR* gene (Answer E) are associated with familial hypocalciuric hypercalcemia and neonatal severe primary hyperparathyroidism. Familial hypocalciuric hypercalcemia is a benign cause of hypercalcemia that is characterized by autosomal dominant inheritance with high penetrance. Inactivating *CASR* mutations make the parathyroid glands less sensitive to calcium, leading to a higher-than-normal serum calcium concentration required to reduce PTH release. In the kidney, there is an increase in tubular calcium and magnesium reabsorption leading to hypercalcemia, hypocalciuria, and frequently high-normal levels of serum magnesium or frank hypermagnesemia. In familial hypocalciuric hypercalcemia, serum PTH concentrations are typically inappropriately normal or high (in about 20% of cases) in the presence of mild hypercalcemia. Patients with familial hypocalciuric hypercalcemia have few symptoms or signs of hypercalcemia, including kidney stones which are rarely reported. Urinary calcium excretion is low in patients with familial hypocalciuric hypercalcemia. Affected patients typically present in childhood with the incidental discovery of mild hypercalcemia, hypocalciuria, normal PTH levels, and high-normal to frankly elevated serum magnesium levels. The patient in this vignette has a suppressed PTH, normal magnesium level, and a history of kidney stones, which makes this diagnosis unlikely.

Educational Objective
Recognize non–PTH-mediated hypercalcemia with elevated 1,25-dihydroxyvitamin D most likely secondary to *CYP24A1* mutations.

UpToDate Topic Review(s)
Regulation of calcium and phosphate balance

Reference(s)

Tebben PJ, Singh RJ, Kumar R. Vitamin D-mediated hypercalcemia: mechanisms, diagnosis, and treatment. *Endocr Rev*. 2016;37(5):521-547. PMID: 27588937

Jacobs TP, Bilezikian JP. Clinical review: rare causes of hypercalcemia. *J Clin Endocrinol Metab*. 2005;90(11):6316-6322. PMID: 16131579

16 ANSWER: A) Very low-calorie diet

A very low-calorie diet (Answer A) is a hypocaloric diet that provides less than 800 kcal/day. Very low-calorie diets are recommended when rapid weight loss is necessary for a specific reason such as undergoing surgery. This approach, under close medical supervision, should be considered in selected patients with a BMI of 30 kg/m² or greater. Women following this diet lose an average of 3.3 to 4.4 lb per week (1.5-2.0 kg) and men lose an average of 4.4 to 5.5 lb per week (2.0-2.5 kg). Over 12 weeks, the average weight loss is 44 lb (20 kg). Most plans include full meal replacements with either protein shakes or bars. Patients are usually followed up every 1 to 2 weeks as they are at increased risk for electrolyte abnormalities, volume depletion, fatigue, constipation, and gallstones.

Pharmacotherapy for obesity will not provide a comparable degree of weight loss in a short period. In studies of phentermine (Answer D), lorcaserin (Answer C), or liraglutide (Answer E), participants achieve weight loss of 8 lb (3.6 kg) at 24 weeks, 8 lb (3.6 kg) at 12 months, and 12.8 lb (5.8 kg) at 12 months, respectively (these values represent weight loss beyond that achieved with diet and lifestyle modification alone).

A low-carbohydrate diet (Answer B) limits carbohydrate intake to less than 60 g of carbohydrate per day without a prescribed energy restriction. A meta-analysis of 6 studies showed weight loss ranged from 7 to 26.5 lb (–3.2 to –12 kg) after 6 months of following a low-carbohydrate diet, which is less weight loss than that achieved with a very low-calorie diet.

Educational Objective
Recommend a very low-calorie diet to achieve rapid weight loss.

UpToDate Topic Review(s)
Obesity in adults: Dietary therapy

Reference(s)

Tsai AG, Wadden TA. The evolution of very-low-calorie diets: an update and meta-analysis. *Obesity (Silver Spring)*. 2006;14(8):1283-1293. PMID: 16988070

Very low-calorie diets. National Task Force on the Prevention and Treatment of Obesity, National Institutes of Health. *JAMA*. 1993;270(8):967-974. PMID: 8345648

Apovian CM, Aronne LJ, Bessesen DH, et al; Endocrine Society. Pharmacological management of obesity: an endocrine Society clinical practice guideline. *J Clin Endocrinol Metab*. 2015;100(2):342-362. PMID: 25590212

Nordmann AJ, Nordmann A, Briel M, et al. Effects of low-carbohydrate vs low-fat diets on weight loss and cardiovascular risk factors: a meta-analysis of randomized controlled trials [published correction appears in *Arch Intern Med*. 2006;166(8):932]. *Arch Intern Med*. 2006;166(3):285-293. PMID: 16476868

17

ANSWER: C) Nocturnal hypoglycemia

This patient's hemoglobin A_{1c} level of 7.3% (56 mmol/mol) is just above her target of less than 7.0% (<53 mmol/mol). If sustained, her current degree of glycemic control places her at a modestly increased risk for long-term diabetes-related microvascular and macrovascular complications. Lowering her hemoglobin A_{1c} must be done cautiously, as she is having frequent hypoglycemia. Reducing the frequency and severity of hypoglycemia is another important treatment goal in patients with type 1 diabetes. Raising glycemic targets has been advocated in patients with recurrent severe hypoglycemia to help restore hypoglycemia awareness. Other interventions that reduce the frequency of hypoglycemia include those that replace insulin in a more physiologic manner, such as insulin pump therapy and accurate adjustment of prandial insulin doses for ingested carbohydrates through carbohydrate counting.

Beginning in 2000, newer basal insulins became available that have longer durations of action and smoother, more predictable insulin profiles leading to less frequent hypoglycemia. These improvements are due to modifications to human insulin, including amino acid deletions, substitutions, and/or additions of side chains, which lead to insulin aggregation in the subcutaneous space and slower, more consistent insulin absorption. Compared with NPH insulin, once-daily insulin glargine and insulin detemir are associated with less nocturnal hypoglycemia. Due to less variable plasma insulin concentrations, insulin degludec and U300 insulin glargine are associated with less nocturnal hypoglycemia (Answer C), while achieving similar hemoglobin A_{1c} levels to those observed with U100 insulin glargine (thus, Answer B is incorrect). No significant differences are seen between insulin degludec and insulin glargine with respect to postmeal glucose levels, which are primarily controlled by prandial insulin (thus, Answer A is incorrect). No long-term studies have been performed that show reduced microvascular complications with insulin degludec when compared with other basal insulins (thus, Answer E is incorrect). Because of a longer duration of action, insulin degludec is recommended to be injected once daily, but not less frequently than once-daily insulin glargine (thus, Answer D is incorrect).

Educational Objective
Recognize differences in actions among existing basal insulins.

UpToDate Topic Review(s)
Management of blood glucose in adults with type 1 diabetes mellitus

Reference(s)
Heller S, Buse J, Fisher M, et al; BEGIN Basal-Bolus Type 1 Trial Investigators. Insulin degludec, an ultra-longacting basal insulin, versus insulin glargine in basal-bolus treatment with mealtime insulin aspart in type 1 diabetes (BEGIN Basal-Bolus Type 1): a phase 3, randomised, open-label, treat-to-target non-inferiority trial. *Lancet*. 2012;379(9825):1489-1497. PMID: 22521071

Ratner RE, Gough SC, Mathieu C, et al. Hypoglycaemia risk with insulin degludec compared with insulin glargine in type 2 and type 1 diabetes: a pre-planned meta-analysis of phase 3 trials. *Diabetes Obes Metab*. 2013;15(2):175-184. PMID: 23130654

18

ANSWER: D) 11β-hydroxylase deficiency

This patient has 11β-hydroxylase deficiency (Answer D). 11β-hydroxylase deficiency is the second most common form of congenital adrenal hyperplasia, accounting for 5% to 8% of cases. Mutations in the *CYP11B1* gene cause deficient conversion of 11-deoxycortisol to cortisol and 11-deoxycorticosterone to corticosterone, resulting in an accumulation of 11-deoxycortisol and 11-deoxycorticosterone (*see image*), as in the vignette. The increase in 11-deoxycorticosterone, with its mineralocorticoid activity, results in hypertension. The increased androgen production results in genital ambiguity and hyperandrogenism in girls, as well as premature pubarche, rapid prepubertal growth, and accelerated bone age in both boys and girls. Hydrocortisone treatment is needed to suppress ACTH and the excess androgen production.

Classic 21-hydroxylase deficiency (Answer B), the most common form of congenital adrenal hyperplasia, blocks conversion of 17-hydroxyprogesterone to 11-deoxycortisol and cortisol, resulting in low levels of both steroids. Cortisol deficiency causes salt wasting and hypotension, in contrast to the hypertension in 11β-hydroxylase deficiency. Similar to what is observed in 11β-hydroxylase deficiency, elevated 17-hydroxyprogesterone then leads to increased production of androstenedione and testosterone, causing ambiguous genitalia in girls and the consequences of hyperandrogenism in girls and boys.

Unlike the neonatal form of congenital adrenal hyperplasia, nonclassic 21-hydroxylase deficiency (Answer A) typically presents at adrenarche or in early adulthood. Women with nonclassic congenital adrenal hyperplasia typically undergo puberty at an early age and have short adult stature and irregular menses.

Women with 3β-hydroxysteroid dehydrogenase deficiency (Answer C) do not make cortisol, aldosterone, or androstenedione. Therefore, they present with salt wasting and adrenal insufficiency. They cannot produce estradiol because they have no androstenedione substrate for aromatization. Therefore, they have amenorrhea and absence of thelarche. Because of absent testosterone production, affected male patients present with hypospadias or more severe genital ambiguity.

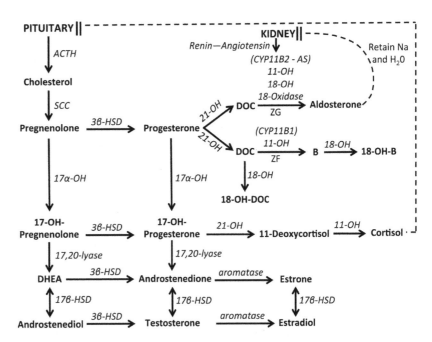

Abbreviations: ACTH, corticotropin; DOC, deoxycorticosterone; SCC, side-chain cleavage enzyme; 11-OH, 11-hydroxylase; 17α-OH, 17α-hydroxylase; 18-OH, 18-hydroxylase; 3β-HSD, 3β-hydroxysteroid dehydrogenase; 17β-HDS, 17β-hydroxysteroid dehydrogenase

Patients with complete 17-hydroxylase deficiency (Answer E) are also deficient in androstenedione, and therefore estradiol, but have excess mineralocorticoids. Therefore, affected girls do not have a recognizable phenotype until puberty when they present with amenorrhea and absence of thelarche. They do not have excess androgens and would not have acne or elevated androgen levels. However, they do have hypertension because of excess corticosterone and deoxycorticosterone.

The therapeutic goals for women with 11β-hydroxylase deficiency are to treat hypertension, maintain regular menses, and alleviate symptoms of androgen excess while avoiding the complications of glucocorticoid replacement. Women with congenital adrenal hyperplasia can develop secondary ovarian androgen excess resulting in elevated testosterone despite appropriate glucocorticoid replacement. Spironolactone can be used to treat the mineralocorticoid-mediated hypertension and to block androgen action at the androgen receptor. Combined hormonal contraception can also be used for hirsutism and acne. Hormonal contraception suppresses ovarian androgens and increases sex hormone–binding globulin, which decreases free testosterone. Hormonal contraception also protects the uterus, preventing endometrial hyperplasia when menses are irregular and prevents pregnancy in patients on spironolactone. Glucocorticoid replacement should not be titrated to suppress the 17-hydroxyprogesterone into the normal range because the 17-hydroxyprogesterone levels tend to be much higher than androgen levels and normalization will result in overtreatment.

Educational Objective
Determine the underlying cause of congenital adrenal hyperplasia.

UpToDate Topic Review(s)
Uncommon congenital adrenal hyperplasias

Reference(s)

White PC, Curnow KM, Pascoe L. Disorders of steroid 11 beta-hydroxylase isozymes. *Endocr Rev.* 1994;15(4):421-438. PMID: 7988480

Speiser PW, White PC. Congenital adrenal hyperplasia. *N Engl J Med.* 2003;349(8):776-788. PMID: 12930931

Soardi FC, Penachioni JY, Justo GZ, et al. Novel mutations in CYP11B1 gene leading to 11 beta-hydroxylase deficiency in Brazilian patients. *J Clin Endocrinol Metab.* 2009;94(9):3481-3485. PMID: 19567537

19 ANSWER: C) Hypogonadism

The autoimmune polyglandular syndromes (APS) comprise a wide spectrum of disorders and are defined by the autoimmune failure of at least 2 glands. APS type 1, or autoimmune polyendocrinopathy candidiasis-ectodermal-dystrophy, is a rare autosomal recessive disease caused by mutations in the autoimmune regulator gene (*AIRE*) that encodes a transcription factor involved in the presentation of tissue-restricted antigens during T-cell development in the thymus. APS type 1 usually presents in childhood, and the diagnosis is generally based on the presence of 2 of the 3 following findings in the classic triad: chronic mucocutaneous candidiasis, hypoparathyroidism, and adrenal insufficiency.

APS types 2 and 3 manifest in adults. APS type 2 is defined by the presence of Addison disease and either type 1 diabetes mellitus or autoimmune thyroid failure or both. APS type 3 is characterized by the presence of autoimmune thyroid disease and autoimmune disorders other than Addison disease or hypoparathyroidism. There is marked overlap in the phenotypes of APS types 2 and 3, and it is important to distinguish them from the much rarer APS type 1. APS types 2 and 3 have a prevalence of 1 in 20,000 and they occur more commonly in women. The incidence peaks between the ages of 20 and 60 years, most commonly in the third and fourth decades.

APS is characterized by lymphocytic infiltration of the affected glands, organ-specific antibodies in the serum, cellular immune defects, and an association with the human leucocyte antigen (HLA) DR/DQ genes or immune response genes. In contrast to APS type 1, the genetic basis of APS types 2 and 3 is much more complex. Genetic susceptibility in APS types 2 and 3 appears necessary although not sufficient to produce the disorder and there is lack of 100% concordance in identical twins. Several genetic loci most likely interact with environmental factors. Susceptibility genes that have been implicated include certain HLA genes, the cytotoxic T-lymphocyte antigen gene (*CTLA4*), and the protein tyrosine phosphatase nonreceptor type 22 gene (*PTPN22*).

This patient has been diagnosed with type 1 diabetes mellitus, autoimmune hypothyroidism, and celiac disease and now presents with features and biochemical findings of hypoadrenalism, consistent with an underlying diagnosis of APS type 2. She is at risk for additional autoimmune endocrine disorders, including hypogonadism (Answer C), as well as nonendocrine autoimmune diseases such as autoimmune gastritis, pernicious anemia, vitiligo, autoimmune hepatitis, and myasthenia gravis. Unlike patients with APS type 1, patients with APS type 2 do not develop mucocutaneous candidiasis (Answer A), and a diagnosis of hypoparathyroidism (Answer D) is very rare. Nonendocrine autoimmune diseases such as Sjogren syndrome (Answer B) and alopecia areata (Answer E) are more common in APS type 3 than in APS type 2 and are therefore not the best answers.

Silent autoantibodies to various organs are common in families with APS type 2 and often there is a prolonged phase of cellular loss preceding autoimmune glandular disease. Antibody screening may be predictive for the development of future autoimmune diseases. Many of the endocrine disorders associated with APS type 2 are adequately treated with hormone replacement therapy. In addition, it is important to screen at-risk individuals for subclinical autoimmune endocrine diseases through regular monitoring of thyroid function and ACTH stimulation tests in order to start replacement therapy when required.

Educational Objective
Assess the risk of autoimmune conditions developing in patients with autoimmune polyglandular syndrome type 2.

UpToDate Topic Review(s)
Causes of primary adrenal insufficiency (Addison's disease)

Reference(s)

Cutolo M. Autoimmune polyendocrine syndromes. *Autoimmun Rev*. 2014;13(2):85-89. PMID: 24055063

Kahaly GJ. Polyglandular autoimmune syndrome type II. *Presse Med*. 2012;41(12 P 2):e663-e670. PMID: 23159534

20 ANSWER: A) No further investigation required

The incidentally discovered adrenal mass is a common endocrine problem. The prevalence varies with age and can be up to 10% in persons older than 70 years. When an adrenal mass is discovered, it is crucial to establish whether it is malignant and/or secreting excess adrenal hormones.

Importantly, adrenal malignancy is rare; only 2% to 5% of incidentalomas are adrenocortical carcinoma. Adrenal metastases are the most common malignant neoplasm of the adrenal gland and have been found in up to

27% of patients with known malignant epithelial tumors at autopsy. However, it is unusual for adrenal metastasis to be the presenting radiologic feature of malignancy; in most cases, the primary lesion has already been identified. While many primary tumors can spread to the adrenal, the most commonly reported are cancers of the lung, colon, breast, pancreas, and kidney.

To assess the malignant potential of an adrenal mass, the image should be carefully evaluated to identify classic features that denote a benign or malignant imaging phenotype. This is particularly pertinent in this case given the recent diagnosis of breast cancer (a malignancy known to have a predilection for metastatic adrenal spread). However, the adenoma shown in the CT image displays all the classic hallmarks of a benign, lipid-rich, adrenal adenoma and is not consistent with a malignant adrenal lesion. The typical radiologic characteristics of different adrenal masses assessed by CT are summarized (*see table*).

Characteristic	Benign adenoma	Adrenal Metastasis	Pheochromocytoma	Adrenocortical Carcinoma
Appearance	Smooth contours, homogeneous	Irregular outline, heterogeneous	Heterogeneous, vascular	Irregular, heterogeneous
Size and location	<4 cm, unilateral	Variable size, often bilateral	Variable, can be bilateral	Usually >>4 cm
Density	Low unenhanced CT attenuation values (<10 Hounsfield units)	High attenuation value (>20 Hounsfield units)	High attenuation value (>20 Hounsfield units)	High attenuation value (>20 Hounsfield units)
Response to intravenous contrast medium	[a] Rapid washout (>50% washout 10 minutes after contrast)	Delayed washout (<50% washout 10 minutes after contrast)	Delayed washout (<50% washout 10 minutes after contrast)	Delayed washout (<50% washout 10 minutes after contrast)

[a] If noncontrast CT demonstrates a small (<4 cm) adrenal mass with a density <10 Hounsfield units, then contrast (and evaluation of washout) is not required.

The adrenal lesion in this vignette is small with low attenuation (lipid rich, with a density of <10 Hounsfield units) and displays rapid washout of intravenous contrast. In addition, the biochemistry also illustrates that this adrenal mass is nonfunctional. Therefore, this benign, nonfunctional lesion requires no further investigation (Answer A).

Given that this lesion is clearly benign, the history of breast cancer is not relevant in this case and adrenal biopsy (Answer B) is unnecessary. Adrenal biopsy should be reserved for patients with a known extra-adrenal malignancy who have an adrenal lesion with indeterminate imaging characteristics and no evidence of catecholamine excess. There is no indication for surgical resection of this mass (Answer C) on the basis of radiologic appearance or biochemical characteristics.

PET scanning with fluorodeoxyglucose (Answer D) is not routinely required in the evaluation of adrenal masses, but it could have been a useful additional tool in this case if the imaging phenotype had been less reassuring. Finally, MRI (Answer E) offers no advantage over CT in the radiologic evaluation of adrenal masses.

The radiologic and clinical follow-up of such masses remains controversial. No prospective studies have been conducted to determine the optimal frequency and duration of follow-up for adrenal incidentalomas. In addition, the radiation exposure related to additional CT scanning should be considered. The recently published European guideline on the management of such masses, however, would suggest that for this small adenoma with benign imaging characteristics, no further routine radiologic follow-up is indicated. However, many clinicians would advocate for another CT in 6 to 12 months to ensure no change in the size or appearance of the adenoma.

Educational Objective
Identify radiologic characteristics typical of benign adrenal adenomas.

UpToDate Topic Review(s)
The adrenal incidentaloma

Reference(s)

Fassnacht M, Arlt W, Bancos I, et al. Management of adrenal incidentalomas: European Society of Endocrinology Clinical Practice Guideline in collaboration with the European Network for the Study of Adrenal Tumors. *Eur J Endocrinol*. 2016;175(2):G1-G34. PMID: 27390021

Nieman LK. Approach to the patient with an adrenal incidentaloma. *J Clin Endocrinol Metab*. 2010;95(9):4106-4113. PMID: 20823463

21

ANSWER: C) Reassess his reproductive axis after stopping testosterone for 4 months

Congenital hypogonadotropic hypogonadism used to be considered a lifelong diagnosis. Several studies indicate that 5% to 15% of affected men recover their reproductive function after treatment normalizes their testosterone levels. For this reason, a trial off testosterone (Answer C) is warranted in this patient to see whether his gonadal function has recovered. The factors associated with reversibility of congenital hypogonadotropic hypogonadism are not known. Reversibility has been described in men with genetic mutations in 9 known genes associated with congenital hypogonadotropic hypogonadism and in men without olfactory structures. Reversibility does not appear to be related to the severity of GnRH deficiency. One clinical feature often associated with reversibility is testicular growth while on testosterone replacement therapy. Another caveat is that the reversibility may only be temporary, so men should be monitored for relapse.

Obtaining a baseline semen analysis (Answer A) is incorrect as testosterone therapy usually causes azoospermia or oligospermia due to suppression of FSH. When assessing a man's fertility potential, he should be off testosterone for several months. Increasing the dosage of testosterone (Answer B), switching to a different type of testosterone therapy (Answer D), or switching to different modality to increase testosterone (Answer E) does not consider the possibility that his reproductive function may have recovered. If his physician determined that he remained hypogonadal, the dosage of testosterone cypionate could be increased to target the midcycle testosterone between 450 and 600 ng/dL (15.6-20.8 nmol/L), which would approximate the 50th percentile according to some studies.

Educational Objective

Recognize that congenital hypogonadotropic hypogonadism may be reversible and recommend periodic treatment withdrawal.

UpToDate Topic Review(s)

Causes of secondary hypogonadism in males

Reference(s)

Boehm U, Bouloux PM, Dattani MT, et al. Expert consensus document: European Consensus Statement on congenital hypogonadotropic hypogonadism-- pathogenesis, diagnosis and treatment. *Nat Rev Endocrinol.* 2015;11(9):547-564. PMID: 26194704

Raivio T, Falardeau J, Dwyer A, et al. Reversal of idiopathic hypogonadotropic hypogonadism. *N Engl J Med.* 2007;357(9):863-873. PMID: 17761590

22

ANSWER: E) Current thyroid-stimulating immunoglobulin titer

Several features of this patient's presentation indicate that he has severe Graves disease. At the time of his initial presentation, he had very high thyroid hormone levels with significant thyroid-stimulating immunoglobulin elevation. TSH receptor antibodies (TRAb) can be assessed by measuring either TSH-binding inhibition immunoglobulin or thyroid-stimulating immunoglobulin. TSH-binding inhibition immunoglobulin assays are competition assays that measure inhibition of binding of either a labeled monoclonal antihuman TSH-receptor antibody or labeled TSH to a recombinant TSH receptor. Bioassays for thyroid-stimulating immunoglobulin measure the ability of simulating antibodies to increase the intracellular level of cAMP in cultured Chinese hamster ovary cells. The thyroid-stimulating immunoglobulin assay was used to assess TRAb levels in the patient described in this vignette. Although his thyroid examination at presentation is not provided, it would be expected that he would have had a large goiter, as well as the described orbitopathy. When a patient such as this is initially treated with methimazole, current recommendations suggest that therapy should be continued for approximately 12 to 18 months.

When considering whether a patient might go into remission after the initial period of thionamide treatment, several factors should be considered. Lower chance of remission is documented in individuals with large goiters and higher free T_4 levels, in men, and in patients who smoke cigarettes. However, the most direct assessment of the likelihood of remission is the degree of TRAb elevation at the end of the initial period of therapy. Those who have low TRAb levels at that time have a greater likelihood of achieving permanent remission, compared with relapse rates of 80% or more in those whose TRAb levels remain persistently elevated. In fact, the current American Thyroid Association Hyperthyroidism Management Guidelines published in 2016 suggest that after 12 to 18 months of methimazole therapy, the medication can be discontinued if TSH and TRAb are normal. Although this patient's TSH concentration is normal, his TRAb levels remain elevated, predicting a reduced likelihood of remission (thus, Answer E is correct).

The patient's concurrent orbitopathy and his initial requirement for a high methimazole dosage to attain euthyroidism might also be associated with lower long-term remission rates. However, the predictive value of these factors is most likely mediated by the degree of TRAb elevation. In other words, patients with high TRAb levels are more likely to have large goiters and coexistent orbitopathy, and they may require higher initial methimazole dosages (thus, Answers B and D are incorrect). This patient's high methimazole dosage may also be due to the treating physician increasing the dosage when the patient was failing to adhere to his medication regimen.

Variable adherence to antithyroidal therapy is certainly a barrier to achieving a euthyroid state. However, this factor has not been directly studied as a risk factor for relapse that is independent of elevated TRAb titers (thus, Answer C is incorrect). Even if a patient undergoes thyroidectomy or radioactive iodine therapy, the patient must still adhere to levothyroxine therapy.

Vitamin D status has been investigated as a factor that may influence the course of autoimmune diseases, such as Hashimoto thyroiditis and Graves disease. Some preliminary studies suggest that 25-hydroxyvitamin D levels may be lower in patients with Graves disease who suffer a relapse than in those who go into remission. However, such data are preliminary (thus, Answer A is incorrect).

Educational Objective
Describe factors that are useful for predicting remission of Graves disease.

UpToDate Topic Review(s)
Thionamides in the treatment of Graves' disease

Reference(s)

Ross DS, Burch HB, Cooper DS, et al. 2016 American Thyroid Association Guidelines for Diagnosis and Management of Hyperthyroidism and Other Causes of Thyrotoxicosis. *Thyroid.* 2016;26(10):1343-1421. PMID: 27521067

Laurberg P, Wallin G, Tallstedt L, Abraham-Nordling M, Lundell G, Torring O. TSH-receptor autoimmunity in Graves' disease after therapy with anti-thyroid drugs, surgery, or radioiodine: a 5-year prospective randomized study. Eur J Endocrinol. *Eur J Endocrinol.* 2008;158(1):69-75. PMID: 18166819

Carella C, Mazziotti G, Sorvillo F, et al. Serum thyrotropin receptor antibodies concentrations in patients with Graves' disease before, at the end of methimazole treatment, and after drug withdrawal: evidence that the activity of thyrotropin receptor antibody and/or thyroid response modify during the observation period. *Thyroid.* 2006;16(3):295-302. PMID: 16571093

23 ANSWER: D) Lower the basal rate for 7 hours after each strenuous run, starting at bedtime

Exercise is recommended for patients with diabetes mellitus to prevent weight gain, improve glycemic control, and reduce cardiovascular risk factors. Patients with type 1 diabetes can safely engage in vigorous exercise such as training for and participating in marathon or half-marathon races or long-distance bicycle races. However, precautions must be taken to maintain the patient's safety. For most patients, the optimal glucose level during exercise is in the range of 120 to 180 mg/dL (6.7-10.0 mmol/L). If the glucose level before exercise is less than 100 to 120 mg/dL (<5.6 mmol/L), the patient should ingest 15 to 30 g of rapid-acting carbohydrate and have carbohydrates readily available during exercise. Intensive exercise should be avoided if the glucose level is greater than 250 mg/dL (>13.9 mmol/L) or if ketosis is present. One study demonstrated that patients with type 1 diabetes who had hyperglycemia, a relative insulin deficiency, and ketosis who underwent a 3-hour bout of exercise (stationary bicycling) developed even higher glucose levels, an increase in glucagon and cortisol, and worsening of ketosis during the exercise. Hyperglycemia can occur in some patients with type 1 diabetes, especially after high-intensity exercise, due to counterregulatory hormone release.

Avoidance of hypoglycemia is key in patients with diabetes who exercise. Hypoglycemia can occur during and for up to 18 hours after moderate or intensive exercise. In one study, 48% of youth experienced nocturnal hypoglycemia during the ensuing night after engaging in a 1-hour bout of afternoon exercise.

If the preexercise meal, the amount and intensity of exercise, and the insulin regimen are kept fairly constant in patients with type 1 diabetes, then glucose responses during and after exercise are predictable and the risk of hypoglycemia is lessened. The patient is this vignette develops intermittent hypoglycemia 5 to 12 hours after strenuous runs. Two possible strategies to avoid hypoglycemia are to add carbohydrates before and after exercise or to lower the insulin infusion rates. As he does not usually have hypoglycemia during or immediately after the run, ingesting carbohydrates to increase glucose before each strenuous run (Answer A) is incorrect. Lowering the basal rate (Answer B) or stopping the pump during the exercise (Answer E) would affect the glucose values during and for several hours after the exercise but would not prevent hypoglycemia that occurs many hours after the exercise. Skipping the premeal bolus of insulin for the meal after the exercise (Answer C) might lead to postmeal hyperglycemia and may or may not prevent hypoglycemia that occurs 5 to 12 hours after the run.

Patients with type 1 diabetes who are on insulin pump therapy can modify the basal rate in response to exercise or increased activity. A study of 16 youth with type 1 diabetes (mean age 13.3 years) treated with insulin pumps in whom standardized afternoon exercise for 60 minutes was conducted showed that a 20% reduction in overnight basal insulin rates significantly reduced the risk of nocturnal hypoglycemia the night following exercise.

The optimal approach in this situation is to have the patient use a lower basal rate starting at bedtime (about 5 to 6 hours after the exercise) and lasting for 7 hours (Answer D). The patient can start with a temporary lower rate of 50% to 75% of the usual basal rate during this time. He can adjust the basal rate accordingly to prevent episodes of nocturnal hypoglycemia that occur late after exercise.

Another treatment option for this patient would be to consider use of a continuous glucose sensor. This would improve the ability to detect hypoglycemia during and after exercise, especially at night when he is most vulnerable to hypoglycemia.

Educational Objective
Manage the effects of exercise on glucose levels in patients with diabetes mellitus.

UpToDate Topic Review(s)
Management of blood glucose in adults with type 1 diabetes mellitus

Reference(s)

Mitchell TH, Abraham G, Schiffrin A, Leiter LA, Marliss EB. Hyperglycemia after intense exercise in IDDM subjects during continuous subcutaneous insulin infusion. *Diabetes Care*. 1988;11(4):311-317. PMID: 3042306

Tsalikian E, Mauras N, Beck RW, et al; Diabetes Research in Children Network Direcnet Study Group. Impact of exercise on overnight glycemic control in children with type 1 diabetes mellitus. *J Pediatr*. 2005;147(4):528-534. PMID: 16227041

Temple MY, Bar-Or O, Riddell MC. The reliability and repeatability of the blood glucose response to prolonged exercise in adolescent boys with IDDM. *Diabetes Care*. 1995;18(3):326-332. PMID: 7555475

Berger M, Berchtold P, Cuppers HJ, et al. Metabolic and hormonal effects of muscular exercise in juvenile type diabetes. *Diabetologia*. 1977;13(4):355-365. PMID: 410693

Taplin CE, Cobry E, Messer L, McFann K, Chase HP, Fiallo-Scharer R. Preventing post-exercise nocturnal hypoglycemia in children with type 1 diabetes. *J Pediatr*. 2010;157(5):784-788.e1. PMID: 20650471

24 ANSWER: A) Subcutaneous asfotase alfa

Hypophosphatasia is a rare, inherited, and sometimes life-threatening metabolic disorder that arises from loss-of-function mutations in the gene that encodes the tissue nonspecific isoenzyme of alkaline phosphatase (*ALPL*). It is characterized by defective mineralization of bone and teeth in the presence of low activity of serum and bone alkaline phosphatase. More than 300 mutations have now been associated with this disorder. Because of impaired mineralization, affected patients manifest rickets, osteomalacia, fractures, early loss of both primary and secondary dentition, as well as other systemic complications such as seizures, respiratory compromise, nephrocalcinosis, myopathy, and chronic pain. Severe forms are typically inherited in an autosomal recessive manner and are associated with a high mortality rate; these cases are often diagnosed in utero or during infancy or childhood. Adults who present later in life are more likely to have dominant-negative mutations and may even be misdiagnosed as having osteoporosis. This is an often unrecognized disorder and it is important to identify because the use of bisphosphonates in these patients has been reported to precipitate fractures.

The phosphate motifs in bisphosphonates (Answer C) have a similar conformation to inorganic pyrophosphate, the natural substrate of tissue nonspecific alkaline phosphatase. Thus, treatment with bisphosphonates is thought to be analogous to "adding fuel to the fire." In adults with hypophosphatasia and osteomalacia treated with bisphosphonates, lateral subtrochanteric femoral pseudofractures have been described. Other osteoporosis medications that would suppress bone turnover or alkaline phosphatase levels such as denosumab (Answer B), raloxifene (Answer D), and calcitonin (Answer E) are also not recommended.

A low alkaline phosphatase concentration is an important surrogate marker for this disease. Additionally, serum concentrations of pyridoxal 5′-phosphate, or vitamin B_6, are elevated due to requirement of tissue nonspecific alkaline phosphatase activity in the extracellular dephosphorylation of this vitamin. This biologically active metabolite of vitamin B_6 is also a sensitive indicator of hypophosphatasia. Treatment of hypophosphatasia focuses on supportive therapy including optimizing bone health and avoiding medications that would exacerbate the disorder, physical therapy and pain management when needed, and orthopedic intervention for fractures. Recombinant enzyme replacement (Answer A) is now approved by the US FDA for patients with infantile- or juvenile-onset disease. Asfotase alfa is a therapy to treat deficient alkaline phosphatase and it thereby reduces the elevated enzyme substrate levels and improves bone mineralization. This enzyme replacement therapy is administered via subcutaneous injection. Clinical trials in patients with perinatal and infantile-onset hypophosphatasia show that treatment leads to a significant improvement in survival compared with survival in historical control patients, as well as significant radiographic improvement. The most common adverse reactions are injection-site reactions. This therapy could be considered for this patient given that she has had early loss of primary dentition and fractures at a young age; however, much less safety and effectiveness data are available for adults with this condition.

Educational Objective
Diagnose hypophosphatasia and recommend appropriate therapy for patients with symptoms that onset before age 18 years.

UpToDate Topic Review(s)
Epidemiology and etiology of osteomalacia

Reference(s)
Whyte MP, Greenberg CR, Salman NJ, et al. Enzyme-replacement therapy in life-threatening hypophosphatasia. *N Engl J Med.* 2012;366(10):904-913. PMID: 22397652

Whyte MP. Hypophosphatasia. In: Valle D, Beaudet AL, Vogelstein B, Kinzler KW, Antonarakis SE, Ballabio A, Gibson K, Mitchell G, eds. *The Online Metabolic and Molecular Bases of Inherited Disease (OMMBID).* Chap 207. New York, NY: McGraw-Hill.

25   ANSWER: D) Long-acting basal insulin once daily

Psychological insulin resistance is a term used to describe patients with diabetes mellitus who are reluctant to start insulin therapy. Psychological insulin resistance affects between 27% and 55% of patients who are insulin-naïve. Patients who are reluctant to start insulin therapy often pressure their physician to prescribe medications that may have additional risks. Patients may also, without telling their physician, alter their diet in order to avoid insulin. This change can certainly be beneficial, but in this vignette a very low-carbohydrate diet together with the addition canagliflozin was a harmful combination.

In cases of psychological insulin resistance, the clinician should ask the patient what part of the insulin injection process is difficult with the goal of providing solutions to the problems. If the difficulty is pain, a simple demonstration of an injection using a short 32-gauge needle may be sufficient to assure the patient that the injection is painless. The patient in this vignette was provided with a basal insulin pen and was shown how to use the pen with short 32-gauge needles (Answer D).

The other listed choices have safety concerns. Inhaled insulin (Answer A) is a new modality that requires baseline pulmonary function testing. Inhaled insulin also covers only prandial insulin needs. A once-weekly injectable glucagonlike peptide 1 agonist (Answer B), such as exenatide or dulaglutide, may be useful in this patient. However, the vignette provides no information regarding her β-cell function or islet-cell antibody status. If she has latent autoimmune diabetes in adults (LADA), she could relapse into ketoacidosis without insulin. The addition of acarbose (Answer E) would have a modest glucose-lowering effect and is not likely to provide additional glucose lowering in a patient already taking 3 oral diabetes medications.

Sodium-glucose cotransporter 2 inhibitors are associated with ketoacidosis, a condition called "euglycemic diabetic ketoacidosis." This patient's recent initiation of canagliflozin and the fact that she never had ketoacidosis before the current episode strongly suggest that this medication is the precipitating factor. The US FDA has included a warning about ketoacidosis in the prescribing information for canagliflozin, dapagliflozin, and empagliflozin.

Educational Objective
Guide a patient with diabetes mellitus and psychological insulin resistance regarding the best way to begin insulin therapy.

UpToDate Topic Review(s)
Insulin therapy in type 2 diabetes mellitus

Reference(s)

Polonsky WH, Jackson RA. What's so tough about taking insulin? Addressing the problem of psychological insulin resistance in type 2 diabetes. *Clinical Diabetes.* 2004;22:147-150.

Peters AL, Buschur EO, Buse JB, Cohan P, Diner JC, Hirsch IB. Euglycemic diabetic ketoacidosis: a potential complication of treatment with sodium-glucose cotransporter 2 inhibition. *Diabetes Care.* 2015;38(9):1687-1693. PMID: 26078479

26 ANSWER: A) A statin

This patient has a very low HDL-cholesterol level. Low HDL-cholesterol is currently defined as a value below 40 mg/dL (<1.04 mmol/L) in men or below 50 mg/dL (<1.30 mmol/L) in women, corresponding to approximately the 50th percentile. Clinical and epidemiologic studies have demonstrated the inverse and independent association between HDL cholesterol and the risk of coronary heart disease. Therefore, low HDL cholesterol is established as a classic independent risk factor and has become part of several multiparametric algorithms used for cardiovascular risk estimation.

HDL-cholesterol levels below 40 mg/dL (<1.04 mmol/L) are often associated with hypertriglyceridemia, obesity, insulin resistance, and diabetes. However, marked HDL-cholesterol deficiency with values below 20 mg/dL (<0.52 mmol/L) is rare and can be associated very high triglyceride levels (>500 mg/dL [5.65 mmol/L]). However, in the absence of severe hypertriglyceridemia, such low HDL-cholesterol levels are associated with perturbations in the HDL metabolic pathways, which is typically a result of impaired HDL biogenesis.

Use of anabolic steroids is commonly associated with low HDL-cholesterol levels. Additionally, a paradoxical reduction in HDL cholesterol can occur with use of fibrates (Answer B) and thiazolidinediones (eg, pioglitazone [Answer D]), either individually or when used in combination. Such reductions are idiosyncratic and typically occur in individuals with baseline HDL-cholesterol levels below 25 mg/dL (<0.65 mmol/L). Polymorphisms in 1 or more genes associated with HDL metabolism may predispose to such an effect. A sudden, dramatic decrease in HDL cholesterol is occasionally precipitated by an underlying hematologic malignancy. However, there is no evidence of such disorders in this patient.

Primary low HDL-cholesterol syndromes as part of monogenic disorders, although rare in the general population, are more frequently observed in individuals with very low HDL-cholesterol levels. Such genetic disorders occur due to mutations in the genes encoding apolipoprotein A-I (the primary protein associated with HDL), ABCA1 (the protein that allows cellular cholesterol to be taken up by apolipoprotein A-I to form HDL particles), or LCAT (the enzyme that esterifies the cholesterol so that it can move into the core of HDL).

Persons with *ABCA1* mutations (leading to Tangier disease) or *LCAT* mutations (fish-eye disease) do not develop premature cardiovascular disease. These individuals typically have characteristic clinical features that can aid in diagnosis. Individuals with *APOA1* mutations, however, are at risk for premature cardiovascular disease. Affected individuals usually have normal levels of LDL cholesterol, triglycerides, and non-HDL cholesterol but very low levels of HDL cholesterol. Similar patterns can often be detected if family members are screened. Family history of premature cardiovascular disease is also usually present (this patient, however, was adopted). It is highly likely that this patient has an *APOA1* mutation. In such patients, measured apolipoprotein A-I levels are typically low. An LDL-cholesterol value less than 70 mg/dL (<1.81 mmol/L) should be targeted, especially for secondary prevention of atherosclerotic cardiovascular disease.

In the setting of primary prevention, as in this patient, statin therapy (Answer A) should be recommended. Optimizing traditional risk factors, subclinical atherosclerosis imaging with coronary artery calcium scanning, or carotid intima-media thickness assessment may also be indicated for risk assessment. Niacin (Answer C) can raise HDL-cholesterol levels, but evidence for benefit in primary cardiovascular prevention is lacking. Prescribing no therapy (Answer E) would be inadequate.

Educational Objective
Manage the risks associated with very low HDL-cholesterol levels.

UpToDate Topic Review(s)
HDL-cholesterol: Clinical aspects of abnormal values

Reference(s)

Rader DJ, deGoma EM. Approach to the patient with extremely low HDL-cholesterol. *J Clin Endocrinol Metab.* 2012;97(10):3399-3407. PMID: 23043194

Schaefer EJ, Anthanont P, Diffenderfer MR, Polisecki E, Asztalos BF. Diagnosis and treatment of high density lipoprotein deficiency. *Prog Cardiovasc Dis.* 2016;59(2):97-106. PMID: 27565770

27 ANSWER E: Pituitary MRI

The first step in the diagnosis of Cushing syndrome is to determine whether the patient has hypercortisolism. The second step is to determine whether the hypercortisolism is ACTH dependent or independent. In ACTH-dependent hypercortisolism, ACTH is not suppressed (it may be normal or high), while in ACTH-independent hypercortisolism, ACTH is low (not necessarily unmeasurable). If the patient has ACTH-dependent hypercortisolism, the third step is to determine the source of the abnormal ACTH secretion.

This patient has an obvious diagnosis of Cushing syndrome, with a typical clinical presentation and frankly elevated 24-hour urinary free cortisol excretion (when 24-hour urinary free cortisol is more than 5 times the upper normal limit, the diagnosis is established). Her ACTH concentration is elevated, indicating that she has ACTH-dependent Cushing syndrome. At this point, no confirmatory test is needed.

In a young woman with ACTH-dependent Cushing syndrome, the most likely etiology is an ACTH-secreting pituitary adenoma (Cushing disease) (even in the presence of hypokalemia). Therefore, the most appropriate next step is pituitary MRI (Answer E). If an obvious adenoma larger than 6 mm is observed, pituitary surgery would be indicated. Although ectopic ACTH syndrome is usually associated with higher ACTH and lower potassium levels than what is observed with Cushing disease, no cutoff exists that can distinguish between the 2 syndromes.

Inferior petrosal sinus sampling (Answer A) measures the ACTH gradient between blood draining from the pituitary and the peripheral levels. This procedure is expensive and not risk-free, and it is reserved for cases in which the pituitary MRI is normal or dubious. It should also be considered in older patients who are at higher risk of ectopic ACTH secretion (eg, heavy cigarette smokers). Bedtime salivary cortisol measurement (Answer B) and the low-dose dexamethasone suppression test (Answer D) are part of the workup for Cushing syndrome, and neither is necessary in this case. The combined dexamethasone–corticotropin-releasing hormone test (Answer C) is sometimes used to distinguish between mild Cushing syndrome and pseudo-Cushing syndrome. The case presented in this vignette is not mild.

Educational Objective
Guide the diagnosis of ACTH-dependent Cushing syndrome.

UpToDate Topic Review(s)
Establishing the cause of Cushing's syndrome

Reference(s)

Nieman LK, Biller BM, Findling JW, et ak. The diagnosis of Cushing's syndrome: an Endocrine Society Clinical Practice Guideline. *J Clin Endocrinol Metab.* 2008;93(5):1526-1540. PMID: 18334580

Nieman LK, Biller BM, Findling JW, et al; Endocrine Society. Treatment of Cushing's syndrome: an Endocrine Society clinical practice guideline. *J Clin Endocrinol Metab.* 2015;100(8):2807-2831. PMID: 26222757

Findling JW, Raff H. Cushing's syndrome: important issues in diagnosis and management. *J Clin Endocrinol Metab.* 2006;91(10):3746-3753. PMID: 16868050

28 ANSWER: B) Intact PTH measurement

The workup of any patient with hypercalcemia begins with measuring intact PTH (Answer B), as this will determine whether the underlying etiology is either dependent on PTH secretion or independent of PTH. The most common cause of PTH-dependent hypercalcemia is primary hyperparathyroidism due to a parathyroid adenoma. Less common causes include multigland parathyroid hyperplasia often associated with multiple endocrine neoplasia syndrome types 1 and 2A, tertiary hyperparathyroidism in patients with chronic renal failure, or parathyroid carcinoma.

Although multiple myeloma can lead to severe hypercalcemia and renal insufficiency, serum protein electrophoresis (Answer A) would not be the best test to order next in this case because the cause of the hypercalcemia must first be determined to be PTH dependent or PTH independent.

Sestamibi scintigraphy (Answer C) is not required now because the patient needs urgent medical management; it should be considered once her condition is stabilized and the presence of a parathyroid-mediated process is established.

This patient's hypercalcemia is unlikely to be due to excessive vitamin D because her phosphate level is on the low end of the reference range. Thus, measuring 25-hydroxyvitamin D (Answer D) is incorrect.

In patients with primary hyperparathyroidism, FNAB of a mass (Answer E) to diagnose a parathyroid adenoma or cancer is not recommended due to technical difficulty in distinguishing benign from malignant processes, possible risk of tumor seeding from the needle tract, and disruption of the tumor causing histopathologic review to be hindered by atypical findings.

Although primary hyperparathyroidism due to a benign adenoma is possible in this case, the severe presentation with a palpable lower neck mass plus a markedly elevated serum calcium level, low phosphate level, renal failure, and bone pain point to the more likely diagnosis of parathyroid carcinoma, a rare cause of primary hyperparathyroidism accounting for less than 1% of cases (accounts for 0.005% of all cancers). More than 90% of parathyroid carcinomas are functional and overproduce PTH. Although findings of very elevated calcium and PTH levels are suggestive of a parathyroid carcinoma, the preoperative establishment of a malignant process is difficult unless metastases to lymph nodes or distant sites are identified. The histopathologic diagnosis of parathyroid carcinoma can also be challenging but includes the following: fibrous bands forming trabecular architecture, capsular invasion, vascular invasion, and mitotic activity in tumor cells. Loss of parafibromin staining is very specific for parathyroid carcinoma but not very sensitive because some parathyroid cancers stain for parafibromin.

The only effective curative treatment is surgery with en bloc resection of the tumor with the ipsilateral thyroid lobe and the lymph nodes in the tracheoesophageal, paratracheal, and upper mediastinal regions. For recurrent disease, management includes medical therapy for treating hypercalcemia (antiresorptive therapies or calcimimetic agent), possible further surgical resection, or radiation. No standard chemotherapy is available.

Educational Objective
Guide the appropriate workup of hypercalcemia, starting with measurement of parathyroid hormone to clarify whether the hypercalcemia is parathyroid-mediated.

UpToDate Topic Review(s)
Parathyroid carcinoma
Diagnostic approach to hypercalcemia

Reference(s)

Goswamy J, Lei M, Simo R. Parathyroid carcinoma. *Curr Opin Otolaryngol Head Neck Surg.* 2016;24(2):155-162. PMID: 26771263

Wei CH, Harari A. Parathyroid carcinoma: update and guidelines for management. *Curr Treat Options Oncol.* 2012;13(1):11-23. PMID: 22327883

29 ANSWER: D) Brain MRI

This patient presents with overt Cushing syndrome. Hypercortisolism is confirmed with a substantially elevated 24-hour urinary free cortisol. To determine the cause of the hypercortisolism, it is first important to distinguish whether the cortisol secretion is ACTH dependent or ACTH independent. The physiologic expectation is that ACTH should be entirely suppressed in the face of autonomous cortisol secretion. Therefore, the elevated ACTH in this case supports an ACTH-dependent cause of hypercortisolism, such as an ACTH-secreting pituitary adenoma or an ectopic source of ACTH (neuroendocrine tumor). These 2 entities can be challenging to distinguish, so a careful stepwise approach is advised to avoid misclassification. ACTH-secreting pituitary adenomas usually express glucocorticoid receptors and can therefore exhibit suppression to higher doses of dexamethasone, whereas neuroendocrine tumors that secrete ACTH usually do not respond to dexamethasone. The failure to suppress cortisol with 1 mg of dexamethasone suggests an ACTH-dependent pathology, but the decrease in cortisol with the higher 8-mg dose of dexamethasone increases the likelihood that this may be an ACTH-secreting adenoma. MRI of the brain with a focus on the pituitary (Answer D) could support this hypothesis by demonstrating a pituitary mass, and subsequent inferior petrosal sinus sampling could be used as confirmatory testing.

Imaging to localize the source of cortisol excess is not recommended until after the aforementioned biochemical workup, mainly to minimize detection of incidental abnormalities that may be red herrings. This patient has a known adrenal adenoma; however, a cortisol-secreting adrenal adenoma(s) or bilateral macronodular hyperplasia with cortisol secretion would typically present with suppression of ACTH and complete failure to respond to low- or high-dose dexamethasone suppression tests. Therefore, the adrenal imaging findings are unrelated to the current presentation. Adrenal venous sampling (Answer E) or abdominal CT to re-image the adrenal glands (Answer A) is not the best next step.

There is no role for imaging to search for a neuroendocrine tumor (Answers B and C) at this time because the most likely etiology is an ACTH-secreting pituitary adenoma.

Educational Objective
Develop an approach to diagnose and localize the source of hypercortisolism and determine the underlying cause of Cushing syndrome.

UpToDate Topic Review(s)
Causes and pathophysiology of Cushing's syndrome

Reference(s)
Nieman LK, Biller BM, Findling JW, et al. The diagnosis of Cushing's Syndrome: an Endocrine Society Clinical Practice Guideline. *J Clin Endocrinol Metab.* 2008;93(5):1526-1540. PMID: 18334580

Lacroix A, Feelders RA, Stratakis CA, Nieman LK. Cushing's syndrome. *Lancet.* 2015;386(9996):913-927. PMID: 26004339

30 ANSWER: B) Switch to NPH insulin at the start of tube feeds and use supplemental scale with regular insulin every 6 hours

Hyperglycemia, defined as fasting blood glucose greater than 126 mg/dL (7.0 mmol/L) or random blood glucose greater than 200 mg/dL (>11.1 mmol/L), is noted in up to 30% of hospitalized patients in the United States. A subset of these patients requires either enteral or parenteral nutrition, which makes their glycemic control worse and thereby increases the risk of hyperglycemia-related complications.

Very few data have been published on the optimal insulin regimen for enteral nutrition. A number of factors must be considered before treatment decisions are made, including the patient's medical history (eg, renal function, history of gastroparesis, ability to consistently adhere to a nutritional plan), type of formula used, and timing and duration of enteral feeding. Only 1 randomized controlled study has evaluated different insulin regimens in patients on continuous enteral tube feeds. This study compared the use of insulin glargine plus regular insulin scale with use of regular insulin scale alone. The blood glucose control in both groups was reported as equivalent; however, 48% of those on just the supplemental scale had NPH insulin added to the regimen. It appears that supplemental insulin alone is insufficient to achieve good control (thus, Answers D and E) are incorrect. Authors of the same randomized controlled trial suggest that insulin glargine may be a safe basal insulin for use with enteral nutrition. This does not, however, address the issue of nocturnal enteral nutrition. A long-acting basal insulin is likely to cause daytime hypoglycemia (thus, Answers A and C are incorrect). An intermediate-acting insulin such as NPH at the start of nocturnal enteral nutrition with regular insulin given every 6 hours based on supplemental scale (Answer B) is the best approach for this patient. The dose of NPH insulin could be 80% of previous total daily dose. Once she goes home, the supplemental insulin will have to be altered to avoid testing and treating at 2 AM.

Educational Objective
Manage hyperglycemia during nocturnal enteral feeding in hospitalized patients.

UpToDate Topic Review(s)
Management of diabetes mellitus in hospitalized patients

Reference(s)

Korytkowski MT, Salata RJ, Koerbel GL, et al. Insulin therapy and glycemic control in hospitalized patients with diabetes and enteral nutrition therapy: a randomized controlled clinical trial. *Diabetes Care.* 2009;32(4):594-596. PMID: 19336639

Gosmanov AR, Umpierrez GE. Management of hyperglycemia during enteral and parenteral nutrition therapy. *Curr Diab Rep.* 2013;13(1):155-162. PMID: 23065369

31 **ANSWER: D) Tyrosine kinase inhibitor therapy**

Radioiodine-refractory differentiated thyroid cancer is a challenging malignancy with a poor prognosis and limited treatment options. Most patients with differentiated thyroid cancer present with tumors confined to the thyroid gland with or without locoregional lymph node involvement. Most patients have disease that is sensitive to radioiodine ablation and have an excellent prognosis with 10-year survival rates greater than 92%. Up to 15% of patients have distant metastases at the time of presentation, and 6% to 20% develop metastases during follow-up. About two-thirds of patients with metastatic differentiated thyroid cancer eventually develop radioiodine-refractory disease, which has a very poor prognosis with 10-year survival rates less than 10%.

There is no consensus definition of what constitutes radioiodine-refractory disease. Current American Thyroid Association thyroid cancer guidelines suggest that refractory disease is indicated by poor avidity of tumors on radioiodine scans and disease progression despite radioactive iodine uptake in the 6 to 12 months after therapy. Poor response to radioiodine therapy is more common in patients older than 40 years and in those with large tumor burden, Hurthle-cell histology, poorly differentiated tumors, or lesions that are fluorodeoxyglucose-avid on PET. Radioiodine-refractory differentiated thyroid cancer often has an indolent phase with stable or slow tumor growth, and such patients who have minimal symptoms can be followed with watchful waiting and serial imaging.

Dramatic advances in our understanding of the mutational landscape and molecular pathways involved in the pathogenesis of differentiated thyroid cancer have resulted in the successful use of a number of targeted therapies. Clinical trials with these agents have advanced the outlook of these patients. The US FDA has approved the use of sorafenib and lenvatinib as first-line agents for the treatment of progressive differentiated thyroid cancer that is refractory to radioiodine.

Sorafenib is an orally active tyrosine kinase inhibitor with multiple targets, including BRAF, VEGFR1, and VEGFR2 (vascular endothelial growth factor receptors 1 and 2), which is used for the treatment of metastatic renal cell and hepatocellular carcinoma. The DECISION trial demonstrated improvements in median progression-free survival (10.8 months) compared with placebo (5.8 months) in patients with radioiodine-refractory locally advanced or metastatic differentiated thyroid cancer. Lenvatinib is an oral tyrosine kinase inhibitor targeting VEGFR1, 2, and 3; FGFR1, 2, 3, and 4 (fibroblast growth factor receptors 1-4); RET (rearranged during transfection); and PDGFR (platelet-derived growth factor). In the SELECT trial, lenvatinib improved median progression-free survival from 3.6 months in the placebo group to 18.3 months in the treatment group. In addition, a number of other multitargeted tyrosine kinase inhibitors that are commercially available have been recognized as viable treatment options for radioiodine-refractory differentiated thyroid cancer and trials are ongoing.

The patient in this vignette was at increased risk of developing thyroid cancer as a consequence of neck irradiation and chemotherapy for Hodgkin lymphoma. He has developed rapidly progressive radioiodine-refractory differentiated thyroid cancer that has not responded to a total ^{131}I dose of 550 mCi, and he has developed non–radioiodine-avid skeletal metastases. In view of extensive bone metastases, he needs referral to an orthopedic colleague for consideration of stabilization of his left hip. He also requires consideration of administration of radiotherapy to the lesions in his spine and ribs. In addition, initiation of tyrosine kinase inhibitor therapy (Answer D) is warranted and the administration of a further dose of radioiodine (Answer A) is unlikely to be successful.

Decreased expression and incorrect targeting of the sodium-iodide symporter to the plasma membrane have been proposed as mechanisms underlying radioiodine-refractory thyroid cancers. A number of approaches aimed to induce redifferentiation of these tumors by increasing the expression of the sodium-iodide symporter, including administration of thalidomide (Answer E), have not shown any significant effects. Traditional cytotoxic systemic chemotherapy (Answer B) has also had minimal effectiveness in patients with metastatic differentiated thyroid cancer. The administration of high-dosage glucocorticoids (Answer C) may be useful in patients with brain metastases, but it is unlikely to be helpful in this patient's management.

Educational Objective
Recommend management options for patients with advanced and rapidly progressive differentiated thyroid cancer.

UpToDate Topic Review(s)
Differentiated thyroid cancer: Overview of management

Reference(s)

Narayanan S, Colevas AD. Current standards in treatment of radioiodine refractory thyroid cancer. *Curr Treat Options Oncol.* 2016;17(6):30. PMID: 27139457

Viola D, Valerio L, Molinaro E, et al. Treatment of advanced thyroid cancer with targeted therapies: ten years of experience. *Endocr Relat Cancer.* 2016;23(4):R185-R205. PMID: 27207700

Haugen BR, Alexander EK, Bible KC, et al. 2015 American Thyroid Association Management Guidelines for Adult Patients with Thyroid Nodules and Differentiated Thyroid Cancer: The American Thyroid Association Guidelines Task Force on Thyroid Nodules and Differentiated Thyroid Cancer. *Thyroid.* 2016;26(1):1-133. PMID: 26462967

32 ANSWER: E) Human menopausal gonadotropin

The patient in the vignette has primary amenorrhea due to GnRH deficiency. Those who present with primary amenorrhea due to GnRH deficiency are referred to as having idiopathic hypogonadotropic hypogonadism or Kallmann syndrome when associated with anosmia. She is an excellent candidate for ovulation induction therapy because patients with hypogonadotropic hypogonadism have high conception rates. Both pulsatile GnRH and exogenous gonadotropin therapy with human menopausal gonadotropins (Answer E) are very effective for these patients. Virtually all women ovulate with either form of therapy and have a good chance of conception, assuming there are no other infertility factors. Human menopausal gonadotropins are highly purified urinary preparations containing both FSH and LH, which are required for normal follicular development. LH is required to stimulate the theca cells to produce androstenedione, which is then aromatized by the granulosa cells into estradiol in the presence of FSH. Pulsatile GnRH stimulates both LH and FSH in a physiologic manner, but the clinical use of pulsatile GnRH is limited by its relative lack of availability.

Recombinant FSH (Answer D), a highly purified FSH preparation, would cause proliferation of granulosa cells and follicle growth. However, in the absence of LH, there would be no androgen precursor to aromatize to estradiol, no increase in estradiol with follicle growth, and no proliferation of the endometrium, making pregnancy impossible.

Clomiphene citrate (Answer C) is occasionally effective in patients with secondary hypothalamic amenorrhea, but it is not useful in a patient with primary amenorrhea resulting from GnRH deficiency. Clomiphene is a selective estrogen receptor modulator with a hypothalamic site of action. In response to clomiphene citrate's blockade of the estrogen receptor in a patient with an intact hypothalamic-pituitary-ovarian axis, there is a compensatory increase in GnRH secretion, and LH and FSH rise. In patients with GnRH deficiency, this would not occur.

Similarly, letrozole (Answer B) would be ineffective in a patient with GnRH deficiency. Letrozole inhibits aromatase, thus decreasing estradiol. This decrease results in a compensatory increase in GnRH secretion due to lack of negative feedback, and LH and FSH also rise. In a patient with GnRH deficiency, the compensatory increase in GnRH secretion would not occur.

Hormone replacement with estradiol and progesterone (Answer A) is appropriate treatment for women with GnRH deficiency who are not interested in pregnancy. Because estradiol and progesterone do not induce ovulation, they are not considered treatment for patients interested in pregnancy.

Educational Objective
Choose the best treatment for a patient with idiopathic hypogonadotropic hypogonadism who desires pregnancy.

UpToDate Topic Review(s)
Isolated gonadotropin-releasing hormone deficiency (idiopathic hypogonadotropic hypogonadism)

Reference(s)

Shoham Z, Smith H, Yeko T, O'Brien F, Hemsey G, O'Dea L. Recombinant LH (lutropin alfa) for the treatment of hypogonadotrophic women with profound LH deficiency: a randomized, double-blind, placebo-controlled, proof-of-efficacy study. *Clin Endocrinol (Oxf)*. 2008;69(3):471-478. PMID: 18485121

Couzinet B, Lestrat N, Brailly S, Forest M, Schaison G. Stimulation of ovarian follicular maturation with pure follicle-stimulating hormone in women with gonadotropin deficiency. *J Clin Endocrinol Metab*. 1988;66(3):552-556. PMID: 3127417

33 ANSWER: E) Stop phentermine and start liraglutide, increasing the dosage as tolerated to 3 mg daily

Medical therapy for obesity is indicated in patients who, despite lifestyle modification, have a BMI greater than 30 kg/m² or those who have a BMI greater than 27 kg/m² with comorbidities such as diabetes, hypertension, or sleep apnea. Drugs used for weight management include serotonin agents, sympathomimetic medications, and medications that alter fat absorption. The choice of agent depends on several factors, including the amount of weight loss desired, presence of comorbidities, adverse effect profile, cost, and patient preference.

This man with a BMI of 38.2 kg/m² attempted lifestyle changes for 6 months without significant effect. Although continuing lifestyle modification (and intensifying these efforts) should always be encouraged, that approach alone (Answer C) may not be sufficient in this patient. He is a candidate for medical therapy and has started phentermine. He has a history of hypertension, and his blood pressure remains uncontrolled on lisinopril, 20 mg daily. Despite his weight loss on phentermine (12-lb [5.5-kg]), the drug should be discontinued because it has not been approved for long-term use as monotherapy, it has not been used long term at this dosage, the patient's persistent hypertension despite taking an ACE inhibitor is a concern, and the insomnia may be due to phentermine use. Thus, simply continuing phentermine at the same dosage (Answer A) is incorrect.

Liraglutide at a dosage of 3 mg daily (Answer E) has been shown to reduce weight by about 5.4% from baseline. Because this patient's hemoglobin A_{1c} level is elevated at 6.9% (52 mmol/mol), initiating liraglutide would address management of both obesity and type 2 diabetes. Stopping phentermine and initiating liraglutide is the best recommendation now.

The addition of a β-adrenergic blocker (Answer B) is not an ideal choice for this patient because these agents have been associated with weight gain.

This patient has a history of depression and is taking a selective serotonin reuptake inhibitor (fluoxetine). The Endocrine Society guidelines recommend caution when prescribing lorcaserin (Answer D) to patients treated with selective serotonin reuptake inhibitors. If a safer alternative is available, it should be considered.

Although not offered as an answer choice, some physicians may consider off-label, long-term use of phentermine with an increased lisinopril dosage for improved blood pressure control in this setting.

Educational Objective
Counsel patients regarding medical therapy for obesity.

UpToDate Topic Review(s)
Obesity in adults: Drug therapy

Reference(s)

Bray GA, Ryan DH. Medical therapy for the patient with obesity. *Circulation*. 2012;125(13):1695-1703. PMID: 22474312

Apovian CM, Aronne LJ, Bessesen DH, et al; Endocrine Society. Pharmacological management of obesity: an Endocrine Society clinical practice guideline. *J Clin Endocrinol Metab*. 2015;100(2):342-362. PMID: 25590212

Saunders KH, Shukla AP, Igel LI, Kumar RB, Aronne LJ. Pharmacotherapy for obesity. *Endocrinol Metab Clin North Am*. 2016;45(3):521-538. PMID: 27519128

34 ANSWER: A) Anastrozole

Men who use and abuse anabolic steroids can be challenging patients for several reasons. First, they are often highly educated on the topic and have more knowledge than the average physician. For this reason, they often dismiss the advice of the medical community or avoid the medical system. Second, these men often are not completely honest about all of the substances that they have taken or continue to take. Men who use and abuse anabolic steroids are usually aware of certain potential adverse effects. One of the most common and bothersome adverse effects is gynecomastia, which occurs because testosterone is converted into estradiol via aromatase. For this reason, many men who use and abuse anabolic steroids take an aromatase inhibitor (Answer A) with the goal of preventing gynecomastia.

Clomiphene citrate (Answer B) is a female fertility medication that is sometimes used off-label for the treatment of male hypogonadism. It would not promote significant muscle growth in a man already taking high dosages of testosterone and other anabolic steroids. Likewise, recombinant FSH (Answer C) is unlikely to further increase the testosterone levels in this case. Recombinant FSH is usually reserved to treat men with hypogonadotropic hypogonadism desiring fertility. While oxandrolone and stanozolol (Answers D and E) are other commonly used anabolic steroids, the man in this vignette is already on a combination of 3 steroids and would be more likely to increase the dosage of his regimen rather than add an additional steroid.

Physicians should use the visit with a patient who is abusing anabolic steroids as an opportunity to counsel the patient regarding serious potential medical and psychiatric adverse effects, including a very low HDL-cholesterol level, erythrocytosis, cardiac events, depression, mania, aggression, infertility, and even premature death.

Educational Objective
Recognize that men who take anabolic steroids often use an aromatase inhibitor to prevent gynecomastia.

UpToDate Topic Review(s)
Use of androgens and other hormones by athletes

Reference(s)

Kutscher EC, Lund BC, Perry PJ. Anabolic steroids: a review for the clinician. *Sports Med.* 2002;32(5):285-296. PMID: 11929356

Pope HG Jr, Katz DL. Psychiatric and medical effects of anabolic-androgenic steroid use. A controlled study of 160 athletes. *Arch Gen Psychiatry.* 1994;51(5):375-382. PMID: 8179461

35   ANSWER: B) Repeated thyroid testing after discontinuation of the patient's supplements

When there is disagreement between the clinical and biochemical assessment of a patient's thyroid status, it is often necessary for the physician to take additional history or perform additional testing to determine whether true thyroid disease exists. It is easier for the physician to recognize that thyroid testing is yielding false results when there is discordance between the TSH and thyroid hormone measurements. Examples of false elevation of serum TSH in a clinically euthyroid patient with normal free T_4 are macro-TSH, anti-animal antibodies, and heterophilic antibodies. Examples of falsely elevated free T_4 in a euthyroid patient with normal TSH include effects of nonesterified free fatty acids, heterophilic antibodies, and iodothyronine antibodies.

In addition to the effects above, which have generally been recognized for many years, a more recently recognized problem with false thyroid test results is due to the use of dietary supplements. Dietary supplements have been gaining popularity, especially with the suggestion of putative health benefits or enhancement of thyroid function that has been promoted in advertising, both online and through social media. Some dietary supplements contain thyroid hormones or thyroid extracts and can cause iatrogenic hyperthyroidism. This situation, however, is easy to recognize, as the hyperthyroidism will be reflected in the TSH and free T_4 or total T_3 results, and the patient would be expected to be symptomatic.

The patient in this vignette appears clinically euthyroid, but the TSH, free T_4, and total T_3 levels all suggest hyperthyroidism. This phenomenon has been described in the literature since at least 2012 and is due to the effects of very large doses of biotin (taken as dietary supplements). The daily requirement for biotin is 30 to 100 mcg. Typically, circulating biotin levels range from 220 to 3000 pg/mL. Over-the-counter biotin supplements are available in retail pharmacies in dosages up to 10 mg. Consumption of these dosages would greatly exceed the daily requirements. High biotin dosages can cause errors in assays that use a biotin-streptavidin signaling system. Biotin has the potential to cause great clinical confusion, as it can lead to a false-positive or false-negative result depending on whether the particular assay being used is a competitive assay or a sandwich assay. In this particular case, the false-negative effect on the TSH assay and the false-positive effect on both free T_4 and total T_3 combined to make a compelling case for the diagnosis of hyperthyroidism. In a recent case report in the literature, the use of large doses of biotin supplements caused not only low TSH, elevated free T_4, and elevated total T_3, but also falsely elevated TSH-binding inhibitory immunoglobulin, understandably leading to an erroneous diagnosis of Graves disease. All laboratory abnormalities resolved with discontinuation of biotin. Thus, the best next step to diagnose this patient's condition is to repeat thyroid testing after discontinuation of her supplements (Answer B). Biotin must be withheld for at least 2 days to prevent its impact on the various assays.

Streptavidin is a protein that binds biotin with high affinity. Because of this tight binding and its small size, biotin has been used in several different immunoassays, including assays for thyroid hormones, TSH, some steroid hormones, and PTH. Using a T_3 assay as an example, light emission from ruthenium once a ruthenium complex binds via biotin to streptavidin on the surface of an electrode is inversely proportional to the T_3 level in the serum sample being measured. The steps in the assay are as follows: (1) T_3 in the sample competes with biotinylated T_3 used in the assay for a T_3 antibody linked to ruthenium, (2) the formed ruthenium-linked T_3 antibody–biotinylated T_3 complex then binds to the streptavidin (3) there is light emission once the ruthenium complex binds to streptavidin. As the T_3 in the serum sample competes with biotinylated T_3 for the ruthenium-linked T_3 antibody, the light emission is inversely proportional to the T_3 in the sample. Excess biotin saturates the streptavidin binding sites, so that little ruthenium-linked T_3 antibody–biotinylated T_3 complex is able to bind. The decreased chemiluminescence is interpreted as high T_3 levels.

A thyroid scan and uptake (Answer C) would not point to the cause of this patient's anomalous thyroid function test results, as her thyroid function is, in fact, normal. However, it would show a normal radioiodine uptake and a normal configuration of uptake within the thyroid gland. Fecal levothyroxine measurement (Answer A) is a rarely used test that may help in the diagnosis of surreptitious levothyroxine ingestion, and it would not be useful here. Urinary iodine (Answer D) would not be helpful unless one was investigating exogenous iodine excess. A T_3 suppression test (Answer E) can be used to investigate autonomous nodules, which are not suspected here.

Educational Objective
Explain the factors that can potentially cause false results in thyroid function testing.

UpToDate Topic Review(s)
Laboratory assessment of thyroid function

Reference(s)

Barbesino G. Misdiagnosis of Graves' disease with apparent severe hyperthyroidism in a patient taking biotin megadoses. *Thyroid.* 2016;26(6):860-863. PMID: 27043844

Elston MS, Sehgal S, Du Toit S, Yarndley T, Conaglen JV. Factitious Graves' disease due to biotin immunoassay interference-a case and review of the literature. *J Clin Endocrinol Metab.* 2016;101(9):3251-3255. PMID: 27362288

Kwok JS, Chan IH, Chan MH. Biotin interference on TSH and free thyroid hormone measurement. Pathology. 2012;44(3):278-280. PMID: 22437752

Wijeratne NG, Doery JC, Lu ZX. Positive and negative interference in immunoassays following biotin ingestion: a pharmacokinetic study. *Pathology.* 2012;44(7):674-675. PMID: 23089740

36 ANSWER: A) Depression

This patient displays a multitude of symptoms suggesting that she has not yet come to terms with her diabetes diagnosis. Patients with diabetes can experience various stages of grief, similar to those experienced by a person dying. She is currently in the anger stage, as she has expressed hating her diagnosis. The next stages would be bargaining, depression, and acceptance. In addition to being angry about her diabetes diagnosis, she is most likely depressed (Answer A). It is possible that she may have a restrictive-type eating disorder (Answer B) and possibly a problem with narcotic abuse (Answer D). Diabulimia is an eating disorder that primarily affects women with type 1 diabetes. It is manifested by consciously omitting insulin in order to cause glycosuria and weight loss. However, of the choices provided, the one that most likely explains her symptoms and cause of diabetic ketoacidosis is depression. In patients with diabetes, depression is associated with poorer diet and nonadherence to diabetes medication. In patients with type 2 diabetes, minor depression is associated with a 1.7-fold increase in mortality, and major depression is associated with a 2.3-fold increase. Symptoms suggestive of depression in this patient are anger, multiple somatic symptoms, fatigue, loss of pleasure in normal activities (anhedonia), and sleep disturbance.

The clinician should ask open-ended questions that allow the patient to vent her frustrations and have her feelings validated. This will also build rapport. A useful starting statement might be something such as, "I can see that you are extremely frustrated about your diabetes." It is also important not to address the factual discrepancies in her story (eg, lack of diabetes education), as this will only cause more distress. The best next step in this patient's case is to empathize with her and to seek the help of a behavioral expert. While endocrinologists can identify depression and eating disorders, they are not trained to treat them. Effective treatment of such patients requires a team approach. In addition to working with a psychiatrist, this patient was referred for weekly visits with a diabetes nurse practitioner who had experience working with patients with depression and eating disorders.

This patient has features of the other listed diagnoses, but none of these can explain her entire symptom complex better than depression. Although she has multiple symptoms, her history does not suggest a factitious disorder (Answer C). She describes having pain "all over," but this is not sufficient to diagnose fibromyalgia (Answer E).

Educational Objective
Identify depression as an underlying cause of treatment nonadherence in patients with diabetes mellitus.

UpToDate Topic Review(s)
Overview of medical care in adults with diabetes mellitus

Reference(s)
Ciechanowski PS, Katon WJ, Russo JE. Depression and diabetes. *Arch Intern Med.* 2000;160(21):3278-3285. PMID: 11088090

Katon WJ, Rutter C, Simon G, et al. The association of comorbid depression with mortality in patient with type 2 diabetes. *Diabetes Care.* 2005;28(11):2668-2672. PMID: 16249537

Young-Hyman D, de Groot M, Hill-Briggs F, Gonzalez JS, Hood K, Peyrot M. Psychosocial care for people with diabetes mellitus: a position statement of the American Diabetes Association. *Diabetes Care.* 2016;39(12):2126-2140. PMID: 27879358

37 ANSWER: A) Alprostadil (intracavernosal injection)

Various types and modalities of medical therapy are available for the treatment of erectile dysfunction. They all act to cause smooth-muscle relaxation by lowering calcium concentrations. A major pathway of penile erection involves the important neurotransmitter nitric oxide, which raises intracellular cyclic guanosine monophosphate (GMP) that activates a specific protein kinase. Phosphodiesterase 5 inhibitors work by blocking the hydrolysis of cyclic GMP to GMP. Another pathway involves prostaglandin E_1, which increases cyclic AMP that activates a different protein kinase.

In general, the phosphodiesterase 5 inhibitors (sildenafil, vardenafil, tadalafil, etc) have been considered first-line therapy for the management of most men with erectile dysfunction because of their effectiveness, ease of administration (oral), and lack of serious adverse effects.

This man's worsening erectile function over time is most likely related to aging, vascular disease, and the effects of longstanding diabetes. A man who is no longer responding to a high dosage of a phosphodiesterase 5 inhibitor is unlikely to dramatically respond to a different medication in this class (Answer C), as their mechanism of action is very similar. One of the most effective second-line treatments is intracavernosal injections of alprostadil (Answer A), which is a synthetic form of prostaglandin E_1. This treatment has few systemic adverse effects as it is administered locally. Nonetheless, men who use it may experience painful erections, priapism, and/or fibrosis. The first injection should be administered by medical personnel to determine the man's response to the medication and to choose an appropriate dose to minimize the risk of adverse effects. Alprostadil can also be administered via a pellet inserted into the distal tip of the urethra. This modality is less effective than the intracavernosal route and may result in urethral bleeding, penile pain, and priapism.

Papaverine (Answer B) is a nonspecific phosphodiesterase inhibitor that is less effective and less commonly used than the second-line therapy already mentioned. Testosterone therapy (Answer D) should only be considered if this man had at least 2 documented low testosterone values. It should be noted that men with normal testosterone levels tend to have a greater response to phosphodiesterase 5 inhibitors than hypogonadal men. In addition, this patient's normal libido makes androgen deficiency unlikely. A vacuum constriction device (Answer E) is not the best answer as it is less effective than intracavernosal injections. A vacuum constriction device consists of a vacuum chamber or cylinder, a pump, and a constriction ring. Once the penis becomes engorged through negative pressure via the pump, a constriction band at the base of the penis prevents blood from leaving to maintain an erection. Potential adverse effects include petechiae and bruising of the penis.

Educational Objective

Identify effective treatments for erectile dysfunction in men who do not respond to phosphodiesterase 5 inhibitors.

UpToDate Topic Review(s)

Treatment of male sexual dysfunction

Reference(s)

Goldfischer ER, Kim ED, Seftel AD, Baygani SK, Burns PR. Impact of low testosterone on response to treatment with tadalafil 5 mg once daily for erectile dysfunction. *Urology*. 2014;83(6):1326-1333. PMID: 24726311.

Lue TF. Erectile dysfunction. *N Engl J Med*. 2000;342(24):1802-1813. PMID: 10853004

McMahon CG. Erectile dysfunction. *Intern Med J*. 2014;44(1):18-26. PMID: 24450519

38 ANSWER: B) Primary polydipsia

When a patient reports frequent urination, one must first rule out that it is not just frequency. This is done by history (amount of fluid the patient drinks) or by measuring the 24-hour urine volume. If polydipsia and polyuria are confirmed (in this case the patient volunteered the high amount of fluid intake and urination), the differential diagnosis must start by excluding osmotic polyuria such as hyperglycemia or hypercalcemia.

This patient has polyuria, a normal calcium level, and an only mildly elevated glucose level. Therefore, his polyuria is not osmotic. He could have either a form of diabetes insipidus (neurogenic or nephrogenic) or primary polydipsia. He is unable to determine when the problem started. In general, patients with diabetes insipidus are able to remember quite precisely when their problem began. More importantly, patients with diabetes insipidus have either high or normal serum osmolality, as they do not overcompensate to bring osmolality into the low range. This patient has somewhat low sodium and serum osmolality, suggesting primary polydipsia. Serum dilution is also suggested by the low uric acid. On the basis of these findings, this patient is unlikely to have diabetes insipidus (either nephrogenic or central [Answers A and C]). He more likely has primary (psychogenic) polydipsia (Answer B). The differential diagnosis is extremely important, as treatment of primary polydipsia with desmopressin would pose great risk of hyponatremia.

Syndrome of inappropriate antidiuretic hormone secretion (Answer D) causes low serum sodium, but it does not manifest as polyuria and polydipsia. The degree of this patient's hyperglycemia (Answer E) is mild and unlikely to cause significant polyuria, as demonstrated by negative glycosuria.

Educational Objective

Distinguish diabetes insipidus from primary polydipsia.

UpToDate Topic Review(s)

Diagnosis of polyuria and diabetes insipidus

Reference(s)

Robertson GL. Diabetes insipidus: differential diagnosis and management. *Best Pract Res Clin Endocrinol Metab*. 2016;30(2):205-218. PMID: 27156759

Wong LL, Verbalis JG. Systemic diseases associated with disorders of water homeostasis. *Endocrinol Metab Clin North Am*. 2002;31(1):121-140. PMID: 12055984

Verbalis JG. Disorders of water metabolism: diabetes insipidus and the syndrome of inappropriate antidiuretic hormone secretion. *Handb Clin Neurol*. 2014;124:37-52. PMID: 25248578

39 ANSWER: A) Evolocumab

On the basis of this patient's clinical features and laboratory values, he has familial hypercholesterolemia (FH), a genetic disorder characterized by very high blood LDL-cholesterol levels. FH is an autosomal dominant disorder caused by mutations in the genes involved in LDL-receptor–mediated cholesterol uptake pathways. The severity of the phenotype depends on residual LDL-receptor activity. FH homozygotes or compound heterozygotes (individuals with 2 mutated *LDLR* alleles) are more severely affected than heterozygotes. The mode of inheritance in this patient is unclear as he was adopted.

A pathognomonic clinical finding in FH, as observed in this patient, is the presence of tendon xanthomas on the extensor tendons of the hands or in the Achilles tendons; such xanthomas can also occur in the triceps and patellar tendons. However, absence of tendon xanthomas does not rule out FH. Secondary causes of hypercholesterolemia, commonly hypothyroidism and renal disease, should be considered and are excluded based on the laboratory test results provided. FH is diagnosed on the basis of clinical findings (if present), family history, and lipid levels. Genetic testing is not widely used for diagnosis in the United States, in part because of cost and lack of insurance coverage.

Treatment of FH involves starting lipid-lowering therapy as early as possible given the increased lifetime risk of premature cardiovascular disease. All patients should be educated about lifestyle management. LDL-cholesterol lowering using statins is first-line therapy, with a goal of at least 50% reduction in LDL-cholesterol levels. Response to statins varies widely in patients with FH and depends on several factors, including residual LDL-receptor activity associated with each genetic variant. Statins increase the functional activity of residual LDL receptors. When LDL-cholesterol–lowering targets cannot be reached by statins alone, other drug therapies should be considered.

Evolocumab (Answer A) is a proprotein convertase subtilisin/kexin type 9 (PCSK9) inhibitor antibody that is currently available for treatment of FH. PCSK9 is a serine protease that is secreted by the liver and targets the LDL receptor for degradation. Thus, the higher the plasma levels of PCSK9, the lower the number of LDL receptors and vice versa. Monoclonal antibodies such as evolocumab and alirocumab bind to PCSK9 and prevent LDL-receptor degradation, leading to more available LDL receptors and therefore lower LDL-cholesterol levels in the blood. When a PCSK9 inhibitor is added to high-intensity statin therapy, up to 100% of the PCSK9 is bound by the antibody, resulting in a 50% reduction in LDL cholesterol. A recent randomized controlled trial of evolocumab vs placebo in individuals with known atherosclerotic cardiovascular disease receiving statin therapy showed a marked reduction in LDL-cholesterol levels and a reduction in cardiovascular risk with the addition of evolocumab. However, the role of PCSK9 inhibition in primary prevention is not known. Nevertheless, this patient should be offered PCSK9 inhibitor therapy due to his markedly elevated LDL-cholesterol levels and genetic hypercholesterolemia. Risk for premature cardiovascular disease is very high. Ezetimibe, niacin, and bile acid sequestrants can all lower LDL-cholesterol levels and work in combination with statins, but their relative effectiveness is lower than that of evolocumab.

Niacin (Answer B), a water-soluble B vitamin, lowers LDL cholesterol and raises HDL cholesterol. Addition of niacin can decrease LDL cholesterol up to 25%. However, in this patient, niacin would not provide sufficient LDL-cholesterol lowering.

Bile acid sequestrants (Answer C) bind to bile salts within the intestinal lumen, preventing their enterohepatic reuptake. This signals further bile salt production, which decreases intracellular cholesterol and up-regulates hepatic LDL receptors. This, in turn, causes increased clearance of circulating LDL cholesterol, levels of which decrease by 10% to 20%. Addition of colesevelam to this patient's regimen would not provide significant LDL-cholesterol lowering.

Fenofibrate (Answer D) is a selective peroxisome proliferator-activated receptor α agonist that lowers triglyceride levels with very modest LDL-cholesterol lowering. In this individual with normal triglyceride levels, there is no indication for fibrate therapy.Lipoprotein apheresis (Answer E) is an extracorporeal method of removing apolipoprotein B–containing lipoproteins from the circulation. Apheresis can improve endothelial function, atherosclerosis, and clinical outcomes, but it is time consuming and expensive, comparable to hemodialysis. Criteria for lipoprotein apheresis in patients receiving maximally tolerated lipid-lowering therapy include an LDL-cholesterol level greater than 500 mg/dL (>12.95 mmol/L) in patients with homozygous FH; an LDL-cholesterol level greater than 300 mg/dL (>7.77 mmol/L) in patients with heterozygous FH; and an LDL-cholesterol level greater than 200 mg/dL (>5.18 mmol/L) in patients with heterozygous FH and atherosclerotic cardiovascular disease. Treatments are given every 1 to 2 weeks and each session takes 3 to 4 hours. However, newer available therapies have reduced the need for apheresis.

Educational Objective
Recommend appropriate management of heterozygous familial hypercholesterolemia.

UpToDate Topic Review(s)
Inherited disorders of LDL-cholesterol metabolism

Reference(s)

Sabatine MS, Giugliano RP, Keech AC, et al; FOURIER Steering Committee and Investigators. Evolocumab and clinical outcomes in patients with cardiovascular disease. *N Engl J Med.* 2017;376(18):1713-1722. PMID: 28304224

Cartier JL, Goldberg AC. Familial hypercholesterolemia: advances in recognition and therapy. *Prog Cardiovasc Dis.* 2016;59(2):125-134. PMID: 27477957

Santos RD, Gidding SS, Hegele RA, et al; International Atherosclerosis Society Severe Familial Hypercholesterolemia Panel. Defining severe familial hypercholesterolaemia and the implications for clinical management: a consensus statement from the International Atherosclerosis Society Severe Familial Hypercholesterolemia Panel. *Lancet Diabetes Endocrinol.* 2016;4(10):850-861. PMID: 27246162

40 ANSWER: A) Ketoconazole

This patient recently started high-dosage ketoconazole (Answer A) as part of his prostate cancer treatment. Ketoconazole is an antifungal agent that binds to cytochrome P450 and inhibits the renal synthesis of 1α-hydroxylase. This drug has been shown to lower serum 1,25-dihydroxyvitamin D levels in healthy patients and in patients with primary hyperparathyroidism. Ketoconazole is used as a second-line treatment for patients with granulomatous disease such as sarcoid whose condition is refractory to prednisone to decrease calcium levels by reducing calcitriol production. The use of this agent is limited by its renal toxicity. Of note, ketoconazole is also used in the treatment of Cushing disease because of its effects on steroid synthesis by inhibiting cytochrome P450 enzymes and significantly reducing cortisol levels.

Prostate cancer frequently metastasizes to bone, and bone metastases are present in nearly all patients with advanced prostate cancer. Metastatic bone disease is generally divided into osteoblastic and osteolytic disease, but most cancers lie within a spectrum of these two extremes. Osteolytic metastases (Answer B) are much more common, however, and are one of the most feared complications of malignancy. They are usually destructive and are much more likely to be associated with pathologic fracture and hypercalcemia (not hypocalcemia). Hypercalcemia occurs when bone destruction is advanced. The bone metastases observed in prostate cancer are primarily osteoblastic, but there is a significant osteolytic component that is mediated by osteoclasts. Hypercalcemia occurs more commonly in patients with osteolytic metastases than in patients with osteoblastic metastases.

Hypercalcemia, not hypocalcemia, can occasionally occur in patients with adrenal insufficiency (Answer C). The mechanisms that contribute to hypercalcemia from adrenal insufficiency include increased bone resorption, volume contraction, and increased proximal tubular calcium reabsorption along with binding of calcium to serum proteins. Cortisol administration corrects the hypercalcemia.

Hypomagnesemia (Answer D) can contribute to low calcium levels; however, this patient was noted to have a normal magnesium level. Magnesium deficiency is common in critically ill patients. Magnesium is an essential cation that has a role in several physiologic processes in the body. Critically low magnesium levels can cause resistance to PTH, diminished PTH release, and subsequent hypocalcemia. Thiazide diuretics (Answer E) can raise, not lower, serum calcium levels by lowering urinary calcium excretion. This propensity for hypercalcemia is pronounced in patients with an underlying increase in bone resorption, such as those with hyperparathyroidism.

Educational Objective

Identify a high ketoconazole dosage as a contributor to hypocalcemia due to the suppression of 1α-hydroxylase, which prevents activation of vitamin D.

UpToDate Topic Review(s)

Etiology of hypocalcemia in adults

Reference(s)

Conron M, Beynon HL. Ketoconazole for the treatment of refractory hypercalcemic sarcoidosis. *Sarcoidosis Vasc Diffuse Lung Dis.* 2000;17(3):277-280. PMID: 11033844.

Hannan FM, Thakker RV. Investigating hypocalcaemia. *BMJ.* 2013;346:f2213. PMID: 23661111

41 ANSWER: E) No further treatment

The synthesis and secretion of the thyroid hormones T_4 and T_3 from follicular cells of the thyroid gland are under direct control of TSH, which is released from the anterior pituitary thyrotrope cells under the control of thyrotropin-releasing hormone. Intracellular thyroid hormone levels are regulated by transporter proteins that facilitate their transport across the cell membrane and by the 3 deiodinating enzymes. Thyroid hormone signaling is predominantly mediated through binding of the bioactive hormone T_3 to the nuclear T_3 receptors. Defects at the level of the thyroid hormone receptors, deiodinases, and transporter proteins result in resistance to thyroid hormone syndromes.

Two genes, *THRA* and *THRB*, encode the thyroid hormone receptors. There are 3 α and 3 β receptor isoforms. All β receptor isoforms (β1, β2, and β3) and the α1 isoform have significant thyroid hormone binding. Thyroid hormone is typically found in a heterodimer with the retinoid X receptor. In the absence of thyroid hormones, the receptors and corepressors bind to the thyroid hormone response elements, thus suppressing transcription. When thyroid hormone binds the thyroid hormone receptor, the corepressors are displaced and coactivators bind, thereby activating the transcriptional effects of thyroid hormone. The intracellular effect of thyroid hormone is at least in part an effect of the tissue distribution of each thyroid hormone receptor.

Mutations in the *THRB* gene represent the first identified and most common cause of resistance to thyroid hormone. It has an estimated prevalence of 1 in 40,000 to 50,000 live births. The typical inheritance pattern is autosomal dominant with the mutant thyroid hormone receptor suppressing the action of the wild-type receptor. More recently, however, some families have been identified with an autosomal recessive inheritance pattern. The symptoms of individuals with *THRB* gene mutations are variable other than presence of a goiter, which is reported in 66% to 95% of cases. Most affected individuals are otherwise asymptomatic, while some have a mixed pattern of clinical features of hypothyroidism and hyperthyroidism because of the continued action of the thyroid hormone receptor α. Most mutations are found in exons 9 and 10, and the clinical phenotype can vary widely even in individuals with the same mutations.

The typical biochemical pattern in patients with a *THRB* mutation is elevated free T_4 and/or free T_3 concentrations in the presence of a nonsuppressed serum TSH level, which often leads to diagnostic confusion. When discordant biochemical findings are present, potential confounding factors should first be considered, including alterations in normal physiology (eg, pregnancy), intercurrent illness (nonthyroidal), and medication usage (eg, levothyroxine, amiodarone, heparin). Once these have been excluded, laboratory artifacts in commonly used TSH or thyroid hormone immunoassays, as well as the presence of heterophilic antibodies and familial dysalbuminemic hyperthyroxinemia, should be screened for, thus avoiding unnecessary further investigation and/or treatment in cases where there is assay interference. Following exclusion of these diagnoses, the main challenge is to make a distinction between a TSH-secreting pituitary adenoma and a loss-of-function mutation in the *THRB* gene. Useful diagnostic tests in this respect are assessment of the α subunit to TSH molar ratio, measurement of the sex hormone–binding globulin concentration, and dynamic testing with measurement of tissue biomarkers and the TSH responsiveness to thyrotropin-releasing hormone, before and after administration of liothyronine (the "T_3 suppression test").

In most patients, the increased endogenous thyroid hormone levels provide adequate compensation for the reduced thyroid hormone sensitivity in the *THRB*-expressing tissues and, thus, treatment is not needed. This patient is asymptomatic, so no further treatment is needed now (Answer E). In contrast, some patients have persistent symptoms such as tachycardia and atrial fibrillation due to apparent thyroid hormone excess in *THRA*-expressing tissues. Symptomatic treatment, such as β-adrenergic blockers for tachycardia, can alleviate these symptoms. The main objective in the treatment of resistance to thyroid hormone is to maintain an acceptable balance between overstimulation of *THRA*-expressing tissues and understimulation of the *THRB*-expressing tissues. The ideal treatment should therefore aim to selectively potentiate T_3 action in the *THRB*-expressing tissues, while keeping the *THRA*-expressing tissues euthyroid. In patients with cardiac decompensation, the use of combined treatment with 3,3′,5-triiodothyroacetic acid (TRIAC) and antithyroid drugs has been successful.

The use of conventional antithyroid drug treatment alone (Answer A) or in combination with levothyroxine (Answer B) induces a decrease in thyroid hormone and a compensatory exaggerated TSH rise, thereby rendering therapy less effective and promoting goiter formation. Goiter usually recurs after thyroidectomy (Answer C) and radioiodine treatment (Answer D), and these are relatively ineffective treatments. Furthermore, levothyroxine replacement following surgery and radioiodine must be administered in supraphysiologic dosages to keep TSH concentrations relatively low, thereby preventing pituitary thyrotroph hyperplasia.

Educational Objective
Recommend management of syndromes of resistance to thyroid hormone.

UpToDate Topic Review(s)
Impaired sensitivity to thyroid hormone

Reference(s)

Groeneweg S, Peeters RP, Visser TJ, Visser WE. Therapeutic applications of thyroid hormone analogues in resistance to thyroid hormone (RTH) syndromes. *Mol Cell Endocrinol.* 2017;pii:S0303-7207(17)30116-30118. PMID: 28235578

Koulouri O, Moran C, Halsall D, Chatterjee K, Gurnell M. Pitfalls in the measurement and interpretation of thyroid function tests. *Best Pract Res Clin Endocrinol Metab.* 2013;27(6):745-762. PMID: 24275187

Dumitrescu AM, Refetoff S. The syndromes of reduced sensitivity to thyroid hormone. *Biochim Biophys Acta.* 2013;1830(7):3987-4003. PMID: 22986150

42 ANSWER: E) Recommend a retinal examination

Pregestational diabetes affects about 2% of all pregnancies and accounts for 15% to 20% of diabetes in pregnancy. The goals of preconception counseling are to optimize glycemic control, diabetes management, optimize management of comorbidities such as hypertension, and manage diabetes-related complications. The purpose of these efforts is to reduce the risk of adverse maternal and fetal outcomes, including congenital malformations, macrosomia in the infant, pregnancy-related complications such as preeclampsia, and progression of microvascular complications in the mother.

Hyperglycemia in pregnancy is a risk factor for progression of microvascular complications, including retinopathy. The recommendation is to identify women with retinopathy before conception, initiate therapy as needed, and follow closely during pregnancy. This young woman should have a retinal examination (Answer E). The in-office nondilated retinal examination is not sufficient for this assessment.

Although pregnancy does not result in new-onset diabetic nephropathy, it can lead to progression of preexisting nephropathy. Risks factors are poorly controlled hypertension, reduced glomerular filtration rate, creatinine concentration greater than 1.5 mg/dL (>132.6 µmol/L), and clinically significant proteinuria (>3 g/24 h). On the basis of this patient's laboratory test results, she does not require protein assessment in a 24-hour urine collection (Answer D).

If a woman is already on insulin pump therapy in the pregestational period, pump use can be continued in pregnancy. However, starting insulin pump therapy as this patient considers pregnancy (Answer A) is not necessary for optimal glycemic management.

The prepregnancy blood pressure goal is 130/80 mm Hg; if the patient has persistently elevated blood pressure, she should be treated with antihypertensive medication acceptable in pregnancy. Labetalol (Answer B) is a pregnancy category C drug, and other agents such as diltiazem, prazosin, or methyldopa would be recommended over labetalol. However, on the basis of her current blood pressure (132/66 mm Hg) treatment is not indicated now.

Patients with type 1 diabetes should be screened for thyroid dysfunction at a preconception counseling visit. If either overt hypothyroidism or subclinical hypothyroidism is documented, levothyroxine replacement should be initiated. The goal TSH value in the first trimester is less than 2.5 mIU/L. This patient's TSH level is normal, so initiating levothyroxine (Answer C) is incorrect.

Educational Objective
Instruct women with type 1 diabetes mellitus regarding preconception planning.

UpToDate Topic Review(s)
Pregestational diabetes: Preconception counseling, evaluation, and management

Reference(s)

American Diabetes Association. Preconception care of women with diabetes. *Diabetes Care.* 2004;27(Suppl 1):S76-S78. PMID: 14693933

Tripathi A, Rankin J, Aarvold J, Chandler C, Bell R. Preconception counseling in women with diabetes: a population-based study in the north of England. *Diabetes Care.* 2010;33(3):586-588. PMID: 20040652

43 ANSWER: E) Cortisol

This patient's presentation is consistent with excess mineralocorticoid activity (severe hypertension, hypokalemia). While this typically raises the concern of excess aldosterone stimulating the mineralocorticoid receptor, it is important to remember that cortisol is also a mineralocorticoid receptor agonist and circulates at a concentration 100- to 1000-fold higher than that of aldosterone. Cortisol (Answer E) is inactivated to cortisone by 11β-hydroxysteroid dehydrogenase 2, which is highly expressed in the kidney and is the reason why aldosterone maintains a high affinity for the mineralocorticoid receptor in this location (*see image*). Glycyrrhizic acid in licorice inhibits this enzyme. In this patient's case, licorice ingestion has prevented the inactivation of cortisol, resulting in massive activation of the mineralocorticoid receptor by cortisol.

The laboratory results reflect suppression of the renin-angiotensin-aldosterone system due to the alternative mineralocorticoid receptor activation. Therefore, the renin-angiotensin-aldosterone system (Answer C) is not contributing to this patient's hypertension or hypokalemia. Mineralocorticoids such as 11-deoxycortisol and deoxycorticosterone are also not contributing to this patient's hypertension because the mechanism does not involve excess secretion of endogenous mineralocorticoids, but rather the inhibition of cortisol inactivation. Although ACTH (Answer D) physiologically stimulates cortisol synthesis, the presentation in this vignette does not require hypercortisolism; even "normal" cortisol levels may induce such a presentation when 11β-hydroxysteroid dehydrogenase 2 is inhibited.

Educational Objective
Explain the mechanism by which glycyrrhizic acid suppresses the renin-angiotensin-aldosterone system due to alternative mineralocorticoid receptor activation.

UpToDate Topic Review(s)
Apparent mineralocorticoid excess syndromes (including chronic licorice ingestion)

Reference(s)
Qunikler M, Stewart PM. Hypertension and the cortisol-cortisone shuttle. *J Clin Endocrinol Metab*. 2003;88(6):2384-2392. PMID: 12788832

Morineau G, Sulmont V, Salomon R, et al. Apparent mineralocorticoid excess: report of six new cases and extensive personal experience. *J Am Soc Nephrol*. 2006;17(11):3176-3184. PMID: 17035606

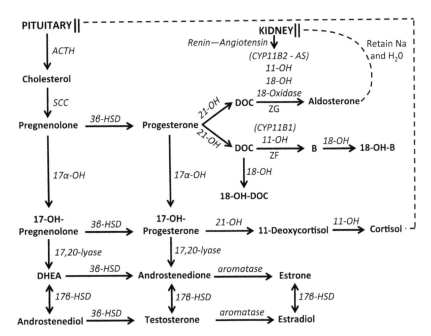

Abbreviations: ACTH, corticotropin; DOC, deoxycorticosterone; SCC, side-chain cleavage enzyme; 11-OH, 11-hydroxylase; 17α-OH, 17α-hydroxylase; 18-OH, 18-hydroxylase; 3β-HSD, 3β-hydroxysteroid dehydrogenase; 17β-HDS, 17β-hydroxysteroid dehydrogenase

44 ANSWER: D) Measure TSH and free T₄

In evaluating pituitary enlargement, one must include pituitary hyperplasia in the differential diagnosis (even if the radiology report does not mention it), particularly if the MRI does not show a discrete adenoma. Such hyperplasia may be physiologic, as seen in young peripubertal girls or boys or in some perimenopausal women, or pathologic, as seen rarely in patients with acromegaly who have GHRH-secreting tumors. This patient does not have an adenoma, but has diffuse pituitary enlargement due to thyrotroph-cell hyperplasia in the setting of severe and most likely longstanding primary hypothyroidism. In this situation, the low thyroid hormone level causes an increase in hypothalamic release of thyrotropin-releasing hormone. This in turn causes an increase in serum TSH and thyrotroph-cell hyperplasia, as well as hyperprolactinemia (because thyrotropin-releasing hormone is also a strong prolactin-releasing factor). The pituitary hyperplasia and the hyperprolactinemia usually resolve in time when euthyroidism is restored with thyroid hormone replacement therapy. No treatment for hyperprolactinemia is needed in these cases. Thus, the best next step in this patient's evaluation is measurement of TSH and free T_4 (Answer D).

IGF-1 measurement (Answer A) would not be useful, as she has no signs or symptoms of acromegaly. Neurosurgical evaluation (Answer B) is not needed, as the pituitary enlargement is typically reversible once TSH normalizes with thyroid hormone replacement therapy. She has no signs or symptoms of adrenal insufficiency, so an ACTH stimulation test (Answer C) is not needed. Neuro-ophthalmologic consultation (Answer E) is not needed given the lack of chiasmatic compression.

Educational Objective
Diagnose thyrotroph hyperplasia and hyperprolactinemia in the setting of primary hypothyroidism.

UpToDate Topic Review(s)
Clinical manifestations of hypothyroidism

Reference(s)

Lee CL, Salvatori R. Visual vignette. Thyrotroph cell hyperplasia. *Endocr Pract*. 2012;18(3):429. PMID: 22592055

Ozbey N, Sariyildiz E, Yilmaz L, Orhan Y, Sencer E, Molvalilar S. Primary hypothyroidism with hyperprolactinaemia and pituitary enlargement mimicking a pituitary macroadenoma. *Int J Clin Pract*. 1997;51(6):409-411. PMID: 9489077

Bhansali A, Sreenivasulu P, Khandelwal N, Masoodi SR. Reversibility of thyrotroph hyperplasia after L-thyroxine replacement therapy in patients with juvenile primary hypothyroidism. *J Pediatr Endocrinol Metab*. 2004;17(4):655-661. PMID: 15198297

Wong AP, Pipitone J, Park MT, et al. Estimating volumes of the pituitary gland from T1-weighted magnetic-resonance images: effects of age, puberty, testosterone, and estradiol. *Neuroimage*. 2014;94:216-221. PMID: 24632090

45 ANSWER: C) Abdominal CT
This case highlights the need to further investigate the cause of deteriorating glucose control in an otherwise healthy elderly patient. The rapid deterioration in her glucose control should raise a flag that something other than nonadherence is at play. Although the patient may have had recent loss of β-cell function, a sudden loss of β-cell function after 20 years of diabetes is unusual. The unexplained weight loss is also an indicator that further testing should be done to assess for possible malignancy.

Various cancers are associated with diabetes. Of these, pancreatic cancer is strongly associated with recent-onset diabetes. In a case-control study, Pannala et al compared the prevalence of diabetes in a cohort of 512 patients with newly diagnosed pancreatic cancer with the prevalence of diabetes in a cohort of age-matched patients without pancreatic cancer. Diabetes was documented in 47% of the patients with pancreatic cancer vs in 7% of age-matched control patients. The patients with pancreatic cancer–associated diabetes tended to have higher fasting blood glucose levels than control patients. Sixty percent of the patients with pancreatic cancer had new-onset diabetes.

Damiano et al prospectively studied 116 patients with new-onset, insulin-dependent diabetes who were 50 years or older with CT imaging of the pancreas. Six patients (5%) had pancreatic adenocarcinoma. Screening CT is not recommended for patients with new-onset diabetes or deterioration of diabetes control. However, given this patient's history of excellent adherence to her regimen and her recent weight loss, the clinician should consider the possibility that her deteriorating diabetes control is secondary to new disease. Abdominal CT (Answer C) is the best next test.

Mammography (Answer A) and a chest CT (Answer D) would identify breast and lung cancer, respectively, but these conditions are not commonly associated with exacerbation of diabetes. A whole-body PET/CT (Answer B), although an excellent test, is not considered the first step in screening for malignancy due to the high expense. Colonoscopy (Answer E) would detect colorectal cancer, which is also not associated with new-onset diabetes or exacerbation of diabetes.

Educational Objective
Investigate the cause of rapidly deteriorating glucose control in an otherwise healthy patient, considering the possibility of malignancy.

UpToDate Topic Review(s)
Clinical manifestations, diagnosis, and staging of exocrine pancreatic cancer

Reference(s)

Cohen DH, LeRoith D. Obesity, type 2 diabetes, and cancer: the insulin and IGF connection. *Endocr Relat Cancer.* 2012;19(5):F27-F47. PMID: 22593429

Pannala R, Leirness JB, Bamlet WR, Basu A, Petersen GM, Chari ST. Prevalence and clinical profile of pancreatic center-associated diabetes mellitus. *Gastroenterology.* 2008;124(4):981-987. PMID: 18395079

Everhart J, Wright D. Diabetes mellitus as a risk factor for pancreatic cancer. A meta-analysis. *JAMA.* 1995;273(20):1605-1609. PMID: 7745774

Teich N. Pancreatic cancer: cause and result of diabetes mellitus. *Gastroenterology.* 2008;134(1):344-345. PMID: 18166361

Damiano J, Bordier L, Le Berre JP, et al. Should pancreas imaging be recommended in patients over 50 years when diabetes is discovered because of acute symptoms? *Diabetes Metab.* 2004;30(2):203-207. PMID: 15223996

46 ANSWER: D) Consumption of bovine thyroid tissue

The patient described in this vignette has hyperthyroidism that is accompanied by both low uptake on a radioactive iodine uptake and scan and also by a low serum thyroglobulin level. These findings exclude endogenous forms of hyperthyroidism such as Graves disease and toxic or hyperfunctioning nodules. Her thyroid examination with the absence of a goiter or palpable nodules is also not suggestive of these diagnoses. An excessive iodine load (Answer A) could potentially cause hyperthyroidism with low uptake on scanning with ^{123}I, but the thyroid examination would be expected to show a goiter or thyroid nodules, which would be consistent with the hyperfunctioning thyroid tissue that was using iodine to make unregulated high levels of thyroid hormone. Serum thyroglobulin would not be expected to be low in a case of exposure to high iodine levels. Sources of exogenous iodine exposure include kelp, medications such as amiodarone, and contrast dye. Iodine-contaminated wells have not been reported as a cause of hyperthyroidism, although water sources at President George H. W. Bush's residences were reportedly tested for iodine after he, his wife, and their dog all developed hyperthyroidism.

The potential causes of hyperthyroidism in an individual with high serum free T_4 levels and low iodine uptake within the thyroid gland include ingestion of thyroid hormone, thyroiditis, and ectopic production of thyroid hormone from a site outside the thyroid gland. Examples of ectopic production of thyroid hormone include struma ovarii and functioning thyroid cancer metastases. These would not be likely diagnoses, as the patient's current episode of hyperthyroidism resolved spontaneously, as did previous similar episodes. There are reports of individuals who have had repeated episodes of viral or silent thyroiditis. However, thyroiditis of any cause is unlikely given the finding of a low serum thyroglobulin. Viral thyroiditis (Answer B) is typically characterized by a tender thyroid gland, and both viral and silent thyroiditis would be expected to be accompanied by an elevated serum thyroglobulin.

A number of chemicals (Answer C) disrupt thyroid gland function. Investigated chemicals include polychlorinated biphenyls, polybrominated diethyl ethers, phthalates, pesticides, and perchlorate. However, the signature of exposure to such chemicals is reduced circulating levels of thyroid hormone, not elevated levels. Consumption of goitrogen-containing vegetables (Answer E) would also be expected to be associated with development of hypothyroidism, not hyperthyroidism. Vegetables such as cabbage and cassava are broken down into products such as thiocyanates, which inhibit iodine uptake into the thyroid gland, thus causing hypothyroidism when taken in very large amounts.

Because thyroid hormones are active when taken orally, contamination of meat with thyroid tissue can cause hyperthyroidism. Such contamination can occur when meat from the neck of slaughtered animals is used in meat products, typically hamburger or sausage. Episodes of "hamburger thyrotoxicosis" have been described following the consumption of thyroid gland–contaminated meat (Answer D). A classic case series of outbreaks of thyrotoxicosis in Minnesota and South Dakota were linked to contaminated meat. The harvesting of meat from the neck region, known as "gullet trimming," has been banned in the United States. Thyrotoxicosis has also been described in deer hunters who unknowingly include thyroid tissue in their venison preparations such as ground venison. The case described in this vignette is similar to a case described in the literature in which an individual living on a farm developed 5 episodes of transient hyperthyroidism over an 11-year period. This was thought to be due to thyroid contamination of meat obtained from cows on the farm.

Educational Objective

Identify the presentation of thyrotoxicosis associated with contamination of meat with thyroid tissue ("hamburger thyrotoxicosis").

Reference(s)

Gore AC, Chappell VA, Fenton SE, et al. Executive summary to EDC-2: the Endocrine Society's Second Scientific Statement on Endocrine-Disrupting Chemicals. *Endocr Rev.* 2015;36(6):593-602. PMID: 26414233

Hedberg CW, Fishbein DB, Janssen RS, et al. An outbreak of thyrotoxicosis caused by the consumption of bovine thyroid gland in ground beef. *N Engl J Med.* 1987;316(16):993-998. PMID: 3561455

Kinney JS, Hurwitz ES, Fishbein DB, et al. Community outbreak of thyrotoxicosis: epidemiology, immunogenetic characteristics, and long-term outcome. *Am J Med.* 1988;84(1):10-18. PMID: 3257352

Parmar MS, Sturge C. Recurrent hamburger thyrotoxicosis. *CMAJ.* 2003;169(5):415-417. PMID: 12952802

47 ANSWER: E) Switch from tenofovir to entecavir

Clinically, this patient has osteomalacia with decreased mineralization of bones noted by radiographic findings of low bone density with thinning of the cortex and multiple areas of fractures in the ribs, spine, pelvis, and ankle with little to no trauma history. The laboratory findings of severe hypophosphatemia with a normal serum calcium, elevated alkaline phosphatase, and an inappropriately low tubular reabsorption of urinary phosphate in the setting of progressive renal insufficiency and hyperchloremic metabolic acidosis are consistent with Fanconi syndrome causing renal phosphate wasting. Tenofovir is a retroviral medication known to cause proximal renal tubular injury and renal insufficiency. Low serum phosphate causes osteomalacia, leading to elevation of alkaline phosphatase and poor mineralization of osteoid and susceptibility to fracture. The most appropriate recommendation is to replace tenofovir with entecavir (Answer E), which is less phosphaturic.

Urinary phosphate wasting can be caused by fibroblast growth factor 23 overproduction in the paraneoplastic syndrome of tumor-induced osteomalacia, but this patient's fibroblast growth factor 23 level is normal, and the normal 1,25-dihydroxyvitamin D level (rather than an inappropriately low level) is not consistent with tumor-induced osteomalacia. Although underlying malignancy with bone metastases can be considered given his history of hepatocellular carcinoma, profound hypophosphatemia should not be present. A bone biopsy was performed in this case and was negative for malignancy. Without any evidence of malignancy, chemotherapy (Answer D) is not warranted. Phosphate replacement (Answer A) is needed, but its effects will not effectively manage his long-term bone health if the underlying agent causing the phosphate wasting (tenofovir) is not replaced. Calcitriol (Answer B) can help with absorption of calcium and phosphate from the gastrointestinal tract, but this effect is not enough to normalize the serum phosphate. Bisphosphonate treatment (Answer C) is not appropriate in this setting of severe hypophosphatemia from renal phosphate wasting. In fact, once tenofovir was replaced with entecavir, this patient's overall phosphate replacement daily dose decreased within 9 months and his bone mineral density improved within a year and continues to improve without any antiresorptive therapy.

Educational Objective

Diagnose the clinical syndrome of tenofovir-induced Fanconi syndrome leading to hypophosphatemia and osteomalacia and recommend appropriate management.

Reference(s)

Gara N, Zhao X, Collins MT, et al. Renal tubular dysfunction during long-term adefovir or tenofovir therapy in chronic hepatitis B. *Ailment Pharmacol Ther.* 2012;35(11):1317-1325. PMID 22506503

Koenig KF, Kalbermatter S, Menter T, Graber P, Kiss D. Recurrent bone fractures due to tenofovir-induced renal phosphate wasting. *Scand J Infect Dis.* 2014;46(3):221-224. PMID 24147545

Ruppe MD, Jan de Beur SM. Disorders of phosphate homeostasis. In: Rosen CJ, Bouillon R, Compston JE, Rosen V, eds. *Primer on the Metabolic Bone Diseases and Disorders of Mineral Metabolism.* 8th ed. Washington, DC: The American Society for Bone and Mineral Research; 2008:601-612.

48

ANSWER: A) Thyroidal metastases from renal cancer

This patient presents with an incidental finding of a retrosternal goiter detected during imaging procedures to determine the stage of renal cell carcinoma. Subsequent biochemical testing has confirmed the presence of subclinical hyperthyroidism with a low but detectable serum TSH level in an asymptomatic patient. Further investigations of the goiter indicate diffuse uptake on an isotope imaging scan and the presence of multiple indeterminate nodules on thyroid ultrasonography based on their hypoechogenicity and increased internal blood flow.

Metastasis to the thyroid gland from nonthyroid sites is an uncommon clinical presentation, and the overall incidence is estimated to be 2%. Renal cell carcinoma and lung cancer are the most common primary tumors in this setting, accounting for 25% and 22%, respectively, of cases reported in the literature. Metastases to the thyroid may be discovered at the time the primary tumor is diagnosed, after preoperative investigation of a neck mass, or on histologic examination of a thyroidectomy specimen. Thyroid metastases and direct infiltration of the thyroid can be difficult to distinguish in patients with locally aggressive cancer of the larynx or upper esophagus. Most patients with thyroid metastasis present with signs and symptoms identical to those of patients with primary thyroid disease. Approximately 70% present with a palpable neck mass and 30% present with an incidental lesion identified on imaging. Thyroid metastasis at an advanced stage within the central neck can result in dysphagia and dysphonia, similar to aggressive thyroid malignancy. Patients often have signs of metastatic disease to other organs.

Despite major improvements in the accuracy of thyroid imaging, including high-resolution ultrasonography, cross-sectional imaging (CT/MRI), and functional imaging (fluorodeoxyglucose-PET scanning), the distinction between primary thyroid lesions and metastases can be difficult. The presence of multiple indeterminate lesions on ultrasonography in a patient with a diagnosis of renal cell carcinoma should raise the suspicion that thyroidal metastases are present (Answer A).

The technetium scan could be consistent with Graves disease (Answer B), but the patient is not overtly hyperthyroid, he does not have an elevated thyroid-stimulating immunoglobulin level, and the thyroid ultrasonographic appearance is not one of Graves disease. Mild toxic nodular hyperthyroidism (Answer E) may be present in patients with multinodular goiter, although the diffuse uptake on the technetium scan without suppression of uptake elsewhere and the finding of multiple indeterminate lesions on ultrasonography would not be consistent with this diagnosis. Similarly, the imaging findings are not consistent with thyroiditis (Answer C) in which reduced uptake on the technetium scan and diffuse (rather than nodular) hypoechogenicity on ultrasonography may be expected. Medullary carcinoma (Answer D) can be associated with pheochromocytoma and hyperparathyroidism in multiple endocrine neoplasia syndromes, but it is not directly linked to renal cell carcinoma.

FNAB of 2 thyroid nodules in this patient was nondiagnostic, but subsequent core biopsies confirmed the presence of metastatic renal cell cancer. He underwent a right nephrectomy and subsequent total thyroidectomy and remains well and free from metastatic disease.

Educational Objective

Diagnose thyroid metastases in a patient with renal cell cancer presenting with multiple suspicious thyroid nodules and subclinical hyperthyroidism.

UpToDate Topic Review(s)

Diagnostic approach to and treatment of thyroid nodules

Reference(s)

Nixon IJ, Coca-Pelaz A, Kaleva AI, et al. Metastasis to the thyroid gland: a critical review. *Ann Surg Oncol.* 2017;24(6):1533-1539. PMID: 27873099

Farina E, Monari F, Tallini G, et al. Unusual thyroid carcinoma metastases: a case series and literature review. *Endocr Pathol.* 2016;27(1):55-64. PMID: 26662609

49

ANSWER: C) Restart high-intensity statin therapy

Cholesteryl ester storage disease (CESD) is a rare autosomal recessive disorder caused by mutations in the gene encoding lysosomal acid lipase (*LIPA*). The resultant markedly decreased activity of the lysosomal acid lipase enzyme leads to progressive accumulation of cholesteryl ester and, to a lesser extent, triglycerides in hepatocytes and macrophages. Lysosomal acid lipase deficiency can present early in life or have a later onset with CESD.

The early-onset infantile form of lysosomal acid lipase deficiency, also known as Wolman disease, is a rare disorder resulting in massive cholesteryl ester accumulation in the liver, spleen, adrenal glands, and macrophages. Affected infants present by 2 to 4 months of age with hepatosplenomegaly and failure to thrive, and death occurs within the first year of life.

In contrast, CESD is an underrecognized subtype of lysosomal acid lipase deficiency that presents after infancy with a highly variable presentation depending on the degree of enzyme deficiency. There is accelerated risk for cardiovascular disease; multiorgan dysfunction; and gradual accumulation of cellular cholesteryl ester in the liver, leading to transaminase elevations, characteristic microvesicular steatosis, and marked dyslipidemia.

Dyslipidemia in CESD is characterized by elevated LDL cholesterol and apolipoprotein B and decreased HDL cholesterol, a pattern similar to that observed in other familial dyslipidemias. LDL-cholesterol levels are variably elevated and can be greater than 190 mg/dL (>4.92 mmol/L). Risk of atherosclerotic cardiovascular disease is very high according to current limited literature from autopsy studies in patients with CESD. Statin therapy (Answer C), alone or in combination with other agents, effectively reduces LDL cholesterol but has little effect on liver dysfunction. Nevertheless, it is imperative to initiate statin therapy in this patient.

Ursodeoxycholic acid (Answer A) is a bile acid occurring naturally in humans. It is used to treat cholestatic liver disease, as it replaces cytotoxic bile acids and decreases liver injury. Liver injury in CESD is not due to bile acid accumulation and hence there is no indication for ursodiol in this patient.

Liver transplant (Answer B) has been used as a treatment in patients with lysosomal acid lipase deficiency who have progressive hepatic deterioration. However, lysosomal acid lipase is widely distributed in tissues and, therefore, liver transplant is not expected to correct all aspects of the enzyme deficiency. Results are mixed, with some cases showing normalization of hepatic function and improvement of hyperlipidemia, growth, and development, while others have less favorable outcomes such as cardiac and renal complications. Thus, liver transplant is not a viable option for this patient. However, liver biopsy to monitor disease progression under the care of a hepatologist is necessary. Additionally, this patient has moderately elevated liver transaminase levels, and alcohol cessation should be strongly encouraged.

Ezetimibe (Answer D), an intestinal inhibitor of NPC1L1 (NPC1 like intracellular cholesterol transporter 1), has been shown to improve liver fat in preclinical studies. Findings of a few small cohort studies in humans suggest that ezetimibe decreases liver fat in obese individuals with steatosis. However, there are no long-term randomized controlled trials indicating benefit of these drugs in fatty liver disease or in CESD.

Enzyme replacement therapy with a recombinant lysosomal acid lipase has recently become available. Recombinant sebelipase alfa (Answer E) was approved for commercial use by the US FDA in December 2015 for the treatment of patients with lysosomal acid lipase deficiency. Recombinant sebelipase alfa offers a disease-specific treatment that could alter the natural course of the disease and reduce the risk of developing its various clinical sequelae. Enzyme replacement therapy should be considered for all individuals diagnosed with lysosomal acid lipase deficiency in addition to a low-fat diet at a daily caloric intake sufficient to maintain or achieve a healthy body weight. However, it requires commitment to lifelong infusion therapy every 1 to 2 weeks. In this man who has a relatively mild manifestation of the disorder, enzyme replacement should be considered eventually, but not necessarily right now. Referral to a geneticist with expertise in lysosomal disorders would be helpful when enzyme replacement therapy is being considered.

Educational Objective
Diagnose and manage cholesteryl ester storage disease.

UpToDate Topic Review(s)
Inborn errors of metabolism: Epidemiology, pathogenesis, and clinical features

Reference(s)
Maciejko JJ. Managing cardiovascular risk in lysosomal acid lipase deficiency. *Am J Cardiovasc Drugs.* 2017;17(3):217-231. PMID: 28197978

Fouchier SW, Defesche JC. Lysosomal acid lipase A and the hypercholesterolaemic phenotype. *Curr Opin Lipidol.* 2013;24(4):332-338. PMID: 23652569

Burton BK, Balwani M, Feillet F, et al. A phase 3 trial of sebelipase alfa in lysosomal acid lipase deficiency. *N Engl J Med.* 2015;373(11):1010-1020. PMID: 26352813

50

ANSWER: C) Daily basal insulin, 22 units; prandial insulin, 7 units; blood glucose target, 140-180 mg/dL (7.8-10.0 mmol/L)

This question addresses how to adjust insulin on the basis of changes in the glomerular filtration rate. Exogenous insulin is primarily eliminated by the kidney. As the glomerular filtration rate decreases, clearance and catabolism of insulin decrease. A common rule of thumb is that the insulin dosage should be reduced by 25% when the estimated glomerular filtration rate decreases to 10 to 50 mL/min per 1.73 m², and the dosage should be reduced by 50% when it decreases to less than 10 mL/min per 1.73 m². The American Diabetes Association recommends a target blood glucose range of 140 to 180 mg/dL (7.8-10.0 mmol/L) for hospitalized patients.

This patient most likely has contrast-induced nephropathy. Diabetes is a major risk factor for this complication, especially when the patient has underlying renal impairment. It is recommended that metformin be held for 24 hours before receiving contrast material. It is not clear in this vignette whether this precaution was taken. Metformin does not increase the risk for contrast-induced nephropathy, but the reduced glomerular filtration rate places a patient on metformin at higher risk for lactic acidosis.

This patient takes 60 units of insulin per day as 70/30 split in 2 doses. Reducing his daily dose by 25% translates to a daily dose of 45 units. If one assumes his appetite is normal, then 50% can be provided as basal insulin (~22 units) and the other 50% can be given as prandial insulin (~7 units per meal). Of the listed choices, Answer C is the closest to this calculation. Answers A and E are too aggressive, and the blood glucose target is also too low in Answer A. Answer B is very close to the desired calculation, but the blood glucose target is too low. Answer D is too conservative.

Educational Objective
Adjust the insulin dosage on the basis of changes in the glomerular filtration rate in patients with diabetes mellitus.

UpToDate Topic Review(s)
Management of hyperglycemia in patients with type 2 diabetes and pre-dialysis chronic kidney disease or end-stage renal disease

Reference(s)
American Diabetes Association. 14. Diabetes care in the hospital. *Diabetes Care.* 2017;40(Suppl 1):S120-S127.

Clement S, Braithwaite SS, Magee MF, et al; American Diabetes Association Diabetes in Hospitals Writing Committee. Management of diabetes and hyperglycemia in hospitals. *Diabetes Care.* 2004;27(2):553-591. PMID: 14747243

Biesenbach G, Raml A, Schmekal B, Eichbauer-Sturm G. Decreased insulin requirement in relation to GFR in nephropathic type 1 and insulin-treated type 2 diabetic patients. *Diabet Med.* 2003;20(8):642-645. PMID: 12873291

Snyder RW, Berns JS. Use of insulin and oral hypoglycemic medications in patients with diabetes mellitus and advanced kidney disease. *Semin Dial.* 2004;17(5):365-370. PMID: 15461745

51

ANSWER: E) Intravenous pamidronate every 3 months

Osteogenesis imperfecta (OI) is an inherited connective tissue disorder of type 1 collagen. The estimated incidence is 1 in 20,000. It is associated with mutations in the *COL1A1* and *COL1A2* genes. Most forms of OI are inherited in an autosomal dominant manner, although autosomal recessive forms have been described. Type 1 collagen is a constituent of bone, ligaments, skin, and sclerae. OI is classified into multiple subtypes on the basis of clinical characteristics. The phenotypic presentation is variable within the same family, and the clinical picture can range from mild, premature osteoporosis to multiple fractures with little or no trauma. It is important to monitor for complications that can develop due to the impairment of type 1 collagen. Patients with OI are prone to early osteoporosis and fracture. Bone densitometry is recommended every 2 years. Bisphosphonates are the mainstay of fracture prevention in children and adults with OI. The most well-studied agent is cyclic pamidronate (Answer E) in children (in mostly uncontrolled studies), which increases bone mineral density, decreases fracture rate, and improves functional status without short-term impairment of bone quality or fracture healing.

Oral alendronate (Answer A) has also been studied in children with severe OI in a randomized controlled trial and it did show a significant increase in lumbar spine bone mineral density compared with that observed with placebo but there was no significant decrease in the incidence of long-bone fractures, bone pain, or disability score.

Additionally, patients with this degree of scoliosis may have difficulty remaining upright for the requisite periods to avoid esophageal irritation following administration of an oral bisphosphonate.

GH therapy (Answer B) has been investigated in children with OI as a potential agent for growth deficiency and improved bone growth. In response to treatment with recombinant human GH injections, patients with OI had an increased bone formation rate and increased linear growth. However, patients with more severe OI type III did not respond to this therapy. Combined treatment with GH and bisphosphonates had a synergistic effect on growth velocity and bone density, but it did not reduce fracture incidence.

Calcitonin (Answer C) has been studied in patients with osteogenesis imperfecta and was not shown to have significant effects in biochemical markers of bone turnover or bone mineral content. Additionally, adverse effects are common with this therapy.

Finally testosterone supplementation (Answer D) has not been studied in patients with OI as a means to reduce fracture incidence.

Educational Objective
Recommend intravenous bisphosphonates to significantly decrease the fracture rate in patients with osteogenesis imperfecta type III/IV.

UpToDate Topic Review(s)
Osteogenesis imperfecta: management and prognosis

Reference(s)

Marom R, Lee YC, Grafe I, Lee B. Pharmacological and biological therapeutic strategies for osteogenesis imperfecta. *Am J Med Genet C Semin Med Genet.* 2016;172(4):367-383. PMID: 27813341

Shapiro JR, Thompson CB, Wu Y, Nunes M, Gillen C. Bone mineral density and fracture rate in response to intravenous and oral bisphosphonates in adult osteogenesis imperfecta. *Calcif Tissue Int.* 2010;87(2):120-129. PMID: 20544187

52 ANSWER: D) Initiate phentermine + topiramate ER
This patient implemented lifestyle modifications and initially lost weight successfully. However, now she is unable to lose additional weight despite attempting to follow a dietary and activity program. Starting a weight-loss medication is indicated in this setting. Because her main barrier in her weight-loss effort seems to be increased appetite, she would benefit from adding an appetite suppressant. Of the listed options, only phentermine + topiramate ER (Answer D) has this effect. Phentermine reduces norepinephrine uptake, and topiramate is a GABA receptor modulator. The addition of this combination pill to a weight-loss program produces a 6.6% to 8.6% weight loss after 1 year.

Initiating metformin (Answer B) would be useful if this patient had diabetes as it would help with glucose control without causing weight gain and could lead to modest weight loss (<5%). Orlistat (which inhibits intestinal lipase causing fat malabsorption) (Answer C) would be a good choice if the patient were still struggling to follow a meal plan and decided to try a low-fat diet. Increasing physical activity (Answer A) will not produce significant weight loss but would be helpful for weight maintenance. While replacing 1 meal each day with a protein bar or shake (Answer E) would decrease her caloric intake for that meal, this approach will not limit her intake at other meals. This patient needs help with appetite control.

Educational Objective
List indications for weight-loss medications.

UpToDate Topic Review(s)
Obesity in adults: Drug therapy

Reference(s)

Garvey WT, Mechanick JI, Brett EM, et al; Reviewers of the AACE/ACE Obesity Clinical Practice Guidelines. American Association of Clinical Endocrinologists and American College of Endocrinology Comprehensive Clinical Practice Guidelines for Medical Care of Patients with Obesity. *Endocr Pract.* 2016;22(Suppl 3):1-203. PMID: 27219496

Kumar RB, Aronne LJ. Efficacy comparison of medications approved for chronic weight management. *Obesity (Silver Spring).* 2015;23(Suppl 1):S4-S7. PMID: 25900871

Apovian CM, Aronne LJ, Bessesen DH, et al; Endocrine Society. Pharmacological management of obesity: an endocrine Society clinical practice guideline. *J Clin Endocrinol Metab.* 2015;100(2):342-362. PMID: 25590212

53 ANSWER: D) Give subcutaneous octreotide

Hypoglycemia occurs 2 to 3 times more often in patients with type 1 diabetes than in patients with type 2 diabetes. However, because many more patients have type 2 diabetes, iatrogenic hypoglycemia is more common in this patient population. A working group of the American Diabetes Association and the Endocrine Society defined a glucose threshold of 70 mg/dL or lower (≤3.9 mmol/L) as indicative of hypoglycemia. Severe hypoglycemia is defined as an episode of hypoglycemia that requires assistance from another individual to actively treat the hypoglycemia or take other corrective actions.

Most patients with type 2 diabetes who develop hypoglycemia are treated with either secretogogues (sulfonylurea or glinide) or, more commonly, insulin. Severe hypoglycemia in patients with type 2 diabetes occurs at rates of 35 to 70 cases per 100 patient-years. In the large, randomized ACCORD trial (Action to Control Cardiovascular Risk in Diabetes) of intensive vs standard glucose-lowering action, patients randomly assigned to the intensive glycemic arm had a 20% higher mortality rate than that of the standard treatment group. In this study, patients who had 1 or more severe hypoglycemic events had higher death rates (hazard ratio, 1.41 [95% confidence interval, 1.03-1.93]), and hypoglycemia was associated with increased cardiovascular mortality.

Older patients are more susceptible to hypoglycemia because of impaired counterregulatory response to hypoglycemia. Other factors that contribute to hypoglycemia include renal dysfunction and impaired autonomic nervous system function. Recurrent hypoglycemia reduces the level at which the adrenergic response to hypoglycemia occurs, leading to lower and lower glucose levels that are not recognized by the patient. Often, the first sign of hypoglycemia in these patients is neuroglycopenia, which is the hallmark of hypoglycemia unawareness. One study found that severe hypoglycemia (glucose ≤50 mg/dL [≤2.8 mmol/L]) that occurs in hospitalized patients with diabetes is associated with increased length of stay and a greater risk of death at 1 year after discharge.

Appropriate acute treatment of severe hypoglycemia in the emergency department or the hospital can include treatment with glucagon or infusion of dextrose (D50). If hypoglycemia recurs, additional D50 can be administered, followed by a continuous intravenous dextrose (D5 or D10) infusion.

In this vignette, the long-acting sulfonylurea glyburide caused inappropriate insulin secretion well after hospital admission, leading to recurrent hypoglycemia. Renal impairment is a contributing factor in this case. After stopping the medication, the best treatment is to administer octreotide (Answer D). Treatment of sulfonylurea-induced hypoglycemia with octreotide is an off-label US FDA indication, but it is very effective and is the treatment of choice in this case. In a prospective, double-blind study, patients with diabetes evaluated in the emergency department after presentation with sulfonylurea-induced hypoglycemia who were treated with octreotide had a mean glucose value 127 mg/dL (7.0 mmol/L) higher than that of placebo-treated patients over the first 8 hours after treatment. Recurrent hypoglycemia rates were lower in the octreotide-treated patients. Octreotide should be given as a 50-mcg subcutaneous injection and can be repeated every 6 hours if hypoglycemia recurs. Most patients with sulfonylurea-induced hypoglycemia need 1 or 2 doses of octreotide to completely resolve hypoglycemia.

Repeated administration of dextrose (D50) as needed (Answer A) has not been effective for this patient and is inappropriate. Administration of glucocorticoids (eg, methylprednisolone) (Answer B) could counter the hypoglycemia but would lead to an overshoot of hyperglycemia and other untoward effects.

Everolimus (Answer C) is a rapamycin analogue that has been used in the treatment of refractory neuroendocrine tumors. One study reported on the use of everolimus in the treatment of hypoglycemia secondary to insulin-secreting neuroendocrine tumors. Treatment of sulfonylurea-induced hypoglycemia with everolimus has not been reported in the literature and therefore is not the treatment of choice in this case. Changing the infusion to D15 (Answer E) may temporarily increase the glucose levels, but the hypoglycemia is likely to recur due to the prolonged action of glyburide.

Once the hypoglycemia has been corrected, the appropriate goal for glycemic control needs to be discussed. Certainly tight glycemic control (hemoglobin A_{1c} <6.5% [<48 mmol/mol]) is not needed and can be potentially dangerous, as in this case. Glyburide has active metabolites that accumulate with increasing degrees of renal insufficiency. Therefore, glyburide should not be restarted in this patient because of the potential for recurrent hypoglycemia. The 2012 Beers list of medicines to be avoided in older adults includes glyburide and sliding-scale insulin as inappropriate treatments. This patient can restart the metformin if renal function has improved by the end of her hospitalization.

Educational Objective
Recommend the optimal treatment of sulfonylurea-induced hypoglycemia.

UpToDate Topic Review(s)
Management of hypoglycemia during treatment of diabetes mellitus

Reference(s)

Seaquist ER, Anderson J, Childs B, Cryer P, Dagogo-Jack S, Fish L, Heller SR, Rodriguez H, Rosenzweig J, Vigersky R. Hypoglycemia and diabetes: a report of a workgroup of the American Diabetes Association and the Endocrine Society. *J Clin Endocrinol Metab*. 2013;98(5):1845-1859. PMID: 23589524

Heller SR, Choudhary P, Davies C, et al, UK Hypoglycaemia Study Group. Risk of hypoglycaemia in types 1 and 2 diabetes: effects of treatment modalities and their duration. *Diabetologia*. 2007;50(6):1140-1147. PMID: 17415551

Bonds DE, Miller ME, Bergenstal RM, et al. The association between symptomatic, severe hypoglycaemia and mortality in type 2 diabetes: retrospective epidemiological analysis of the ACCORD study. *BMJ*. 2010;340:b4909. PMID: 20061358

Turchin A, Matheny ME, Shubina M, Scanlon JV, Greenwood B, Pendergrass ML. Hypoglycemia and clinical outcomes in patients with diabetes hospitalized in the general ward. *Diabetes Care*. 2009;32(7):1153-1157. PMID: 19564471

Fasano CJ, O'Malley G, Dominici P, Aguillera E, Latta DR. Comparison of octreotide and standard therapy versus standard therapy alone for the treatment of sulfonylurea-induced hypoglycemia. *Ann Emerg Med*. 2008;51(4):400-406. PMID: 17764782

Kulke MH, Bergsland EK, Yao JC. Glycemic control in patients with insulinoma treated with everolimus. *N Engl J Med*. 2009;360(2):195-197. PMID: 19129539

American Geriatrics Society 2012 Beers Criteria Update Expert Panel. American Geriatrics Society updated Beers Criteria for potentially inappropriate medication use in older adults. *J Am Geriatr Soc*. 2012;60(4):616-631. PMID: 22376048

54 ANSWER: D) Administer stress-dose steroids

The evaluation of adrenal function must be done with a clear understanding of the situation in which a sample for cortisol measurement was collected. For example, a low cortisol collected in the middle of the night may be normal in a patient with normal circadian rhythm, but not in a situation of acute stress. Also, because total cortisol is generally measured, some adjustment must be made on the basis of the (presumed) cortisol-binding globulin levels, which are increased by oral estrogen and are reduced in malnourished patients (in general correlating with serum albumin). Therefore, in a patient who has been in the intensive care unit for a long time, cortisol levels may be lower than they would have been at the beginning of hospital admission simply due to reduced binding protein. Unfortunately, an exact formula is not available to perform an accurate correction of cortisol based on albumin level.

This patient was admitted to the hospital recently and was healthy before the head trauma, so his nutritional status and cortisol-binding globulin levels should be normal. He is acutely sick, requiring pressors to maintain blood pressure. In such a situation, his serum cortisol should be maximally stimulated, above 20 μg/dL (>551.8 nmol/L). Furthermore, even a low cortisol-binding globulin could not explain such a low cortisol level. Therefore, the baseline serum cortisol value of 3.9 μg/dL (107.6 nmol/L) is diagnostic of adrenal insufficiency (assuming that he had not received synthetic glucocorticoid therapy that would have suppressed his hypothalamic-pituitary-adrenal axis) (thus, Answer E is incorrect). Because he had head trauma, his adrenal insufficiency is most likely due to acute traumatic brain injury. He was healthy before the accident, so it would take several weeks of reduced ACTH secretion to cause adrenal atrophy that would result into a reduced serum response during an ACTH stimulation test. This is the reason why his cortisol peak was normal. Results from a test that assesses the whole hypothalamic-pituitary-adrenal axis (such as an insulin tolerance test) would already be abnormal, but a stimulation test is not necessary here. Therefore, the most appropriate next step is to administer stress-dose steroids (Answer D).

Measuring serum aldosterone (Answer A) would not help because it would most likely be normal in this case of secondary adrenal insufficiency. The result from a 1-mcg ACTH stimulation test (Answer B) would also most likely be normal. Fludrocortisone (Answer C) is not needed in the setting of secondary adrenal insufficiency. Furthermore, even if this were primary adrenal insufficiency, stress-dose hydrocortisone would have enough mineralocorticoid activity, so the addition of a mineralocorticoid would be unnecessary.

Educational Objective
Explain how results from ACTH stimulation testing may be normal in patients with recent-onset central adrenal insufficiency.

UpToDate Topic Review(s)
Diagnosis of adrenal insufficiency in adults

Reference(s)

Wagner AK, McCullough EH, Niyonkuru C, et al. Acute serum hormone levels: characterization and prognosis after severe traumatic brain injury. *J Neurotrauma*. 2011;28(6):871-888. PMID: 21488721

Ospina NS, Al Nofal A, Bancos I, et al. ACTH stimulation tests for the diagnosis of adrenal insufficiency: systematic review and meta-analysis. *J Clin Endocrinol Metab*. 2016;101(2):427-434. PMID: 26649617

Venkatesh B, Cohen J. The utility of the corticotropin test to diagnose adrenal insufficiency in critical illness: an update. *Clin Endocrinol (Oxf)*. 2015;83(3):289-297. PMID: 25521173

Hamrahian AH, Oseni TS, Arafah BM. Measurements of serum free cortisol in critically ill patients. *N Engl J Med*. 2004;350(16):1629-1638. PMID: 15084695

55 ANSWER: E) Shorter height

Clinicians should suspect the diagnosis of 46,XX testicular disorder of sex development (also referred to as 46,XX male syndrome) in men with primary hypogonadism, small testes (mean bitesticular volume of 4 mL), and shorter height than that of men with Klinefelter syndrome (47,XXY). Karyotype analysis distinguishes between the 2 conditions.

46,XX testicular disorder of sex development is an uncommon cause of male hypogonadism with a reported prevalence of 1 in 20,000 newborn males. More than 250 cases have been described in the literature. Men with 46,XX testicular disorder of sex development resemble men with Klinefelter syndrome in many ways. Phenotypically, both groups have normal male genitalia but very small testes and high rates of gynecomastia (thus, Answers C and D are incorrect). An important phenotypic difference between the 2 groups is height—men with 46,XX testicular disorder of sex development have a mean height of 66.5 in (169 cm) (which is similar to that of healthy women), whereas men with Klinefelter syndrome have a mean height of 72 in (183 cm) (which is slightly above that of men without Klinefelter syndrome) (thus, Answer E is correct). Phenotypically, men with 46,XX testicular disorder of sex development also have high rates of maldescended testes.

From an endocrine perspective, men with 46,XX testicular disorder of sex development and men with Klinefelter syndrome both have low levels of total and free testosterone coupled with elevated levels of LH and FSH (thus, Answer A is incorrect). Men with either cause of hypogonadism have similar BMIs, although men with 46,XX testicular disorder of sex development are shorter and weigh less (thus, Answer B is incorrect).

Most men with 46,XX testicular disorder of sex development have Y-chromosome material (including the *SRY* gene) on the paternal X chromosome and lack the AZF region, which is needed for spermatogenesis. Consequently, they are infertile and semen analysis shows azoospermia. During puberty, they are eugonadal for their age. The condition most often results from abnormal exchange of genetic material between chromosomes during paternal meiosis (with the translocation leading to misplacement of the *SRY* gene onto an X chromosome). Epigenetically, affected patients also have a high rate of skewed inactivation patterns of androgen receptor alleles.

Educational Objective
Identify the typical phenotype and endocrine profile of men with 46,XX testicular disorder of sex development (46,XX male syndrome).

Reference(s)

de la Chapelle A. Analytic review: nature and origin of males with XX sex chromosomes. *Am J Hum Genet.* 1972;24(1):71-105. PMID: 4622299

Vorona E, Zitzmann M, Gromoll J, Schüring AN, Nieschlag E. Clinical, endocrinological, and epigenetic features of the 46,XX male syndrome, compared with 47,XXY Klinefelter patients. *J Clin Endocrinol Metab.* 2007;92(9):3458-3465. PMID: 17579198

Wu QY, Li N, Li WW, et al. Clinical, molecular and cytogenetic analysis of 46,XX testicular disorder of sex development with SRY-positive. *BMC Urol.* 2014;14:70. PMID: 25169080

56 ANSWER: A) Fasting somatostatin

Approximately 1% to 2% of patients with hyperglycemia have secondary forms of diabetes. Autoimmune or secondary diabetes should be considered in this patient because of the age of onset and his relatively low BMI. A number of etiologies can lead to secondary diabetes and should be considered: pancreatic disorders, endocrinopathies, medication- or toxin-induced diabetes, and genetic syndromes. The etiology of the hyperglycemia can vary from reduced insulin secretion to increased insulin resistance to increased glucagon release leading to glycogenolysis and gluconeogenesis. In this 64-year-old previously healthy man, there is no reason to suspect a genetic syndrome. There is no known history of toxin exposure or drug use that could cause hyperglycemia. Pancreatic insufficiency or an endocrinopathy should be considered.

The triad of diabetes, diarrhea/steatorrhea, and cholelithiasis makes somatostatinoma the most likely cause of secondary diabetes. Thus, measuring fasting somatostatin (Answer A) is the best next step. Somatostatinomas are rare tumors, occurring in 1 in 40 million individuals. They can be located in the pancreas, duodenum, and rarely the jejunum. About 45% occur in the setting of multiple endocrine neoplasia syndromes. About 10% of patients with neurofibromatosis type 1 have somatostatinomas.

There is marked overlap between the presentations of glucagonoma and somatostatinoma. Both can present with weight loss and diarrhea. The average age of onset for both is in the fifth decade of life. However, the presence of cholelithiasis makes somatostatinoma more likely. About 70% of persons with glucagonoma have necrolytic migratory erythema, which is absent in this patient. Therefore, measuring plasma glucagon (Answer B) is incorrect.

Cortisol excess is associated with insulin resistance and glucose intolerance, but only 10% to 15% of affected patients develop overt diabetes. In this vignette, there is no mention of proximal muscle weakness, striae, edema, or other laboratory findings such as hypokalemia that would suggest cortisol excess. Therefore, measuring 24-hour urinary cortisol excretion (Answer C) is incorrect.

Acromegaly can also be associated with glucose intolerance and, in a small subset of patients, with overt diabetes. This patient's clinical presentation is not consistent with acromegaly. The symptom onset was recent, while the clinical features of acromegaly (eg, hyperhidrosis, soft-tissue swelling) are typically progressive over years. Therefore, measuring IGF-1 (Answer D) is incorrect.

Finally, hemochromatosis can be associated with diabetes mellitus. Clinical manifestations include liver disease (hepatomegaly early in the disease), skin hyperpigmentation, arthropathy, hypogonadism, and cardiomyopathy, none of which are described in this patient. The course of the disease is also slower than what this patient has experienced. Therefore, measuring transferrin saturation and ferritin (Answer E) is incorrect.

Educational Objective

Evaluate new-onset hyperglycemia in older individuals and consider secondary causes of diabetes.

Reference(s)

Ganda O. Prevalence and incidence of secondary and other types of diabetes. In: *Diabetes in America.* Chapter 5. 2nd ed. Available at: http://niddk.nih.gov.

Anderson CW, Bennett JJ. Clinical presentation and diagnosis of pancreatic neuroendocrine tumors. *Surg Oncol Clin N Am.* 2016;25(2):363-374. PMID: 27013370

57 ANSWER: D) Prolonged bisphosphonate use

This patient's history of prolonged bisphosphonate use along with a clinical prodrome of pain localized to the femoral shaft are suggestive of impending fracture seen with atypical femoral fractures. Additionally, the x-ray of the right femur shows areas of typical lateral cortical thickening that cause a "beaking" or "flaring" effect adjacent to areas of transverse fracture lines (*see image, white arrows*), which eventually evolve and propagate medially and ultimately lead to a complete fracture. The slightly elevated alkaline phosphatase seen in this patient is associated with her bone anomaly.

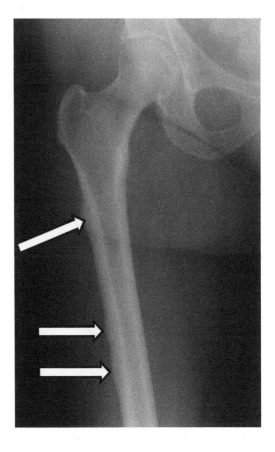

The precise incidence of medication-related atypical femoral fracture related to duration of bisphosphonate use (Answer D) is unknown, but in some studies, it is reported to range from 38.9 cases/100,000 person-years (with 6 to 8 years of bisphosphonate use) to 107.5/100,000 person-years (with more than 10 years of bisphosphonate use). The median duration of bisphosphonate use in patients with atypical femoral fracture is 7 years. A prodrome of persistent thigh or groin pain is common (70% of cases). A complete fracture is associated with sudden onset of severe pain associated with little or no trauma. If a patient on bisphosphonate therapy reports persistent thigh or groin pain, it is recommended to obtain plain radiographs of the symptomatic hip, including full diaphysis of the femur and the contralateral hip. If the radiograph is negative but clinical suspicion remains high, a technetium bone scan or MRI of the femur should be performed. In patients with incomplete subtrochanteric/femoral shaft fractures associated with pain, as in this case, prophylactic reconstruction nail fixation is recommended. If there is minimal pain, conservative therapy with limited weight bearing with crutches or a walker for 2 to 3 months is recommended. In patients with low bone mass (osteopenia) and no other high risks for fracture, a drug holiday from bisphosphonate therapy should be considered after 5 years of use. The Task Force of the American Society for Bone and Mineral Research emphasizes that the incidence of atypical femoral fracture associated with bisphosphate therapy for osteoporosis is very low, especially when compared with the number of vertebral, hip, and other fractures that are prevented by bisphosphonate therapy.

This patient does not have tumor-induced osteomalacia (Answer A) because her phosphate and 1,25-dihydroxyvitamin D levels are not low. She does not have osteomalacia from vitamin D deficiency (Answer E) because her calcium and phosphate levels are normal. Mastocytosis (Answer B) is incorrect because she has no anemia and does not report any urticaria or rash. The radiologic findings on the femoral x-ray are not consistent with Paget disease of bone (Answer C).

Educational Objective
Recognize the clinical presentation of impending atypical femoral fracture due to prolonged bisphosphonate use.

UpToDate Topic Review(s)
Risks of bisphosphonate therapy in patients with osteoporosis

Reference(s)

Gedmintas L, Solomon DH, Kim SC. Bisphosphonates and risk of subtrochanteric, femoral shaft, and atypical femur fracture: a systematic review and meta-analysis. *J Bone Miner Res.* 2013;28(8):1729-1737. PMID: 23408697

Shane E, Burr D, Ebeling PR, et al. Atypical subtrochanteric and diaphyseal femoral fractures: second report of a task force of the American Society for Bone and Mineral Research. *J Bone Miner Res.* 2014;29(1):1-23. PMID: 23712442

Toro G, Ojeda-Thies C, Calabro G, et al. Management of atypical femoral fracture: a scoping review and comprehensive algorithm. *BMC Musculoskelet Disord.* 2016;17:227. PMID: 27215972

58 ANSWER: E) Area A of the nodule shows nuclear features of papillary thyroid cancer

The histologic specimen shown in the vignette (reprinted from Gupta N, Dasyam AK, Carty SE, et al. *J Clin Endocrinol Metab*. 2013;98[5]:E914-E922) contains areas with 3 different characteristics. Area C shows features of benign thyroid tissue. There are thyroid follicles lined by cuboidal epithelium surrounding a lumen filled with pink homogeneous colloid. The interstitium has a rich vascular supply. The interstitium also contains C cells, which secrete calcitonin, but they are not visible without immunohistochemical staining. Normal-appearing round to oval follicles lined by flattened epithelium and filled with colloid are also shown in this figure (*see image 1*).

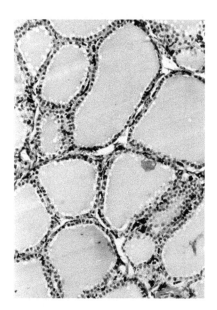

Image 1. Reprinted courtesy of www.pathologyoutlines.com (normal thyroid histology chapter, AFIP images) available at: http://www.pathologyoutlines.com/topic/thyroidhistology.html.

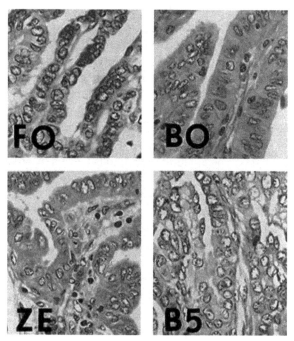

Image 2. Reprinted courtesy of www.pathologyoutlines.com (papillary thyroid cancer chapter, AFIP stained images with different fixatives: FO = formalin, BO = bouins, ZE = zenkers, B5 = mercury based fixative). Available at: http://www.pathologyoutlines.com/topic/thyroidpapillarycytology.html.

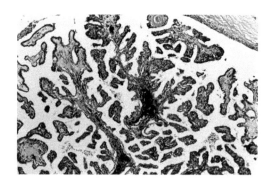

Image 3. Reprinted courtesy of www.pathologyoutlines.com (papillary thyroid cancer chapter, AFIP images). Available at: http://www.pathologyoutlines.com/topic/thyroidpapillarycytology.html.

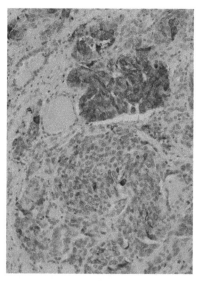

Image 4. Reprinted courtesy of www.pathologyoutlines.com (medullary thyroid cancer chapter, AFIP stained images). Available at: http://www.pathologyoutlines.com/topic/thyroidmedullary.html.

In contrast, Area A of the histologic specimen has the classic nuclear features of papillary thyroid cancer (thus, Answer E is correct and Answer A is incorrect). The spectrum of nuclear features that can be seen in papillary thyroid cancer include overlapping nuclei, enlarged nuclei, orphan Annie nuclei (consisting of optically clear or ground-glass chromatin), eosinophilic intranuclear inclusions, longitudinal nuclear grooves, and distinct micronuclei (*see image 2*). Cytoplasmic features include dense cytoplasm and distinct cell borders.

In a lower-power magnification (*see image 3*), the branching papillae with fibrovascular cores and associated follicles in classic papillary thyroid cancer can be seen.

As discussed, Area C shows benign-appearing thyroid tissue. The patient's third FNAB most likely sampled Area A, as this has clear nuclear features of papillary thyroid cancer (thus, Answer D is incorrect).

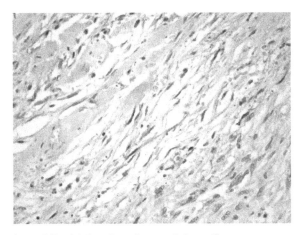

Image 5. Reprinted courtesy of www.pathologyoutlines.com (anaplastic thyroid cancer chapter, AFIP images). Available at: http://www.pathologyoutlines.com/topic/thyroidUndiff.html.

None of the nodule's areas depicted in the vignette show features of medullary thyroid cancer or anaplastic thyroid cancer (thus, Answers B and C are incorrect). Medullary thyroid cancer may be difficult to detect using FNAB specimens. There is abundant cellularity. Cells occur singly or in small clusters and may be spindle-shaped or plasmacytoid. Nuclei are eccentric and there may be binucleation and multinucleation. The specimen stains for calcitonin as shown (*see image 4*).

Anaplastic thyroid cancer is very cellular with pleomorphic tumor cells. The cells are spindle shaped or polygonal (*see image 5*) and are associated with necrosis and mitoses.

Area B is interesting in that it shows borderline nuclear features of papillary thyroid cancer. These 3 different histologic patterns within 1 nodule explains why there were 3 different opinions rendered about the results of the patient's 3 different FNAB cytology specimens. Presumably, the 3 FNABs sampled Areas C, B, and A, respectively. This particular specimen was found to have a *RAS* mutation in all 3 areas. The variant of papillary thyroid cancer, in this case, was the follicular variant, thus explaining why the classic branching papillae were not seen.

Educational Objective
Identify the nuclear features of papillary thyroid cancer.

UpToDate Topic Review(s)
Thyroid biopsy

Reference(s)
Cibas ES, Ali SZ. The Bethesda System for reporting thyroid cytopathology. *Thyroid.* 2009;19(11):1159-1165. PMID: 19888858

Rosai J. Tumors of the Thyroid Glands. Fasicle 21. *AFIP Atlas of Tumor Pathology, 4th Series.* Armed Forces Institute of Pathology, 2015.

Gupta N, Dasyam AK, Carty SE, et al. RAS mutations in thyroid FNA specimens are highly predictive of predominantly low-risk follicular-pattern cancers. *J Clin Endocrinol Metab.* 2013;98(5):E914-E922. PMID: 23539734

59 ANSWER: E) No change to her current regimen

Treatment of high blood pressure in persons with diabetes mellitus reduces the risk of cardiovascular disease, stroke, and renal dysfunction. Epidemiologic studies of patients with diabetes show increased cardiovascular event rates and mortality when blood pressure is above 115/75 mm Hg. Reductions in cardiovascular events, stroke, renal dysfunction, and diabetes-related deaths have been documented when blood pressure is lowered to less than 140/90 mm Hg. A meta-analysis of trials of adults with type 2 diabetes showed no further reduction of mortality or myocardial infarction with additional blood pressure lowering to below 130/80 mm Hg. A modest reduction in stroke rates was observed but with increased adverse treatment effects, including hypotension and syncope.

Antihypertensive medications are associated with an increased risk of serious fall injuries in elderly persons. Therefore, current American Diabetes Association guidelines recommend a blood pressure treatment target of less than 140/90 mm Hg for most patients with diabetes. Lower targets (less than 130/80 mm Hg) may be considered for patients at high risk for a cardiovascular event and those with proteinuria, if this can be achieved without increased adverse treatment effects. More aggressive blood pressure lowering would put this older patient with osteoporosis, peripheral neuropathy, and episodic orthostatic light-headedness at an increased risk for falls and fractures. A standard blood pressure treatment target of less than 140/90 mm Hg is appropriate, so continuing her current regimen (Answer E) is the best recommendation.

For patients with diabetes who do not have proteinuria, medications in the ACE inhibitor, angiotensin receptor blocker, thiazide diuretic, and calcium-channel blocker classes all improve cardiovascular outcomes. Studies have not shown improved treatment outcomes when changing from hydrochlorothiazide to a calcium-channel blocker (Answer D), and such a change would remove the protective effect of a thiazide diuretic on bone density. Adding an ACE inhibitor to an angiotensin receptor blocker (Answer B) is contraindicated given the increased risk of hyperkalemia and acute kidney injury. Clonidine (Answer C) has not been shown to reduce cardiovascular events in patients with diabetes, and its addition in this case would not provide further benefit. In addition to increasing her fall risk, the addition of amlodipine to achieve a lower blood pressure (Answer A) could also worsen her peripheral edema.

Educational Objective
Manage blood pressure in patients with diabetes mellitus.

UpToDate Topic Review(s)
Treatment of hypertension in patients with diabetes mellitus

Reference(s)

Adler AI, Stratton IM, Neil H, et al. Association of systolic blood pressure with macrovascular and microvascular complications of type 2 diabetes (UKPDS 36): prospective observational study. *BMJ*. 2000;321(7258):412-419. PMID: 10938049

Emdin CA, Rahimi K, Neal B, Callender T, Perkovic V, Patel A. Blood pressure lowering in type 2 diabetes: a systematic review and metaanalysis. *JAMA*. 2015;313(6):603-615. PMID: 25668264

Tinetti ME, Han L, Lee DS. et al. Antihypertensive medications and serious fall injuries in a nationally representative sample of older adults. *JAMA Intern Med*. 2014;174(4):588-595. PMID: 24567036

60 ANSWER: C) Albers-Schonberg disease, autosomal dominant osteopetrosis (gain-of-function mutation in the gene encoding a chloride channel [CLCN7])

This patient's increased bone density is due to osteopetrosis. Osteopetrosis refers to a group of disorders caused by impairment of osteoclast-mediated bone resorption. Two major clinical forms have been described. The first is the autosomal dominant adult (benign) type (so-called Albers-Schonberg disease) that is associated with increased bone mass and fractures often diagnosed in youth. The hereditary forms in humans are due to mutations in the gene encoding the osteoclast-specific subunit of the vacuolar proton pump (*TCIRG1*), loss-of-function mutations in the gene encoding chloride channel 7 (*CLCN7*), or rarely mutations in the gene encoding carbonic anhydrase II (*CA2*). The most common form is related to mutations in *CLCN7* (Answer C). This chloride channel is necessary for osteoclast acidification. All of these disorders lead to paralysis of the osteoclast and failed bone resorption. Because of impaired bone quality, affected patients experience fragility fractures despite increased bone density. Cranial nerve entrapment and impaired hematopoiesis due to compromised medullary space are also observed. Laboratory abnormalities include anemia, elevation in the brain isoenzyme of creatine kinase, lactate dehydrogenase isoenzymes, and aspartate transaminase levels, as well as increased acid phosphatase released from defective osteoclasts. Rarely, hypocalcemia and secondary hyperparathyroidism occur. This disorder has radiographic features of dense, sclerotic bones and a characteristic picture-frame appearance of vertebral bodies. Given the onset in his teens and his family history, this patient has the autosomal dominant form.

The second form of osteopetrosis is the autosomal recessive infantile (malignant) type that is typically fatal during infancy or early childhood if untreated (Answer B). This patient's age of onset and family history do not support an autosomal recessive form. Affected children present with recurrent infections. Spontaneous bruising and bleeding are common problems because of excessive bone in the marrow spaces. Hypersplenism and hemolysis may exacerbate severe anemia. Eruption of the dentition is delayed. There is compression of cranial nerves with blindness and deafness. Blindness can also be caused by retinal degeneration or raised intracranial pressure. Neurologic involvement is present in some patients, independent of nerve compression. Bones are dense on radiographic examination but are fragile. Untreated children usually die during the first decade of life as a result of hemorrhage, pneumonia, severe anemia, or sepsis. Bone marrow transplant is the main therapeutic option.

Another cause of increased bone density is an inherited gain-of-function mutation in the gene encoding the LDL receptor-related protein 5 (*LRP5*) (Answer A), also referred to as type 1 autosomal dominant osteopetrosis or Worth syndrome. This autosomal dominant disorder is associated with increased trabecular and cortical bone mass without an increased propensity for fracture. *LRP5*, along with *LRP6*, mediates canonical WNT signaling when complexed with frizzled receptors. WNT signaling functions in osteoblast-mediated bone formation. The typical skeletal phenotype includes a dense skull base, thickened cortices of long bones, wide jaw, and torus palatinus. Fragility fractures do not typically occur, and alkaline phosphatase levels are normal. Patients may also experience headaches, cranial nerve palsies, hearing loss, mandibular osteomyelitis, pseudotumor cerebri, and type 1 Chiari malformation from encroachment of thickened bone. Loss-of-function mutations in the *LRP5* gene cause osteoporosis-pseudoglioma syndrome, which is characterized by congenital blindness and extremely severe childhood-onset osteoporosis with fractures.

Tumor-induced osteomalacia (Answer D) is not associated with high bone mass but rather with bone loss. Severe hypophosphatemia with osteomalacia occurs as an acquired disorder in association with a tumor of mesenchymal origin. Tumor-induced osteomalacia, also called oncogenic hypophosphatemic osteomalacia, is due to the tumor production of fibroblast growth factor 23, which inhibits phosphate transport in renal epithelial cells and produces both hypophosphatemia and reduced calcitriol. Increased fibroblast growth factor 23 activity also occurs in patients with X-linked hypophosphatemia and autosomal dominant hypophosphatemic rickets.

Paget disease of bone (Answer E) is a derangement in bone metabolism that causes focal areas of sclerotic bone seen on radiographs. This disorder does not cause generalized increase in bone mass. Paget disease is caused by increased bone resorption resulting in focal areas of impaired bone quality with increased vascularity and an increased predisposition to fracture in affected areas. The average age at diagnosis is in the fifth decade of life with a slight predilection for men. Paget disease is rarely seen in persons younger than 40 years. Osteoclasts in pagetic bone are abnormal, with a bizarre appearance. They are multinucleated and are present in excessive numbers. This leads to abnormal deposition of lamellar bone that is characteristically described as mosaic in appearance. Most patients with Paget disease are asymptomatic and the diagnosis is made after an elevated alkaline phosphatase concentration is detected on routine laboratory evaluation or abnormalities are noted on radiographs. Paget disease can affect any bone, but it is most typically seen in the skull, spine, pelvis, and long bones.

Educational Objective
Determine the underlying etiology of adult-onset autosomal dominant osteopetrosis.

UpToDate Topic Review(s)
Skeletal dysplasias: specific disorders

Reference(s)
Whyte MP. Sclerosing bone disorders. In Favus MJ, ed. *Primer on the Metabolic Bone Diseases and Disorders of Mineral Metabolism*. 6th ed. Philadelphia, PA: Lippincott-Raven; 2006:398-414.

61 **ANSWER: D) Polycystic ovary syndrome**
This patient has polycystic ovary syndrome (Answer D). Polycystic ovary syndrome is the most common endocrinopathy in women of reproductive age, affecting 8% to 10% of this population. Her symptoms fulfill the Rotterdam criteria. She has irregular menstrual cycles and hyperandrogenism, as evidenced by both clinical symptoms (acne) and biochemical findings (elevated DHEA-S level). Other disorders causing irregular menstrual cycles are ruled out. These include hyperprolactinemia (prolactin level is normal), thyroid disease (TSH level is normal), and primary ovarian insufficiency (FSH level is normal). Disorders that cause hyperandrogenism are also excluded. A 17-hydroxyprogesterone level less than 200 ng/dL (<6.1 nmol/L) between 7 and 9 AM, when ACTH

peaks, is inconsistent with nonclassic congenital adrenal hyperplasia (Answer A). Cushing syndrome (Answer E) is unlikely because the patient does not appear to have other clinical features of excess cortisol production such as moonlike facies, hypertension, muscle wasting, or abdominal striae. Ovarian androgen-producing tumors (Answer B) present with profound phenotypic changes of virilization, such as deepening of the voice, clitoral enlargement, male-pattern balding, and male-pattern hirsutism developing over the course of months. In addition, testosterone levels are typically greater than 200 ng/dL (>6.9 nmol/L) in the setting of ovarian androgen-secreting tumors. Adrenal adenomas (Answer C) and carcinomas that secrete only androgens are rare and also present over a short timeframe with virilization, which is inconsistent with this patient's presentation.

Polycystic ovary syndrome presents less commonly with an isolated DHEA-S elevation than with elevated testosterone. Therefore, measuring DHEA-S may not be necessary if the patient has a long course inconsistent with an adrenal tumor, or if the patient has an elevated testosterone level or clinical hyperandrogenism. Some guidelines also suggest that elevated DHEA-S is unlikely to change management. Elevated DHEA-S has been reported in 10% of women with polycystic ovary syndrome. The DHEA-S level is inversely related to BMI and age, and would therefore more likely be high in a young, thin patient. Elevated DHEA-S is not caused by increased activity of the hypothalamic-pituitary-adrenal axis. Rather, it is thought to be caused by primary increased output from the steroidogenic cells. Distinguishing polycystic ovary syndrome with an elevated DHEA-S level from an adrenal adenoma or carcinoma should not be difficult because symptoms are less severe and develop over years as opposed to months. In addition, the DHEA-S levels would be expected to be higher (for example, >700 µg/dL [>19.0 µmol/L]) in the setting of adrenal adenoma or carcinoma. However, not all tumors will sulfate DHEA and levels are not always high. Measurement of 24-hour urinary 17-ketosteroid excretion may better identify adrenal adenomas and carcinomas in patients with concerning symptoms because it captures DHEA, estrone, and androstenedione, which are primarily produced by the adrenal gland.

Educational Objective
Diagnose polycystic ovary syndrome and adrenal hyperandrogenism.

UpToDate Topic Review(s)
Diagnosis of polycystic ovary syndrome in adults

Reference(s)

Kumar A, Woods KS, Bartolucci AA, Azziz R. Prevalence of adrenal androgen excess in patients with the polycystic ovary syndrome (PCOS). *Clin Endocrinol (Oxf)*. 2005;62(6):644-649. PMID: 15943823

Cordera F, Grant C, van Heerden J, Thompson G, Young W. Androgen-secreting adrenal tumors. *Surgery*. 2003;134(6):874-880. PMID: 14668717

Rotterdam ESHRE/ASRM-Sponsored PCOS consensus workshop group. Revised 2003 consensus on diagnostic criteria and long-term health risks related to polycystic ovary syndrome (PCOS). *Hum Reprod*. 2004;19(1):41-47. PMID: 14688154

62 ANSWER: D) Oral contraceptive use

Hypertriglyceridemia is often associated with disorders that independently increase plasma triglyceride concentrations, such as type 2 diabetes, obesity, excessive alcohol consumption, hypothyroidism, or concomitant use of certain drugs. When one or more of these factors is present, hypertriglyceridemia is termed secondary. However, secondary hypertriglyceridemia often has an underlying genetic component. This implies that persons who develop very high triglyceride levels often have inherited defects that confer susceptibility, which becomes clinically expressed in the presence of an external (secondary) stress. Establishing whether there is a strong secondary factor underlying dyslipidemia is important because this knowledge guides intervention.

Addition of specific drugs can result in triglyceride elevations. Oral estrogens such as ethinyl estradiol, usually prescribed with progestogen as oral contraceptives (Answer D), increase the production rate of apolipoprotein B–containing lipoproteins. Estrogen stimulates hepatic triglyceride synthesis and decreases hepatic lipase and lipoprotein lipase activity, which can raise triglyceride levels. In women with normal baseline triglycerides, oral estrogen therapy increases triglycerides by about 10 to 15 mg/dL (0.11 to 0.17 mmol/L). In the setting of a genetic defect, marked hypertriglyceridemia and possibly pancreatitis can ensue. These effects are not seen with use of transdermal estrogen. This patient's family history is suggestive of a strong genetic component, and oral contraceptive use is the most likely factor contributing to her hypertriglyceridemia. Continued use of oral contraceptives should be reconsidered in this patient.

Polycystic ovary syndrome (Answer A) is a condition that is associated with various metabolic dysregulation, including insulin resistance, hypertriglyceridemia, and low HDL cholesterol. However, the degree of triglyceride elevation seen in polycystic ovary syndrome is typically less than that observed in this patient.

Abdominal obesity (Answer B) is associated with modestly increased triglyceride levels and decreased HDL-cholesterol levels, which are features of the metabolic syndrome. Underlying insulin resistance is a likely contributor to the dyslipidemia. The degree of triglyceride elevation in this case is beyond that expected for obesity alone, and instead suggests that there is an underlying genetic component, although her obesity may well be a contributor.

Alcohol overuse (Answer C) increases hepatic VLDL triglyceride synthesis in obese individuals. However, there is no indication of excessive use of alcohol in this patient.

Lipid abnormalities in hypothyroidism (Answer E) can be manifested as hypercholesterolemia, hypertriglyceridemia, or a mixed pattern. A decrease in lipoprotein lipase activity is found in overt hypothyroidism, decreasing the clearance of triglyceride-rich lipoproteins. Therefore, patients with overt hypothyroidism may also present with elevated triglyceride levels associated with increased levels of VLDL and occasionally fasting chylomicronemia. A TSH value of 5.2 mIU/L is mildly abnormal and could be classified as subclinical hypothyroidism, a setting in which most patients have normal lipid levels.

Educational Objective
Identify contributing factors to secondary hypertriglyceridemia in a young woman.

UpToDate Topic Review(s)
Hypertriglyceridemia

Reference(s)
Berglund L, Brunzell JD, Goldberg AC, et al; Endocrine Society. Evaluation and treatment of hypertriglyceridemia: an Endocrine Society clinical practice guideline. *J Clin Endocrinol Metab*. 2012;97(9):2969-2989. PMID: 22962670

63 ANSWER: E) Initiate a bisphosphonate drug holiday and reassess DXA and clinical parameters in 1 to 2 years

Despite the significant benefits of bisphosphonates in reducing risk of vertebral, hip, and nonvertebral fractures, serious complications such as osteonecrosis of the jaw and atypical femoral fractures have been reported with their use. These adverse effects are most likely associated with cumulative intake of these drugs. The overall risk of medication-related osteonecrosis of the jaw is low (0.38-21 cases per 10,000 patients), as is the risk of medication-related atypical femoral fractures (3.2-50 cases/100,000 person-years). However, these are serious, harmful complications, and drug holidays should be considered in the appropriate clinical setting. The American Association of Clinical Endocrinologists' guidelines indicate that a drug holiday is reasonable after 4 to 5 years of bisphosphonate therapy in patients at moderate risk of fractures and after 10 years for patients at high risk, but the guidelines do not define these risk groups. The National Osteoporosis Guideline Group recommends a drug holiday for patients who have no personal fracture history, have a low FRAX risk of fracture, and have a hip T score greater than –2.5. The American Society for Bone and Mineral Research task force developed the following guidelines for postmenopausal women treated with oral bisphosphonates for 5 or more years or with intravenous bisphosphonates for 3 or more years:

- If the patient sustained any insufficiency-related fractures before or during therapy, the provider should reassess the benefits and risks and consider continuing the bisphosphonate or changing to alternative therapy.

- If there is no personal history of insufficiency-related fracture but the patient has a low hip T score less than –2.5 or a high fracture risk, the provider should consider continuing the bisphosphonate for up to 10 years or changing to alternative therapy.

- If there is no personal history of insufficiency-related fracture and the patient has a hip T score greater than −2.5 or is not at high fracture risk, a drug holiday should be considered with reassessment every 2 to 3 years (Answer E).

There is no consensus on how long to maintain a drug holiday, and the recommendation is to continue monitoring at appropriate intervals for risk factors or bone loss.

This patient has never sustained a fracture, has a hip T score of −2.3, and has been on bisphosphonate therapy for more than 10 years; thus, there is no indication to change to a different medical therapy (Answers A, B, and C). Additionally, teriparatide is not recommended in a patient with a history of irradiation to the skeleton (chest wall in this case) due to the potential risk of osteosarcoma. Given the lack of high-risk features for fractures, there is no reason to continue alendronate (Answer D).

In patients who have been on long-term bisphosphonate therapy, a complete physical examination should include an oral exam to assess for gingival health and exposed bone (especially in patients who smoke cigarettes). The patient should also be asked about lateral thigh pain, which could be a prodrome for atypical femoral fracture. Before initiating a drug holiday, the clinician should obtain vertebral imaging to exclude the presence of recent subclinical fractures that would preclude the initiation of a drug holiday. Bone turnover marker assessment may be informative in determining when medication should be restarted; ongoing studies are evaluating the utility of assessing bone turnover markers in this setting.

Educational Objective
Implement a bisphosphonate drug holiday after 10 years of use in a postmenopausal woman if there are no high-risk features present.

UpToDate Topic Review(s)
The use of bisphosphonates in postmenopausal women with osteoporosis

Reference(s)

Adler RA, El-Haij Fuleihan G, Bauer DC, et al. Managing osteoporosis in patients on long-term bisphosphonate treatment: report of a task force of the American Society for Bone and Mineral Research. *J Bone Miner Res.* 2016;31(1):16-35. PMID: 26350171

Compston J, Bowring C, Cooper A, et al; National Osteoporosis Guideline Group. Diagnosis and management of osteoporosis in postmenopausal women and older men in the UK: National Osteoporosis Guideline Group (NOGG) update 2013 [published corrections appear in *Maturitas.* 2013;76(4):387 and *Maturitas.* 2014;77(2):195]. *Maturitas.* 2013;75(4):392-396. PMID: 23810490

Reid IR. Short-term and long-term effects of osteoporosis therapies. *Nat Rev Endocrinol.* 2015;11(7):418-428. PMID: 25963272

Watts NB, Bilezikian JP, Camacho PM, et al. American Association of Clinical Endocrinologists medical guidelines for clinical practice for the diagnosis and treatment of postmenopausal osteoporosis: executive summary of recommendations. *Endocr Pract.* 2010;16(6):1016-1019. PMID: 21216723

64 ANSWER: D) Reduced lifespan of red blood cells due to hemolysis caused by his stenotic aortic valve

Although hemoglobin A_{1c} measurement is an excellent marker of overall glycemic control, the test has several pitfalls. The relative accuracy of hemoglobin A_{1c} measurement vs other methods to assess glycemic control, such as fructosamine measurement or continuous glucose monitoring, is commonly called the "glycation gap." Any condition that shortens the lifespan of erythrocytes or that causes increased red blood cell turnover falsely lowers hemoglobin A_{1c} and widens the glycation gap. This is due to a shortened time that the erythrocyte is exposed to glucose. Intravascular hemolysis occurs when the erythrocyte crosses a stenotic aortic valve. The mechanism is thought to be due to shear stress. Thus, aortic stenosis in a native valve has the capacity to falsely lower hemoglobin A_{1c} (Answer D). Other conditions that are associated with falsely increased or decreased hemoglobin A_{1c} values are shown (*see table*).

Although heart surgery can transiently increase glucose in the immediate postoperative period (Answer A), glucose levels generally return to preoperative levels by the second postoperative day following routine cardiac surgery. The use of salicylates and opioids can falsely increase, not decrease, hemoglobin A_{1c} (Answer B). While nonadherence to his diabetes regimen (Answer C) may explain a transient loss of diabetes control, it does not explain his postoperative glucose value of 250 mg/dL after 2 days of therapy with intravenous insulin. Although vasopressor medications used in the immediate postoperative period (eg, norepinephrine, vasopressin, etc) can suppress β-cell function, there is no evidence that cardiac surgery per se (Answer E) has an adverse effect on β-cell function.

Conditions That Falsely Increase or Decrease Hemoglobin A₁c

Condition	Effect on Hemoglobin A₁c	Mechanism
Red cell transfusion	↑ or ↓	High glucose in storage medium increases hemoglobin A₁c; dilution effect decreases hemoglobin A₁c
Hemoglobin variants	↑ or ↓	Reduced red blood cell lifespan decreases hemoglobin A₁c; interference with assay increases or decreases hemoglobin A₁c
Pregnancy	↓	Decreased red blood cell lifespan
Uremia	↓	Decreased red blood cell lifespan
Aortic stenosis	↓	Turbulence across valve shears red blood cells, reduced lifespan
Vitamin E, ribavirin, interferon alfa	↓	Reduced glycation, hemolysis
Splenomegaly	↓	Decreased red blood cell lifespan
Anemia from acute or chronic blood loss	↓	Increased red blood cell production
Chronic opioid ingestion	↑	Mechanism uncertain
Chronic salicylate ingestion	↑	Possible assay interference
Chronic EtOH ingestion	↑	Formation of acetaldehyde-hemoglobin A1
Iron, B₁₂, folate deficiency	↑	Increased red blood cell lifespan
Asplenia	↑	Increased red blood cell lifespan

Educational Objective

Identify factors that may falsely increase or decrease hemoglobin A₁c values.

UpToDate Topic Review(s)

Estimation of blood glucose control in diabetes mellitus

Reference(s)

Radin MS. Pitfalls in hemoglobin A1c measurement: when results may be misleading. *J Gen intern Med.* 2014;29(2):388-394. PMID: 24002631

Sugiura T, Okumiya T, Kubo T, Takeuchi H, Matsumura Y. Evaluation of intravascular hemolysis with erythrocyte creatine in patients with aortic stenosis. *Int Heart J.* 2016;57(4):430-433. PMID: 27357437

Nayak AU, Holland MR, Macdonald DR, Nevill A, Singh BM. Evidence of consistency of the glycation gap in diabetes. Diabetes Care. 2011;34(8):1712-1716. PMID: 21715524

Furnary AP, Zerr KJ, Grunkemeier GL, Starr A. Continuous intravenous insulin infusion reduces the incidence of deep sternal wound infection in diabetic patients after cardiac surgical procedures. *Ann Thoracic Surg.* 1999;67(2):352-360. PMID: 10197653

65 **ANSWER: C) Measure 24-hour urinary free cortisol**

While this young patient with modest weight gain, hypertension, and impaired glucose tolerance has no pathognomonic clinical signs of Cushing syndrome, screening for cortisol excess was justified. However, clinical suspicion is low given the absence of significant striae, thin bruised skin, or proximal myopathy. It is, therefore, surprising that the overnight dexamethasone suppression test result is suggestive of cortisol excess. In normal individuals, early-morning plasma cortisol should suppress to less than 1.8 μg/dL (<50 nmol/L) after 1 mg of dexamethasone is administered between 11 PM and midnight the night before. In this case, the abnormal result merits additional evaluation. Given the low clinical suspicion, additional biochemical screening tests should be performed before further investigation and imaging to determine the underlying cause of cortisol excess. Imaging studies (Answers A and B) would be premature before confirmation of hypercortisolism.

The Endocrine Society Clinical Practice Guideline for the diagnosis of Cushing syndrome suggests a number of first-line tests in the initial screening for cortisol excess: the 1-mg overnight dexamethasone suppression test, 2-day low-dose dexamethasone suppression test, late-night salivary cortisol measurement, or 24-hour urinary free cortisol measurement. Given that this patient has an abnormal result from one test (1-mg overnight dexamethasone suppression test), as well as minimal clinical evidence of cortisol excess, another test to confirm or dispute this result is warranted.

This patient is taking carbamazepine, which is known induce hepatic CYP3A4 enzymes that increase the metabolism of dexamethasone and potentially lead to a false-positive result. Therefore, any further screening test that uses dexamethasone (eg, low-dose dexamethasone suppression test [Answer D]) would be similarly affected. Other inducers of hepatic CYP3A4 that can cause false-positive results in this setting include mitotane, rifampicin, barbiturates, and phenytoin. Lamotrigine does not affect dexamethasone metabolism in this way, so repeating the test after stopping lamotrigine (Answer E) would not be helpful. Moreover, it is inadvisable to stop an anticonvulsant medication without consulting the patient's neurologist.

Measurement of 24-hour urinary cortisol excretion (Answer C) provides a direct and robust index of cortisol secretion and is unaffected by concomitant medication. It is therefore the most sensible next test to exclude cortisol excess in this patient who is unable to undergo dexamethasone suppression testing. Late-night salivary cortisol measurement would also be useful, but it is not offered as an answer choice.

Educational Objective
Select appropriate screening tests for cortisol excess and describe the potential for concomitant medication to interfere with dexamethasone.

UpToDate Topic Review(s)
Establishing the diagnosis of Cushing's syndrome

Reference(s)

Nieman LK, Biller BM, Findling JW, et al. The diagnosis of Cushing's syndrome: an Endocrine Society Clinical Practice Guideline. *J Clin Endocrinol Metab.* 2008;93(5):1526-1540. PMID: 18334580

Ma RC, Chan WB, So WY, Tong PC, Chan JC, Chow CC. Carbamazepine and false positive dexamethasone suppression tests for Cushing's syndrome. *BMJ.* 2005;330:(7486):299-300. PMID: 15695278

66 ANSWER: A) LH, ↓; testosterone, ↓; TSH ↓; free T$_4$↓

Iron overload (due to multiple blood transfusions or hereditary hemochromatosis) can result in excessive iron deposition in multiple endocrine tissues including the pituitary, thyroid, pancreas, and gonads, leading to cellular damage and endocrine failure. The key to understanding this question is in recalling the relative frequency of various forms of endocrine dysfunction seen in iron overload.

Diabetes mellitus is the most common endocrine complication in this setting and is described in 50% of individuals with hemochromatosis. Indeed, this patient has an elevated random plasma glucose value, which is suggestive of diabetes mellitus but this requires confirmation. Pituitary dysfunction is described in approximately one-third of cases. Iron accumulation is mostly in the anterior pituitary; involvement of the posterior pituitary is rare. Secondary hypogonadism is the next most common endocrine abnormality in hereditary hemochromatosis, causing decreased libido and impotence in men. Other pituitary deficiencies may occur but more rarely. Primary hypogonadism, presumably due to testicular iron deposition, can also occur but this is much less common.

The clinical picture in this vignette is most consistent with gonadal failure (thus, Answer D [normal gonadal function] is incorrect). The patient's testicular volume is currently normal due to the relatively recent onset of gonadal failure, and he was able to undergo puberty. For reasons outlined above, secondary hypogonadism as depicted by the hormonal pattern in Answers A or C is more likely than primary hypogonadism as depicted in Answers B or E.

This patient has clinical evidence of hypothyroidism. Both primary and secondary hypothyroidism, have been described in hemochromatosis and other disorders of iron overload. Secondary thyroid dysfunction due to pituitary infiltration is more common (Answers A or B).

In summary, this man presents with clinical evidence of hypogonadism and hypothyroidism. Given that these conditions probably developed because of pituitary iron overload, the most likely biochemical findings are secondary gonadal and thyroid deficiencies, which are shown only in Answer A.

Educational Objective

Identify the usual pattern of pituitary hormone loss in iron overload syndromes such as hemochromatosis or transfusion-dependent anemia.

UpToDate Topic Review(s)

Clinical manifestations and diagnosis of hereditary hemochromatosis

Reference(s)

Walton C, Kelly WF, Laing I, Bu'lock DE. Endocrine abnormalities in idiopathic haemochromatosis. *Q J Med*. 1983;52(205):99-110. PMID: 6683854

Kelly TM, Edwards CQ, Meikle AW, Kushner JP. Hypogonadism in hemochromatosis: reversal with iron depletion. *Ann Intern Med*. 1984;101(5):629-632. PMID: 6435491

Livadas DP, Sofroniadou K, Souvatzoglou A, Boukis M, Siafaka L, Koutras DA. Pituitary and thyroid insufficiency in thalassaemic haemosiderosis. *Clin Endocrinol (Oxf)*. 1984;20(4):435-443. PMID: 6424975

67 ANSWER: B) Undergo comprehensive nutritional evaluation and continue postbariatric micronutrient replacement with an added prenatal vitamin

Approximately 80% of patients who undergo bariatric surgery are women and 50% of these women are of childbearing age. Patients who consider pregnancy after bariatric surgery present a distinct set of challenges and require a management plan tailored to individual needs. Thus, usual prenatal care (Answer E) may be inadequate.

A consensus statement published in 2013 recommends a comprehensive postoperative nutritional assessment after Roux-en-Y gastric bypass surgery, which includes iron studies and measurement of vitamin B_{12}, folic acid, 25-hydroxyvitamin D, PTH, vitamin A, copper, zinc, selenium, and thiamine. The consensus statement also recommends nutritional surveillance and screening during pregnancy (each trimester), which includes iron studies and measurement of folic acid, vitamin B_{12}, calcium, and fat-soluble vitamins. Expert opinion suggests that women considering pregnancy after bariatric surgery switch from a multivitamin to a prenatal vitamin and continue to take any previously prescribed micronutrient supplementation. Further titration of dosages can be undertaken on the basis of test results. Thus, the best recommendation for this patient is summarized in Answer B.

This patient has a history of gestational diabetes. Although her weight loss after bariatric surgery reduces her risk for gestational diabetes and preeclampsia in future pregnancies, she should still be monitored. Screening for diabetes is important as soon as pregnancy is confirmed. In this patient population, hemoglobin A_{1c} measurement may be the preferred method to screen for pregestational diabetes because patients who undergo Roux-en-Y bypass often do not tolerate oral glucose tolerance testing (Answer C). For this reason, some providers avoid this method of assessment, even during pregnancy, and prefer to rely on blood glucose trends and averages.

Metformin (Answer D) has been shown to prevent gestational diabetes in women with polycystic ovary syndrome who had gestational diabetes in a previous pregnancy. However, the ability of metformin to prevent gestational diabetes in future pregnancies in women without polycystic ovary syndrome is unclear. An ongoing clinical trial in the United Kingdom (PRoDroME) is investigating this question.

The consensus statement published in 2013 recommends that women who undergo bariatric surgery delay pregnancy for 12 to 18 months after the operation, although the evidence to support this recommendation is poor. While there is concern about inadequate absorption and theoretically decreased effectiveness of oral contraceptive pills in this patient population, a systematic review did not demonstrate decreased effectiveness. Therefore, an oral contraceptive pill may be a reasonable option if she chooses to delay pregnancy. Pregnancy, however, is not contraindicated after bariatric surgery (thus, Answer A is incorrect).

In obese women, weight loss before pregnancy improves a number of infant and maternal outcomes such as macrosomia, maternal hypertension and gestational diabetes, and rates of cesarean delivery, etc. However, there is some concern for increased risk of small-for-gestational-age infants in woman who have lost a clinically significant amount of weight before conception (which includes women who have undergone bariatric surgery). More data are needed to determine whether the rates of small-for-gestational-age infants are higher than in the general population and how the degree and timing of weight loss are associated with this increased risk.

Educational Objective

Make recommendations regarding the management of pregnancy after bariatric surgery.

UpToDate Topic Review(s)
Fertility and pregnancy after bariatric surgery

Reference(s)

Kominiarek MA. Preparing for and managing a pregnancy after bariatric surgery. *Semin Perinatol.* 2011;35(6):356-361. PMID: 22108087

Mechanick JI, Youdim A, Jones DB, et al; American Association of Clinical Endocrinologists; Obesity Society; American Society for Metabolic & Bariatric Surgery. Clinical practice guidelines for the perioperative nutritional, metabolic, and nonsurgical support of the bariatric surgery patient—2013 update: cosponsored by American Association of Clinical Endocrinologists, The Obesity Society, and American Society for Metabolic & Bariatric Surgery. *Obesity (Silver Spring).* 2013;21(Suppl 1):S1-S27. PMID: 23529939

68 ANSWER: C) Perform an ACTH stimulation test

Diabetes insipidus that is not related to recent pituitary surgery does not resolve. Therefore, in this patient, the resolution of polydipsia and polyuria must have another explanation. Adrenal insufficiency can mask diabetes insipidus by reducing the glomerular filtration rate and possibly slowing the catabolism of vasopressin. Indeed, in patients with hypopituitarism and diabetes insipidus, polyuria and polydipsia may manifest only after glucocorticoid replacement therapy is instituted.

Serum and urinary sodium measurement (Answer A) would not help determine the diagnosis. Serum sodium is often normal in patients with diabetes insipidus who have an intact thirst mechanism and access to water. In general, urinary sodium measurement is not helpful in the diagnosis of diabetes insipidus. Furthermore, in this case the polyuria resolved. Vasopressin measurement (Answer B) is often not reliable and rarely assists in the workup of diabetes insipidus. A formal water deprivation test (Answer D) is not needed, as the patient already had a diagnosis of diabetes insipidus, and at present he no longer has polyuria. Desmopressin will most likely need to be re-started (Answer E) after glucocorticoid replacement therapy is initiated, but at this point it is not needed. The most important issue now is to determine why his diabetes insipidus has resolved and whether he has developed adrenal insufficiency. This can be accomplished with an ACTH stimulation test (Answer C) or morning cortisol and ACTH measurement. The diagnosis is very important to make, particularly in view of his upcoming hernia repair, for which he would need stress dose steroids. This patient turned out to have developed secondary adrenal insufficiency. Biopsy of the stalk mass documented a germinoma.

Other causes of reduced urination (such as renal damage) should be considered, but this would be unlikely in this case, as the patient had noted reduced urination for several weeks.

Educational Objective
Explain how adrenal insufficiency can mask diabetes insipidus.

UpToDate Topic Review(s)
Diagnosis of adrenal insufficiency in adults

Reference(s)

Ahmed ABJ, George BC, Gonzalez-auvert C, Dingman JF. Increased plasma arginine vasopressin in clinical adrenocortical insufficiency and its inhibition by glucosteroids. *J Clin Invest.* 1967;46:111-123. PMID: 6018744

Non L, Brito D, Anastasopoulou C. Neurosarcoidosis-associated central diabetes insipidus masked by adrenal insufficiency. *BMJ Case Rep.* 2015;2015. pii: bcr2014206390. PMID: 25612752

69 ANSWER: E) Y-chromosome microdeletion testing

Infertility may be defined as failure to achieve a clinical pregnancy after 12 months or more of regular, unprotected sexual intercourse. Male infertility is a complex condition; more than 2000 genes have been associated with normal spermatogenesis. The cause of male-factor infertility is identified in only 20% to 30% of cases. Therefore, most cases of male-factor infertility are considered idiopathic.

Normal spermatogenesis requires the presence of certain genes within the azoospermia factor (AZF) regions (AZFa, AZFb, and AZFc) on the Y chromosome. The Y chromosome contains 8 palindromic sequences that replicate through intrapalindromic homologous arm-to-arm recombination. Y-chromosome microdeletions result from errors in this recombination. Ordering Y-chromosome microdeletion testing (Answer E) is the best next step in this patient's evaluation, as 10% of men with nonobstructive azoospermia and 5% of men with severe oligospermia have Y-chromosome microdeletions. Andrology and urology organizations recommend Y-chromosome microdeletion testing in men with a total motile sperm count of less than 5 or 10 million. Depending on the degree of the oligospermia, some men with Y-chromosome microdeletions father children naturally, but many require assisted reproductive technologies such as intracytoplasmic sperm injection. Men found to have Y-chromosome microdeletions should be offered genetic counseling, as the deletions will be passed to male offspring.

Chromosome aneuploidy analysis (Answer A) uses fluorescent in situ hybridization to evaluate for the presence of aberrant numbers of chromosomes. This test is not advisable as a screening tool due to the low rates of sperm chromosome aneuploidy, as well as the high cost.

DNA fragmentation analysis (Answer B) is a technique to assess spermatozoa for single- and double-strand DNA breaks. Although DNA fragmentation is often higher in subfertile men, controversies exist regarding its predictive value for fertility or outcomes with assisted reproductive techniques.

Fructose is produced in the seminal vesicles and provides energy for sperm. The absence of fructose in semen would signify a lack of seminal vesicles or an obstruction of the vas deferens. Semen fructose measurement (Answer C) would not yield helpful information in a man with palpable vas deferens and 4 million mobile sperm on semen analysis.

Testicular biopsy (Answer D) is incorrect because less invasive testing would be advised first.

Educational Objective
Appropriately recommend Y-chromosome microdeletion testing in men with infertility.

UpToDate Topic Review(s)
Evaluation of male infertility

Reference(s)

Hamilton JA, Cissen M, Brandes M, et al. Total motile sperm count: a better indicator for the severity of male factor infertility than the WHO sperm classification system. *Hum Reprod*. 2015;30(5):1110-1121. PMID: 25788568

Hotaling J, Carrell DT. Clinical genetic testing for male factor infertility: current applications and future directions. *Andrology*. 2014;2(3):339-350. PMID: 24711280

Hotaling JM. Genetics of male infertility. *Urol Clin North Am*. 2014;41(1):1-17. PMID: 24286764

70 ANSWER: C) Initiate a continuous glucose monitor

Hypoglycemic unawareness is a common problem in patients with tightly controlled type 1 diabetes mellitus and is a major risk factor for severe hypoglycemia requiring assistance. Recurrent hypoglycemia reduces the normal counterregulatory hormone response of glucagon and epinephrine secretion to low glucose levels, and decreases hypoglycemia awareness. Antecedent hypoglycemia was identified in the Diabetes Control and Complications Trial as the most common predictor of a future severe hypoglycemic event.

While this patient's hemoglobin A_{1c} level has run consistently in a good range, favorable mean glucose levels are occurring at the expense of recurrent hypoglycemia. Prevention of future severe hypoglycemia, a potentially life-threatening complication of insulin therapy, should be the primary concern at the time of this visit. Strict avoidance of hypoglycemia for periods as short as 3 days improves hypoglycemia awareness for up to 3 months and reduces the risk of future hypoglycemia, and it is therefore one treatment option at this juncture.

Continuous glucose monitors (Answer C) should be considered for patients with persistent hypoglycemia unawareness, given this tool's potential to alert patients to unrecognized hypoglycemia. Continuous glucose monitors have been shown to lower hemoglobin A_{1c} levels in adults and children with type 1 diabetes and to reduce the frequency of severe hypoglycemia among adult patients with hypoglycemia unawareness. A hybrid continuous glucose monitor and insulin pump device is now available that communicates with and automatically suspends the basal insulin infusion when the glucose level is low and unrecognized. Use of this device reduces the amount of time spent in hypoglycemia overnight. Initiating a continuous glucose monitor would be expected to reduce this patient's risk of a severe hypoglycemic reaction in the future.

Excessive insulin dosing to correct high glucose levels can lead to hypoglycemia. A change in this patient's insulin sensitivity factor from 40 (1 unit of glulisine to lower glucose 40 mg/dL [2.2 mmol/L]) to 20 (1 unit of glulisine to lower glucose 20 mg/dL [1.1 mmol/L]) (Answer A) would double the amount of insulin given to correct high glucose levels and would increase the risk of hypoglycemia.

In the setting of set premeal insulin glulisine doses, this patient's low glucose variability suggests that he is successfully maintaining similar carbohydrate content in his meals from day to day. A change to carbohydrate counting (Answer B) would not be expected to reduce his risk of hypoglycemia. If he were commonly eating meals with different amounts of carbohydrates, adjustment of his insulin glulisine bolus based on the calculated carbohydrate content of the meal would reduce glucose variability and rates of postprandial hypoglycemia.

In adults, studies comparing continuous subcutaneous insulin infusion (insulin pumps) with basal insulin analogue glargine and lispro-based multiple daily injection regimens show small reductions in hemoglobin A_{1c} with insulin pumps (Answer D), but not in total or severe hypoglycemia. In these studies, fasting glucose levels are similar in the 2 groups as a result of insulin titration protocols that target a fasting glucose goal.

Insulin degludec is a basal insulin with a considerably longer duration of action and lower pharmacodynamic variability than either insulin glargine or insulin detemir. Studies comparing these basal insulins in patients with type 1 diabetes have shown similar control of hemoglobin A_{1c}, but less nocturnal hypoglycemia with insulin degludec than with insulin glargine or insulin detemir. A change from degludec to detemir (Answer E) would not be expected to reduce rates of severe hypoglycemia.

In this vignette, the severe hypoglycemia occurred after a day of increased physical activity, which is known to enhance insulin sensitivity and lower glucose levels. Although not listed as an option here, increasing carbohydrate intake or lowering insulin doses before or during exercise also reduce the likelihood of hypoglycemia.

Educational Objective
Recommend interventions to reduce the occurrence of severe hypoglycemia in patients with type 1 diabetes mellitus.

UpToDate Topic Review(s)
Management of hypoglycemia during treatment of diabetes mellitus

Reference(s)

Dagogo-Jack S, Rattarasarn C, Cryer PE. Reversal of hypoglycemia unawareness, but not defective glucose counter regulation, in IDDM. *Diabetes.* 1994;43(12):1426-1434. PMID: 7958494

Yeh HC, Brown TT, Maruthur N, et al. Comparative effectiveness and safety of methods of insulin delivery and glucose monitoring for diabetes mellitus: a systematic review and meta-analysis. *Ann Intern Med.* 2012;157(5):336-347. PMID: 22777524

Choudhary P, Ramasamy S, Green L, et al. Real-time continuous glucose monitoring significantly reduces severe hypoglycemia in hypoglycemia-unaware patients with type 1 diabetes. *Diabetes Care.* 2013;36(12):4160-4162. PMID: 24103902

Bergenstal RM, Klonoff DC, et al; ASPIRE In-Home Study Group. Threshold-based insulin-pump interruption for reduction of hypoglycemia. *N Engl J Med.* 2013;369(3):224-232. PMID: 23789889

71 **ANSWER: E) Periodic monitoring of the patient's thyroid nodules and serum TSH**
Historically, radiation therapy was used to treat benign conditions such as thymic abnormalities, tinea capitis, adenoid or tonsillar hypertrophy, and acne. While this is no longer acceptable therapy because of the risks, radiation therapy is still used for childhood cancers such as lymphoma, neuroblastoma, Wilms tumor, and acute lymphoblastic leukemia.

The thyroid is one of the most radiation-sensitive tissues in the body. The risk of subsequent thyroid problems is inversely related to the patient's age and directly related to the radiation dose. This patient received radiation therapy to the neck at a young age. She is therefore at increased risk of developing hypothyroidism, thyroid nodules, and thyroid cancer. The risk of thyroid cancer is greatest in those who were exposed to radiation therapy before age 15 years. One study evaluated individuals who had received a median dose of 3500 cGy for treatment of Hodgkin lymphoma and were a median age of 14 years at diagnosis and a median age of 30 years at follow-up. Compared with sibling controls, the relative risk of hypothyroidism was 17.1 and the relative risk of thyroid nodules was 27. The radiated individuals also had an observed rate of thyroid cancer that was 18-fold greater than that expected, using the SEER database as the comparator. In another study of children up to age 14 years, the standardized incidence ratio for thyroid cancer was 52 with 6.5 years of follow-up.

The thyroid cancer histologies associated with radiation therapy for Hodgkin lymphoma are usually papillary and follicular histologies, not medullary thyroid cancer. There is lack of agreement about when calcitonin should be measured as part of the evaluation of thyroid nodules. One study found that medullary thyroid cancer was identified by a screening calcitonin measurement in 0.44% of patients. The American Thyroid Association guidelines for the management of thyroid nodules recommends neither for nor against routine calcitonin measurement. Measurement of calcitonin (Answer C) could be considered for patients who have nodules with suspicious cytology that does not appear to be consistent with papillary cancer. This is not the situation in this vignette.

This patient underwent FNAB of her hypoechoic nodule measuring 1.6 × 2.0 × 1.3 cm. The likelihood of malignancy in a nodule with adequate sampling that is read as cytologically benign is 1% to 3%. The clinical characteristics of benign and malignant radiation-induced thyroid nodules do not seem to be different from those in non–radiation-exposed individuals, and the performance and accuracy of FNAB seem to be similar in the 2 populations. Given the benign cytology, this patient's thyroid nodules can be followed (Answer E), rather than proceeding with either thyroidectomy (Answer A) or lobectomy (Answer D). FNAB of subcentimeter nodules is generally not recommended. This patient, however, did undergo such a biopsy with cytologic findings consistent with Hashimoto thyroiditis, which fits with the patient's positive TPO antibody titers.

This patient is at considerable risk of developing hypothyroidism based on her radiation exposure and positive TPO antibody titer. Hypothyroidism usually develops at a mean of 7 years after the diagnosis of Hodgkin lymphoma, and it is more likely to occur in women and in those who received higher radiation doses. Development of TPO antibodies is variably associated with radiation exposure. This patient is currently euthyroid despite her positive TPO antibodies. Although she may need to be treated with levothyroxine in the future to maintain a normal serum TSH level, there is no clear need to initiate levothyroxine now given that her TSH is currently normal. TSH suppression therapy (Answer B), using levothyroxine to lower TSH levels below the normal range to avoid potential stimulation of thyroid nodules, has variable effectiveness and carries potential cardiac and skeletal risks. It is therefore not recommended.

This patient does require periodic monitoring of her TSH levels and thyroid nodules. There are no specific guidelines regarding the frequency of monitoring a patient such as this one, but initial annual monitoring, with decreased frequency if stability is seen, might be reasonable. She is at risk of developing hypothyroidism; the risk of developing hypothyroidism 20 years after a diagnosis of Hodgkin lymphoma is 30% to 50%. She also needs follow-up by physical examination and thyroid ultrasonography to monitor the size and characteristics of her thyroid nodules. In one study of a cohort of patients with Hodgkin lymphoma, the median time to develop thyroid cancer was 15.5 years with a range of 5 to 26 years.

Educational Objective
Determine the appropriate management of thyroid disorders in an individual who has received radiation therapy to the neck.

UpToDate Topic Review(s)
Radiation-induced thyroid cancer

Reference(s)

Haugen BR, Alexander EK, Bible KC, et al. 2015 American Thyroid Association Management Guidelines for Adult Patients with Thyroid Nodules and Differentiated Thyroid Cancer: the American Thyroid Association Guidelines Task Force on Thyroid Nodules and Differentiated Thyroid Cancer. *Thyroid*. 2016;26(1):1-133. PMID: 26462967

Maule M, Scelo G, Pastore G, et al. Risk of second malignant neoplasms after childhood leukemia and lymphoma: an international study. *J Natl Cancer Inst*. 2007;99(10):790-800. PMID: 17505074

Sklar C, Whitton J, Mertens A, et al. Abnormalities of the thyroid in survivors of Hodgkin's disease: data from the Childhood Cancer Survivor Study. *J Clin Endocrinol Metab*. 2000;85(9):3227-3232. PMID: 10999813

Elisei R, Bottici V, Luchetti F, et al. Impact of routine measurement of serum calcitonin on the diagnosis and outcome of medullary thyroid cancer: experience in 10,864 patients with nodular thyroid disorders. *J Clin Endocrinol Metab*. 2004;89(1):163-168. PMID: 14715844

72 ANSWER: A) Small-bowel resection

Patients with inflammatory bowel disease, including ulcerative colitis and Crohn disease, are at increased risk for osteopenia, osteoporosis, fracture, and nephrolithiasis. Nearly 20% of adult patients with inflammatory bowel disease are diagnosed with renal stones at some point in their lifetime. In patients with Crohn disease who have also had resection of the terminal ileum, the incidence of associated nephrolithiasis is much higher. Small-bowel resection (Answer A) can result in malabsorption of fatty acids and bile salts, which thereby increase oxalate absorption and excretion. This is a result of increased binding of free calcium to fatty acids in the intestinal lumen and increased colonic permeability of oxalate induced by exposure of the colon to nonabsorbed bile salts. Other clinical situations that can likewise increase the risk of calcium oxalate stones by the same mechanism include surgical bowel resection or diversion (eg, bariatric surgery) or cystic fibrosis.

Other factors that predispose patients with inflammatory bowel disease to kidney stone formation include diarrheal fluid losses that reduce urine volume and lead to a metabolic acidosis, with a low urine pH and a marked decrease in citrate excretion. A decrease in excretion of urinary inhibitors of crystal formation is another mechanism that can promote kidney stone development. Citrate acts in the tubular lumen by combining with calcium to form a nondissociable but soluble complex. As a result, there is less free calcium available to combine with oxalate. In addition, citrate also appears to inhibit the important process of crystal formation (thus, Answer E is incorrect).

Likewise, magnesium also affects the supersaturation of urine with respect to calcium oxalate and may also contribute to stone development when there is a deficiency, so magnesium supplementation would not be expected to increase stone formation (thus, Answer D is incorrect).

Avoidance of calcium supplementation can be a common mistake in patients with malabsorption and kidney stones. Moderate calcium supplementation inhibits intestinal oxalate absorption. A randomized controlled trial of men with hypercalciuria showed that a diet higher in calcium with restricted intake of oxalate was associated with a lower rate of stone recurrence than a low-calcium diet alone (thus, Answer B is incorrect).

High-dosage steroids decrease intestinal calcium absorption, decrease bone formation, increase bone resorption, and decrease renal calcium reabsorption. Physiologic replacement of glucocorticoids has not been shown to increase the incidence of kidney stones in patients with inflammatory bowel disease (thus, Answer C is incorrect).

Educational Objective
Describe metabolic abnormalities leading to calcium oxalate stones in patients with inflammatory disease, including those with bowel resections.

UpToDate Topic Review(s)
Evaluation of the adult patient with established nephrolithiasis and treatment if stone composition is unknown

Reference(s)
Gaspar SR, Mendonca T, Oliveira P, Oliveira T, Dias J, Lopes T. Urolithiasis and Crohn's disease. *Urol Ann.* 2016;8(3):297-304. PMID: 27453651

McConnell N, Campbell S, Gillanders I, Rolton H, Danesh B. Risk factors for developing renal stones in inflammatory bowel disease. *BJU Int.* 2002;89(9):835-841. PMID: 12010224

73 ANSWER: B) Metformin and a fibrate

This patient has a longstanding history of marked hypertriglyceridemia—that is, triglyceride levels greater than 1000 mg/dL (>11.30 mmol/L). Marked hypertriglyceridemia results when patients who have an underlying familial form of dyslipidemia develop another condition that results in secondary hypertriglyceridemia. Such common secondary causes include untreated or uncontrolled diabetes, hypothyroidism, use of drugs that can raise triglycerides (eg, β-adrenergic blockers and thiazides), or excessive alcohol consumption. Because pancreatitis is a major and life-threatening complication when triglycerides are higher than 1000 mg/dL, there is an immediate need to decrease his triglycerides. Although not all individuals with very high triglyceride levels develop pancreatitis, from a practical standpoint, it is best to maintain levels at less than 1000 mg/dL—ideally as low as possible. There are no set targets for triglyceride levels other than to reduce the risk of pancreatitis by decreasing levels below 1000 mg/dL. Patients with severe hypertriglyceridemia should be advised to abstain from alcohol.

The focus of treatment is triglyceride-lowering agents to maintain triglycerides at an acceptable level. Fibrates (Answer B) are the recommended first-line agents in patients at risk for triglyceride-induced pancreatitis. Fibrates lower triglycerides by activating peroxisome proliferator–activated receptor α, increasing lipoprotein lipase activity, and increasing catabolism of triglycerides. These agents works particularly well in individuals with marked hypertriglyceridemia (20%-50% reduction, sometimes up to 70%). Available fibrates in the United States include gemfibrozil (twice-daily dosing) and fenofibrate (once-daily dosing).

Statins (Answers A and D) are indeed the first-line agents for cardiovascular risk reduction in patients with diabetes. They are primarily cholesterol-lowering agents and they only modestly decrease triglyceride levels. Thus, statins would not be able to lower this patient's triglycerides to a safe level. Statin therapy should, however, be considered after attempting triglyceride-lowering therapy. However, the role of combination therapy for reducing cardiovascular risk is unclear.

Fish oil (Answers C and E), as concentrated eicosapentaenoic acid and docosahexaenoic acid, has modest effects on triglycerides with reductions up to 50%. Fish oil, when used in high dosages, reduces triglycerides by decreasing VLDL synthesis and increasing its catabolism. However, in marked hypertriglyceridemia it is seldom beneficial and is not considered first-line therapy. Reversal of the secondary cause of hypertriglyceridemia is also necessary, and in this patient it would involve treatment of diabetes. In this setting, normalizing blood glucose levels is important because hyperglycemia exacerbates hypertriglyceridemia. Metformin is the first-line agent for treatment of type 2 diabetes and its use is indicated in this patient. Hence, treatment with metformin and fenofibrate is the best choice. Metformin also has modest beneficial lipid-lowering effects, including lowering triglycerides and LDL cholesterol and raising HDL cholesterol, although it would not be expected to decrease markedly elevated triglycerides as in this patient. Insulin therapy is the alternative option, and it would be indicated to help lower triglycerides rapidly, especially in the setting of a very high hemoglobin A_{1c} level (>9% [>75 mmol/mol]), acute pancreatitis, or symptoms suggestive of impending pancreatitis. However, for the reasons already stated, statins and fish oil (as listed in Answers D and E with insulin) are not effective in triglyceride reduction.

Educational Objective
Recommend appropriate therapy in a patient with combined hyperlipidemia and diabetes mellitus.

UpToDate Topic Review(s)
Hypertriglyceridemia

Reference(s)

Smellie WS. Hypertriglyceridaemia in diabetes. *BMJ*. 2006;333(7581):1257-1260. PMID: 17170417

Berglund L, Brunzell JD, Goldberg AC, Goldberg IJ, Stalenhoef A. Treatment options for hypertriglyceridemia: from risk reduction to pancreatitis. *Best Pract Res Clin Endocrinol Metab*. 2014;28(3):423-437. PMID: 24840268

74 ANSWER: B) Stop cabergoline once pregnant

This patient has had an excellent clinical, biochemical, and radiologic response to cabergoline (a dopamine agonist) used to treat her prolactinoma. The main question relates to the safety of dopamine agonists during pregnancy and when or if they should be discontinued in women who wish to become pregnant.

The main aims of prolactin-lowering therapy in this patient were to restore pituitary-gonadal function and allow spontaneous ovulation, as well as to shrink her macroadenoma to minimize the consequence of pituitary expansion during pregnancy. Stopping therapy suddenly now (Answer A) would put her at risk for relapse given her visible adenoma on MRI and the fact that her serum prolactin remains at the high end of the normal range on her current cabergoline dosage. While the Endocrine Society clinical practice guideline for the management of prolactinoma suggests that therapy can be withdrawn after 2 years if there has been a response to treatment, this should be done gradually with dosage tapering and monitoring of serum prolactin. This may be an option if the patient accepts that there is a risk of recurrence of hyperprolactinemia. However, even if this were embarked upon, the cabergoline dosage should be gradually reduced to 0.25 mg twice weekly (thus, Answer D is incorrect).

Both cabergoline and bromocriptine effectively manage hyperprolactinemia. However, cabergoline is often the drug of first choice because it is more effective than bromocriptine and is better tolerated. While there is more accumulated experience with bromocriptine in pregnancy, both drugs are considered safe. The incidence of miscarriage and congenital malformations associated with each drug is no higher than in the general population. As a result of greater experience, some clinicians may favor the use of bromocriptine to treat prolactin excess when pregnancy is desired, although many would use cabergoline. Regardless, in the setting of a microprolactinoma, there is no requirement to continue dopamine agonist therapy once the patient is pregnant (thus, Answer C is incorrect).

It is unusual for dopamine agonist therapy to be continued throughout pregnancy (Answer E) and it is not warranted in this case. Very rarely, treatment may be resumed during pregnancy if an adenoma expands sufficiently to result in visual field impairment. The chance that an increase in the size of a lactotroph adenoma will be clinically important depends on the size of the adenoma before pregnancy. For a microadenoma such as the one described in this vignette, the risk is very low. One review of 12 studies involving 658 patients with microprolactinomas showed that only 2.7% exhibited a symptomatic increase in adenoma size during pregnancy. The only other circumstance in which continuation of dopamine agonist therapy in pregnancy may be prudent is in women who have macroadenomas that are invasive or abutting the optic chiasm and who have not had prepregnancy debulking surgery or radiotherapy.

Therefore, the best course of action is to advise the patient to stop her cabergoline once pregnant (Answer B). Continuation of therapy until that time ensures ongoing fertility, but the small size and position of her microadenoma (away from the optic chiasm) indicate that ongoing treatment during pregnancy is not justified.

Educational Objective
Guide the management of microprolactinoma in a woman seeking to become pregnant.

UpToDate Topic Review(s)
Management of lactotroph adenoma (prolactinoma) during pregnancy

Reference(s)

Melmed S, Casanueva FF, Hoffman AR, et al; Endocrine Society. Diagnosis and treatment of hyperprolactinemia: an Endocrine Society clinical practice guideline. *J Clin Endocrinol Metab.* 2011;96(2):273-288. PMID: 21296991

Molitch ME. Prolactinoma in pregnancy. *Best Pract Res Clin Endocrinol Metab.* 2011;25(6):885-896. PMID: 22115164

75 ANSWER: E) No additional therapeutic interventions

This patient has multiple risk factors for cardiovascular-related death, including advanced heart failure, obstructive sleep apnea, and uncontrolled diabetes. Although optimizing his diabetes therapy with insulin will most likely reduce the risk of microvascular complications, insulin therapy (Answer A) has not been shown to reduce macrovascular events in patients with type 2 diabetes. In contrast, findings from the ACCORD trial (Action to Control Cardiovascular Risk in Diabetes) suggest that aggressive therapy with multiple diabetes medications may increase mortality risk.

Empagliflozin and liraglutide reduce the risk for cardiovascular death in adults with type 2 diabetes. However, empagliflozin (Answer C) should only be used in patients with an estimated glomerular filtration rate of 45 mL/min per 1.73 m^2 or greater. The drug should not be initiated if the estimated glomerular filtration rate is below this value and it is contraindicated for patients with an estimated glomerular filtration rate less than 30 mL/min per 1.73 m^2. Thus, this patient is beyond the window of benefit for empagliflozin. Liraglutide (Answer D) is contraindicated in this patient with a history of pancreatitis. In the PROactive study, pioglitazone (Answer B) was shown to reduce cardiovascular events, but the drug is contraindicated in patients with advanced heart failure.

Therefore, no additional medications can be recommended to reduce this patient's risk for cardiovascular-related death (Answer E). The best management for this patient is to optimize his diabetes therapy and encourage him to achieve modest weight loss.

Educational Objective
Explain the benefits and limitations of medical therapy to reduce the risk of cardiovascular-related death in patients with diabetes mellitus.

UpToDate Topic Review(s)
Prevention of cardiovascular events in those with established disease or at high risk

Reference(s)

Accord Study Group, Gerstein HC, Miller ME, et al. Long-term effects of intensive glucose lowering on cardiovascular outcomes. *N Engl J Med.* 2011;364(9):818-828. PMID: 21366473

Dormandy JA, Charbonnel B, Eckland DJ, et al; PROactive Investigators. Secondary prevention of macrovascular events in patients with type 2 diabetes in the PROactive study (PROspective pioglitazone Clinical Trial In macrovascular Events): a randomized controlled trial. *Lancet.* 2005;366(9493):1279-1289. PMID: 16214598

Zinman B, Wanner C, Lachin JM, et al. Empagliflozin, cardiovascular outcomes, and mortality in type 2 diabetes. *N Engl J Med.* 2015;373(22):2117-2128. PMID: 26378978

ORIGIN Trial Investigators, Gerstein HC, Bosch J, et al. Basal insulin and cardiovascular and other outcomes in dysglycemia. *N Engl J Med.* 2012;367(4):319-328. PMID: 22686416

76 ANSWER: B) Thyroid ultrasonography

Cowden syndrome or PTEN hamartoma syndrome is a relatively rare autosomal dominant disorder characterized by multiple hamartomas throughout the body. Affected patients have an increased lifetime risk of several carcinomas, including breast (50%-85% lifetime risk), thyroid (30%-40% lifetime risk), endometrial (25%-30% lifetime risk), colorectal (5%-10% lifetime risk), and renal cell carcinoma (up to 30%-35% lifetime risk). Cowden syndrome is estimated to occur in 1 in 200,000 persons, although the condition is most likely underdiagnosed. Cowden syndrome is the prototype of the PTEN hamartoma tumor syndrome disorders and is linked to germline mutations in the *PTEN* tumor suppressor gene. Molecular genetic testing can be performed to assess for *PTEN* mutations. However, new prospective research identified disease-causing mutations in only 25% of affected individuals.

A number of consensus diagnostic criteria should be used as the mainstay of diagnosis. An operational diagnosis can be made on the basis of the following:

(a) 3 or more major criteria, but 1 must be macrocephaly, Lhermitte-Duclos disease (a benign slow-growing hamartoma), or gastrointestinal hamartomas

(b) 2 major and 3 minor criteria

Operational diagnosis in a family in which 1 individual meets the above criteria or has a *PTEN* mutation can be made on the basis of the following:

(a) Any 2 major criteria
(b) 1 major and 2 minor criteria
(c) 3 minor criteria

Major Criteria	Minor Criteria
Breast cancer	Autism spectrum disorder
Endometrial cancer (epithelial)	Colon cancer
Thyroid cancer (follicular)	Esophageal glycogenic acanthosis
Gastrointestinal hamartomas (≥3)	Lipomas
Lhermitte-Duclos disease	Mental subnormality (IQ ≤75)
Macrocephaly (head circumference ≥ 97 percentile)	Renal cell carcinomas
Macular pigmentation of penis	Testicular lipomatosis
Multiple mucocutaneous lesions (any of): • Multiple trichilemmomas (≥3) • Acral keratoses (≥3) • Mucocutaneous neuromas (≥3) • Oral papillomas (≥3)	Papillary or follicular variant thyroid cancer Thyroid adenoma or multinodular goiter Vascular anomalies (including multiple intracranial developmental venous anomalies)

The patient in this vignette has 2 major clinical criteria (macrocephaly and mucocutaneous lesions) and 1 minor criterion (autism spectrum disorder) in addition to the finding of a *PTEN* mutation in 2 first-degree relatives. Therefore, the diagnostic criteria for Cowden syndrome are fulfilled.

Both benign and malignant thyroid tumors occur in patients with Cowden syndrome; however, due to the prevalence of these conditions in the general population, their presence has a low predictive value for identifying those who have *PTEN* mutations. Follicular thyroid cancers appear overrepresented in *PTEN* mutation carriers compared with the occurrence in the general population; thus, this is included as a major criterion, with papillary thyroid cancer and benign thyroid nodules considered to be minor criteria.

The most critical management aspect of Cowden syndrome is surveillance for early cancer detection, resulting in improved overall survival. All patients with Cowden syndrome should undergo annual thyroid ultrasonography (Answer B) and dermatologic evaluation once the diagnosis has been established. Women should receive annual mammography and breast MRI beginning at age 30 years along with annual transvaginal ultrasonography (Answer E) and blind suction endometrial biopsies. These screening measures may be undertaken 5 to 10 years before any known diagnosis in the family of a particular type of carcinoma (whichever is earlier) and it would therefore be appropriate to request regular breast and endometrial imaging in this patient once she is 25 years old (she is too young now). Prophylactic mastectomy or prophylactic hysterectomy may also be considered after appropriate counseling. All adults with Cowden syndrome should have a colonoscopy (Answer D) beginning at age 35 years, as well as renal imaging every 2 years, beginning at age 40 years. This patient is too young for these tests now. The routine use of imaging modalities such as total body CT (Answer A) and ^{18}F-fluorodeoxyglucose PET imaging (Answer C) is not recommended.

Educational Objective
Recommend appropriate screening investigations in a patient with Cowden syndrome.

UpToDate Topic Reviews
PTEN hamartoma tumor syndrome, including Cowden syndrome

Reference(s)

Gosein MA, Narinesingh D, Nixon CA, Goli SR, Maharaj P, Sinanan A. Multi-organ benign and malignant tumors: recognizing Cowden syndrome: a case report and review of the literature. *BMC Res Notes.* 2016;9:388. PMID: 27488391

Pilarski R, Burt R, Kohlman W, Pho L, Shannon KM, Swisher E. Cowden syndrome and the PTEN hamartoma tumor syndrome: systematic review and revised diagnostic criteria. *J Natl Cancer Inst.* 2013;105(21):1607-1616. PMID: 24136893

77   ANSWER: A) Ectopic production of 1α-hydroxylase

In the evaluation of any patient with hypercalcemia, the most important initial measurement is intact PTH. If inappropriately elevated in the setting of hypercalcemia, the etiology is due to a PTH-mediated process, most commonly primary hyperparathyroidism from a single-gland parathyroid adenoma or less often multigland hyperplasia often from multiple endocrine neoplasia syndrome types 1 and 2A or tertiary hyperparathyroidism in patients with chronic kidney failure. In this patient, the intact PTH is appropriately suppressed; thus, this is a non–PTH-mediated process. Additionally, ectopic production of authentic PTH (Answer B) is a rarely reported cause of hypercalcemia of malignancy.

With an appropriately suppressed intact PTH, the differential is broader and includes malignancy-associated hypercalcemia, medications (eg, overingestion of vitamin D or vitamin A supplements, hydrochlorothiazide), granulomatous diseases (fungal infections, tuberculosis, sarcoidosis), hyperthyroidism, adrenal insufficiency, pheochromocytoma, or prolonged immobilization. In this patient with newly diagnosed large B-cell lymphoma, the suspicion is high for malignancy-associated hypercalcemia. Malignancy-associated hypercalcemia is associated with 4 mechanisms: (1) ectopic production of PTHrP causing humoral hypercalcemia of malignancy, (2) secretion of cytokines or osteoclast-activating factors causing local osteolysis-mediated hypercalcemia, (3) overproduction of 1,25-dihydroxyvitamin D due to activation of 1α-hydroxylase by lymphoma of all types, and (4) ectopic production of authentic PTH (which is extremely rare, described in a few case reports).

In this case, because of the elevated phosphate level and the recent diagnosis of large B-cell lymphoma, the suspicion is high for overproduction of 1,25-dihydroxyvitamin D from 1α-hydroxylase activation by lymphoma cells (Answer A). Understanding the underlying mechanism is critical because it can guide medical therapy, as steroids are effective in suppressing 1α-hydroxylase activity to decrease production of active vitamin D and increase intestinal absorption of calcium and phosphate.

Humoral hypercalcemia of malignancy due to PTHrP production is the most common category of malignancy-associated hypercalcemia (80% of cases) and it is typically associated with squamous-cell cancers of the lung, head/neck, esophagus, and cervix or with breast cancer, among other solid tumors. PTHrP is a poor stimulus for 1α-hydroxylation compared with PTH; thus, 1,25-dihydroxyvitamin D is typically low or normal in patients with humoral hypercalcemia of malignancy. The phosphate level is typically normal or at the low end of normal, which is not the case in this patient's laboratory assessment. Thus, PTHrP overproduction (Answer E) is not the cause of hypercalcemia in this patient. Local osteolytic hypercalcemia is the second most common category mediating malignancy-associated hypercalcemia, typically associated with multiple myeloma, some forms of lymphoma, leukemia, or breast cancer.

Prolonged immobilization (Answer C) can lead to increased osteoclastic activity, which in turn mediates hypercalcemia and at times hyperphosphatemia; however, there is no indication of prolonged immobilization or illness in this patient to account for this degree of hypercalcemia.

Fibroblast growth factor 23 is a phosphaturic factor that is overproduced in autosomal dominant hypophosphatemic rickets or tumor-induced osteomalacia, a paraneoplastic syndrome typically associated with indolent mesenchymal tumors. Overproduction of fibroblast growth factor 23 (Answer D) leads to significant hypophosphatemia due renal phosphate wasting. However, this patient's phosphate level is elevated.

Educational Objective
Recognize the clinical presentation of vitamin D–mediated hypercalcemia due to ectopic production of 1α-hydroxylase in a patient with large B-cell lymphoma.

UpToDate Topic Review(s)
Hypercalcemia of malignancy: Mechanisms

Reference(s)
Rosner MH, Dalkin AC. Onco-nephrology: the pathophysiology and treatment of malignancy-associated hypercalcemia. *Clin J Am Soc Nephrol.* 2012;7(10):1722-1729. PMID: 22879438

Stewart AF. Clinical practice. Hypercalcemia associated with cancer. *N Engl J Med.* 2005;352 (4):373-379. PMID: 15673803

78 ANSWER: D) Order a glucagon GH stimulation test

Radiation therapy to several areas of the brain and skull base can cause hypopituitarism. This is not limited to patients whose pituitary is the primary target; it can also affect patients who receive radiation to contiguous areas. Even patients who receive brain radiation for gliomas that are far from the pituitary can develop hypopituitarism. GH deficiency is the most common pituitary deficit occurring after radiation-induced pituitary damage.

Patients who undergo radiation therapy for nasopharyngeal carcinoma are at high risk of hypopituitarism. As for other radiation therapies, the pituitary deficit may occur several years after radiation is completed. His adrenal and gonadal axes are normal. However, particularly in male patients, GH deficiency can be present despite normal serum IGF-1 levels. Because postradiation hypopituitarism is primarily due to hypothalamic damage, it may take time for the GH-secreting cells of the pituitary to atrophy. Therefore, a test that directly stimulates the somatotroph cells (such as the GHRH stimulation test) may be normal in the first few years after radiation despite the presence of real GH deficiency. This patient may have developed GH deficiency that would not be detected by a GHRH + arginine test (thus, Answer E is incorrect). Conversely, a stimulus that tests the whole axis (such as the insulin tolerance test, and presumably glucagon [Answer D]) would be abnormal at an earlier time.

IGF-1 is bound to IGFBP3 and acid-labile subunit. Despite the secretion of both proteins being GH-dependent, IGFBP3 (Answer A) and acid-labile subunit are not useful in diagnosing adult-onset GH deficiency. Similarly, measurement of free IGF-1 (still used mainly in research settings) (Answer B) is not a useful assessment in the diagnosis of adult-onset GH deficiency. There is no literature on the use of the nighttime GH secretion profile (Answer C) in the diagnosis of acquired adult-onset GH deficiency.

Educational Objective

Explain how growth hormone deficiency can occur in patients with a normal insulinlike growth factor 1 level and why a stimulation test that directly stimulates the pituitary gland may be falsely negative in patients with early postradiation growth hormone deficiency.

UpToDate Topic Review(s)

Growth hormone deficiency in adults

Reference(s)

Appelman-Dijkstra NM, Malgo F, Neelis KJ, Coremans I, Biermasz NR, Pereira AM. Pituitary dysfunction in adult patients after cranial irradiation for head and nasopharyngeal tumours. *Radiother Oncol.* 2014;113(1):102-107. PMID: 25236713

Agha A, Sherlock M, Brennan S, et al. Hypothalamic-pituitary dysfunction after irradiation of nonpituitary brain tumors in adults. *J Clin Endocrinol Metab.* 2005;90(12):6355-6360. PMID: 16144946

Darzy KH, Aimaretti G, Wieringa G, Gattamaneni HR, Ghigo E, Shalet SM. The usefulness of the combined growth hormone (GH)-releasing hormone and arginine stimulation test in the diagnosis of radiation-induced GH deficiency is dependent on the post-irradiation time interval. *J Clin Endocrinol Metab.* 2003;88(1):95-102. PMID: 12519836

Svensson J, Johannsson G, Bengtsson BA. Insulin-like growth factor-I in growth hormone-deficient adults: relationship to population-based normal values, body composition and insulin tolerance test. *Clin Endocrinol (Oxf).* 1997;46(5):579-586. PMID: 9231054

79 ANSWER: A) Adrenal insufficiency

This patient presents with progressive fatigue, weight loss, and anorexia and has an apparently normal morning cortisol level; however, the accompanying ACTH is markedly elevated. Given the clinical findings suggestive of adrenal insufficiency and the history of an autoimmune thyroid disorder, this patient's presentation is most consistent with primary adrenal insufficiency (Addison disease) (Answer A). Although a morning cortisol level of 17 µg/dL (469.0 nmol/L) may at first seem appropriate and reassuring, it must be interpreted in the context of the clinical presentation and the ACTH value. In this case, the most reasonable interpretation is that she was only able to secrete a seemingly normal morning cortisol concentration when she was stressed despite supraphysiologic concentrations of ACTH. These findings suggest that the patient has not lost all of her adrenocortical reserve, and that the diagnosis is relatively early primary adrenal insufficiency. When diagnosing primary adrenal insufficiency this early in its course, a normal-appearing cortisol value may be falsely reassuring and an elevated ACTH value can suggest diminished adrenocortical reserve in the right clinical context. Treatment of hypothyroidism with levothyroxine can increase the basal metabolic rate, including hepatic metabolism and renal clearance of cortisol, and thus this intervention may have precipitated the presentation of adrenal insufficiency. Autoimmune disorders of the thyroid and adrenal are frequently co-associated in patients with autoimmune polyglandular syndromes; however, given the rarity of primary adrenal insufficiency, patients should not be routinely screened unless they have suggestive symptoms or signs. Although hypothyroidism is most commonly associated with primary adrenal insufficiency, Graves disease can also occur.

Celiac disease (Answer D) is an autoimmune disease that is a part of the autoimmune polyglandular syndromes and this patient should be screened for this disorder; however, there is no evidence to suggest that the current presentation is most likely due to malabsorption. The current laboratory values may suggest a mild overreplacement of levothyroxine (Answer B), but they are not consistent with marked thyrotoxicosis or hypothyroidism. There is no evidence to suggest that the patient's radioactive iodine ablation was unsuccessful (Answer C) since the TSH rose appropriately following the procedure. No signs or symptoms are present to suggest that she has Cushing disease (Answer E). Although the ACTH value is high, her clinical presentation is more concerning for adrenal insufficiency, not hypercortisolism.

Educational Objective

Diagnose primary adrenal insufficiency in a patient with an autoimmune thyroid disorder.

UpToDate Topic Review(s)

Causes of primary adrenal insufficiency (Addison's disease)

Reference(s)

Bornstein SR. Predisposing factors for adrenal insufficiency. *N Engl J Med.* 2009;360(22):2328-2339. PMID: 19474430

Bornstein SR, Allolio B, Arlt W, et al. Diagnosis and treatment of primary adrenal insufficiency: an Endocrine Society Clinical Practice Guideline. *J Clin Endocrinol Metab.* 2016;101(2):364-389. PMID: 26760044

80 ANSWER: E) Referral to a dietitian for guidance on a supervised and restricted diet

Prader-Willi syndrome is the most common form of obesity caused by a genetic syndrome. The underlying genetic defect is the absence of paternal expression of the Prader-Willi syndrome critical region on the long arm of chromosome 15 (an imprinted region). At birth, affected infants are hypotonic and have feeding difficulties, but as they get older they develop progressive hyperphagia and obesity. The cornerstone for weight control in these patients includes institution of a low-calorie diet, rigorous supervision, regular exercise, restricted access to food, and psychological and behavioral counseling for the patient and family. Therefore, a referral to a dietitian to discuss a supervised low-calorie, well-balanced diet should be offered to this patient (Answer E).

Pharmacologic and surgical strategies to assist with weight loss have been studied in this population, but none has been shown to control hyperphagia. An open-label study in which topiramate (Answer C) was administered to patients with Prader-Willi syndrome showed that it did not significantly alter appetite or decrease BMI. Patients with Prader-Willi syndrome have leptin levels similar to those without syndromic obesity; therefore, they are not leptin deficient and prescribing leptin (Answer D) is incorrect. A case series of patients with Prader-Willi syndrome who underwent bariatric surgery showed that within 2 to 5 years after biliopancreatic diversion (Answer A), nearly half of the patients regained weight. Regarding Roux-en-Y gastric bypass (Answer B), 63% of patients with Prader-Willi syndrome were described as having poor weight-loss response, 23% had complications, and 47% required surgical revision. These procedures did not achieve the expected weight loss and were associated with high morbidity. Thus, they are currently not recommended as treatment options for patients with Prader-Willi syndrome.

Endocrinopathies associated with Prader-Willi syndrome include GH deficiency, hypogonadism, adrenal insufficiency, hypothyroidism, type 2 diabetes, and osteoporosis.

Educational Objective
Counsel families regarding weight-loss strategies appropriate for patients with Prader-Willi syndrome.

UpToDate Topic Review(s)
Clinical features, diagnosis, and treatment of Prader-Willi syndrome

Reference(s)

Irizarry KA, Miller M, Freemark M, Haqq AM. Prader Willi syndrome: genetics, metabolomics, hormonal function, and new approaches to therapy. *Adv Pediatr.* 2016;63(1):47-77. PMID: 27426895

Goldstone AP, Holland AJ, Hauffa BP, Hokken-Koelega AC, Tauber M;, speakers contributors at the Second Expert Meeting of the Comprehensive Care of Patients with PWS. Recommendations for the diagnosis and management of Prader-Willi syndrome [published correction appears in *J Clin Endocrinol Metab.* 2008;93(11):4183-4197]. *J Clin Endocrinol Metab.* 2008;93(11):4183-4197. PMID: 18697869

Irizarry KA, Bain J, Butler MG, et al. Metabolic profiling in Prader-Willi syndrome and nonsyndromic obesity: sex differences and the role of growth hormone. *Clin Endocrinol (Oxf).* 2015;83(6):797-805. PMID: 25736874

Scheimann AO, Butler MG, Gourash L, Cuffari C, Klish W. Critical analysis of bariatric procedures in Prader-Willi syndrome. *J Pediatr Gastroenterol Nutr.* 2008;46(1):80-83. PMID: 18162838

81 ANSWER: E) Acetaminophen

Continuous glucose monitoring (CGM) has been available to aid self-management of diabetes since 1999. Continuous glucose sensors are placed subcutaneously and measure glucose in the interstitial fluid. Glucose levels are reported every 5 to 10 minutes on a continuous basis. Despite steady improvements in technology, glucose sensors do not yet have the accuracy to function as standalone devices for treatment of diabetes. Multiple daily fingerstick glucose measurements are required to calibrate the current generation of CGM and to verify that sensor glucose readings are reliable. Next-generation continuous glucose sensors are being developed that require infrequent fingerstick calibration (once daily) or no calibration and will most likely be available for clinical use in the next few years. Sensor-augmented pump therapy is another recent innovation that has a low-glucose suspend feature to interrupt insulin infusion from the pump when the glucose level falls below a programmed threshold. CGM is expensive, and insurance approval for reimbursement of the cost of the sensor and supplies is needed before initiation.

Continuous glucose sensors have been shown to improve glycemic control in patients with type 1 diabetes in several large randomized controlled trials. In the STAR-3 randomized trial, frequent use of CGM (on average, wearing the sensor for 6 or more days per week) was more effective in lowering aggregate glucose levels than intermittent use of the sensor.

CGM is an appropriate therapeutic option in the treatment of patients with hypoglycemia unawareness as in this vignette. A number of studies have shown a reduction in mild and nocturnal hypoglycemia in patients using CGM compared with usual glucose monitoring with capillary glucose testing. At least one randomized controlled trial with sensor-augmented pump therapy using automated insulin suspension demonstrated a significant reduction in the risk of severe hypoglycemia with these devices compared with standard insulin pump therapy alone.

A potential problem with the accuracy of CGM is interfering substances. Acetaminophen can lead to factitious elevation in CGM glucose levels. A recent study of 10 nondiabetic participants reported CGM glucose readings obtained after ingestion of 1 g of acetaminophen that ranged from 85 to 400 mg/dL (4.7-22.2 mmol/L), and this was attributed to interference by acetaminophen. The peak elevation in glucose of 180 mg/dL (10.0 mmol/L) above baseline levels occurred approximately 1 hour after ingestion of acetaminophen. Plasma glucose values remained steady at about 90 mg/dL (5.0 mmol/L) in participants who did not receive acetaminophen. Given this information, acetaminophen (Answer E) most likely caused falsely elevated glucose levels as measured by CGM in this patient. Ibuprofen (Answer A), cefuroxime (Answer B), losartan (Answer C), and atorvastatin (Answer D) have not been reported to lead to spurious glucose levels with CGM use.

Educational Objective
Identify medications that can potentially interfere with the accuracy of continuous glucose sensors.

UptoDate Topic Review(s)
Blood glucose self-monitoring in management of adults with diabetes mellitus

Reference(s)

Juvenile Diabetes Research Foundation Continuous Glucose Monitoring Study Group, Tamborlane WV, Beck RW, et al. Continuous glucose monitoring and intensive treatment of type 1 diabetes. *N Engl J Med.* 2008;359(14):1464-1476. PMID: 18779236

Bergenstal RM, Tamborlane WV, Ahmann A, et al; STAR 3 Study Group. Effectiveness of sensor-augmented insulin-pump therapy in type 1 diabetes [published correction appears in *N Engl J Med.* 2010;363(11):1092]. *N Engl J Med.* 2010;363(4):311-320. PMID: 20587585

Juvenile Diabetes Research Foundation Continuous Glucose Monitoring Study Group, Beck RW, Buckingham B, et al. Factors predictive of use and benefit from continuous glucose monitoring in type 1 diabetes. *Diabetes Care.* 2009;32(11):1947-1953. PMID: 19675206

Ly TT, Nicholas JA, Retterath A, Lim EM, Davis EA, Jones TW. Effect of sensor-augmented insulin pump therapy and automated insulin suspension vs standard insulin pump therapy on hypoglycemia in patients with type 1 diabetes: a randomized clinical trial. *JAMA.* 2013;310(12):1240-1247. PMID: 24065010

Basu A, Veettil S, Dyer R, Peyser T, Basu R. Direct evidence of acetaminophen interference with subcutaneous glucose sensing in humans: a pilot study. *Diab Technol Ther.* 2016;18(Suppl 2):S243-S247. PMID: 26784129

82 ANSWER: B) Increase the octreotide dosage to 30 mg every 4 weeks

Clearly, surgery has not cured this patient's acromegaly and there is persistent biochemical evidence of GH excess, as well as residual, surgically incurable, disease in his cavernous sinus. Therefore, alternative, nonsurgical treatment options must be considered.

First-line medications available for the management of residual or recurrent acromegaly are somatostatin analogues (octreotide or lanreotide) or the GH receptor antagonist pegvisomant. Octreotide and lanreotide are equally effective in the management of acromegaly. Most studies demonstrate IGF-1 normalization in up to 50% of patients and these agents can reduce pituitary adenoma size by up to 50% in approximately one-third of patients. Either octreotide or lanreotide should be started at its lowest dosage (20 mg monthly for octreotide and 90 mg monthly for lanreotide). At least 2 (and often 3) doses are required before assessment of biochemical response is recommended, so the timing of GH and IGF-1 evaluation in this case is ideal. This patient has had a good response to octreotide with an approximate 30% reduction in IGF-1, although his IGF-1 and GH levels remain above the normal range, so the best course of action is to increase the octreotide dosage to 30 or 40 mg once monthly (Answer B) with further assessment of GH/IGF-1 after another 3 months.

Pegvisomant competes with endogenous GH for binding at its receptor and blocks peripheral production of IGF-1. This is also a highly effective agent in achieving IGF-1 normalization, although subsequent clinical studies of its effectiveness suggest this occurs less frequently (in approximately 60%) than in the original landmark studies that documented IGF-1 normalization in 97% of patients. Serum GH cannot be used to monitor the treatment effectiveness because pegvisomant inhibits the action of GH rather than its secretion. Pegvisomant (Answer C) would be a reasonable alternative to a somatostatin analogue in this case if the patient failed to respond to or was unable to tolerate the maximum octreotide dosage.

Similarly, combination therapies consisting of somatostatin analogues with either pegvisomant or the dopamine agonist cabergoline (Answers D and E) are not yet indicated in this patient who is on low-dosage octreotide treatment. Such therapies can be considered in patients who have failed to respond to maximum dosages of somatostatin analogue and are recommended by the Endocrine Society clinical practice guideline in such circumstances. However, some reports suggest that the combination of octreotide and pegvisomant is no more effective than pegvisomant alone.

Pituitary radiotherapy (Answer A) should be reserved for cases of residual or recurrent acromegaly in patients for whom medical therapy has failed or who have significant residual disease threatening the optic chiasm. Moreover, this patient's young age, the risk of central hypogonadism, and the risk of secondary intracranial tumors make radiation therapy an unattractive option.

Educational Objective
Describe alternative treatment options and follow-up for patients with acromegaly not completely cured by surgery.

UpToDate Topic Review(s)
Treatment of acromegaly

Reference(s)

Katznelson L, Laws ER, Melmed S, et al. Acromegaly: an Endocrine Society clinical practice guideline. *J Clin Endocrinol Metab.* 2014;99(11):3933-3951. PMID: 25356808

Trainer PJ, Drake WM, Katznelson L, et al. Treatment of acromegaly with the growth hormone-receptor antagonist pegvisomant. *N Engl J Med.* 2000;342(16):1171-1177. PMID: 10770982

Trainer PJ, Ezzat S, D'Souza GA, Layton G, Strasburger CJ. A randomized, controlled, multicentre trial comparing pegvisomant alone with combination therapy of pegvisomant and long-acting octreotide in patients with acromegaly. *Clin Endocrinol (Oxf).* 2009;71(4):549-557. PMID: 19438906

83 **ANSWER: B) Depressive symptoms, improve; body weight, increase; ovaries, hyperplasia**
Many, but not all, transgender men seek hormone therapy with testosterone for masculinization. Transgender men often desire a lower voice, facial and body hair, increased strength, and cessation of menses. Other effects include acne, increased hemoglobin, increased sexual desire, and clitoral growth and pain. It is important to be able to counsel transgender men about the effects of testosterone that they may not know about, including potential risks. On therapy, serum testosterone should be targeted to the median testosterone level ±100 ng/dL (±3.5 nmol/L) of a cisgender man of the same age.

Testosterone therapy has been associated with a reduction in gender dysphoria (thus, Answers D and E are incorrect). This improvement in gender dysphoria is broadly related to cross-sex hormone therapy in general, as transgender women also experience a reduction in gender dysphoria with estrogen and antiandrogen therapy.

The first 1 to 2 years of testosterone therapy in transgender men is associated with an average weight gain of 4.8 to 7.7 lb (2.2-3.5 kg) depending on the formulation and dosage used (thus, Answers A and E are incorrect). There is usually a gain of lean mass accompanied by loss of fat mass.

The effects of testosterone on the reproductive system of transgender men can be complex. Testosterone therapy is associated with reduced serum concentrations of estrogen, LH, and FSH. Menses usually stop by 6 months with the intramuscular esters, but this process may take up to a year and occasionally requires the addition of a progestin. Testosterone therapy is associated with stromal hyperplasia of the ovaries, which are typically larger than those of nontransgender women (thus, Answers A, C, and E are incorrect). Histologically, the ovaries of transgender men on testosterone resemble those of women with polycystic ovary syndrome ($\geq$12 antral follicles per ovary). It is important to counsel transgender men that pregnancy may be possible if they discontinue testosterone therapy, assuming that they have not had a hysterectomy or oophorectomy. Transgender men who become pregnant should not receive testosterone therapy as testosterone is a category X medication that may cause fetal harm.

The changes most likely to occur with initiation of testosterone therapy in this patient are improved depressive symptoms, increased body weight, and ovary hyperplasia (Answer B).

Educational Objective
Explain the effects of testosterone therapy in transgender men.

UpToDate Topic Review(s)
Transgender men: Evaluation and management

Reference(s)

Grynberg M, Fanchin R, Dubost G, et al. Histology of genital tract and breast tissue after long-term testosterone administration in a female-to-male transsexual population. *Reprod Biomed Online.* 2010;20(4):553-558. PMID: 20122869

Hembree WC, Cohen-Kettenis P, Gooren L, et al; Endocrine Society. Endocrine treatment of gender-dysphoric/gender-incongruent persons: an Endocrine Society clinical practice guideline. *J Clin Endocrinol Metab.* 2017 [Epub ahead of print] PMID: 28945902

Irwig MS. Testosterone therapy for transgender men. *Lancet Diabetes Endocrinol.* 2017;5(4):301-311. PMID: 27084565

84 ANSWER: A) Sitagliptin

This patient has newly diagnosed diabetes, which remains uncontrolled following hospital discharge. Initiation of antihyperglycemic therapy is warranted. The presence of stage 4 renal insufficiency greatly influences which agent can be safely used. Renal insufficiency leads to reduced clearance of insulin and many diabetes medications, thus increasing the risk of hypoglycemia and drug toxicity.

Compared with sulfonylureas, dipeptidyl-peptidase 4 inhibitors are associated with a reduced risk of hypoglycemia because of glucose-dependent insulin secretion. Sitagliptin (Answer A) requires a dosage adjustment based on the degree of renal insufficiency, but it can be safely used in this patient and it is the best therapeutic recommendation in this setting. Another dipeptidyl-peptidase 4 inhibitor, linagliptin, does not require dosage adjustment based on renal function.

Of the listed options, only pioglitazone (Answer D) does not have unchanged drug or active metabolites that are renally cleared. However, thiazolidinediones must be used with caution in the setting of renal insufficiency given salt and water retention and the increased risk of congestive heart failure associated with their use. In this patient with ischemic heart failure, pioglitazone should be avoided.

Metformin (Answer E) is eliminated unchanged primarily by the kidneys, but metformin levels become significantly elevated when the estimated glomerular filtration rate falls below 30 mL/min per 1.73 m^2. Higher metformin levels lead to inhibition of pyruvate dehydrogenase, increased metabolism of pyruvate to lactate, and increased risk of lactic acidosis. In 2016, the US FDA announced a change to metformin's labeling in response to data supporting the safety of metformin in persons with mild to moderate renal insufficiency. The FDA's recommendation is to start metformin only if the glomerular filtration rate is greater than 45 mL/min per 1.73 m^2, to continue metformin with periodic assessment of the risks when it falls between 30 and 45 mL/min per 1.73 m^2, and to stop metformin should it fall below 30 mL/min per 1.73 m^2. Metformin is therefore contraindicated in this patient who has a glomerular filtration rate of 28 mL/min per 1.73 m^2.

Of all second-generation sulfonylureas, glyburide (Answer B) carries the highest risk of hypoglycemia, which may be prolonged in patients with renal insufficiency. This increased risk is due to the presence of active metabolites that are renally cleared. Glyburide is not recommended when the estimated glomerular filtration rate falls below 60 mL/min per 1.73 m^2.

In persons with baseline renal insufficiency, the osmotic diuresis associated with sodium-glucose cotransporter 2 inhibitors (Answer C) may lead to volume depletion and rarely hypotension and worsening renal function. Initiation of canagliflozin is not recommended when the estimated glomerular filtration rate is below 45 mL/min per 1.73 m^2 and is contraindicated when it is below 30 mL/min per 1.73 m^2.

Educational Objective
Select an oral hypoglycemic agent in a patient with uncontrolled diabetes and renal failure.

UpToDate Topic Review(s)
Dipeptidyl peptidase-4 (DPP-4) inhibitors for the treatment of type 2 diabetes mellitus

Reference(s)
Hahr AJ, Molitch ME. Management of diabetes mellitus in patients with chronic kidney disease. *Clin Diabetes Endocrinol.* 2015;1(2):2-9.

Inzucchi SE, Lipska KJ, Mayo H, Bailey CJ, McGuire DK. Metformin in patients with type 2 diabetes and kidney disease: a systematic review. *JAMA.* 2014;312(24):2668-2675. PMID: 25536258

85 ANSWER: A) Reassure her that no further treatment is needed

In a patient with hypercalcemia and an inappropriately normal (rather than suppressed) intact PTH level, the most common cause is primary hyperparathyroidism due to a single-gland parathyroid adenoma. A less common cause is multigland hyperplasia often associated with multiple endocrine neoplasia types 1 or 2A. However, per the fourth International Workshop Guidelines for the Management of Asymptomatic Primary Hyperparathyroidism, the workup of patients who have hypercalcemia with elevated or inappropriately normal intact PTH should include 24-hour urine analysis for calcium and creatinine excretion, primarily to rule out the rare hereditary disorder of familial hypocalciuric hypercalcemia. Familial hypocalciuric hypercalcemia is an autosomal dominant disorder of high penetrance that accounts for approximately 2% of patients with asymptomatic hypercalcemia. An inactivating mutation in the calcium-sensing receptor gene (*CASR*) causes the receptor (CaSR) on the parathyroid glands and kidneys to be less sensitive to calcium activation. This defect leads to continued secretion of PTH, even in the setting of hypercalcemia. Thus, laboratory testing demonstrates a slightly higher-than-normal serum calcium level and a normal to mildly elevated intact PTH level. In the kidney, *CASR* mutations cause increased tubular reabsorption of calcium, which leads to low urinary calcium excretion. The diagnosis is confirmed by calculating the fractional excretion of calcium with the following equation:

$$\text{(urine calcium concentration} \times \text{serum creatinine concentration)} \div$$
$$\text{(serum calcium concentration} \times \text{urine creatinine concentration)}$$

Familial hypocalciuric hypercalcemia is likely if the fractional excretion of calcium ratio is less than 0.01. In this case, the fractional excretion of calcium ratio is 0.004, which is consistent with familial hypocalciuric hypercalcemia. Affected patients should be counseled to not undergo parathyroid surgery (Answer B), as this is a clinically benign disorder with no association with renal stone development, osteoporosis, fractures, or renal insufficiency. Additionally, parathyroidectomy is not curative in most cases of familial hypocalciuric hypercalcemia. Thus, this patient should be reassured that no further treatment is needed (Answer A). Genetic testing for *CASR* mutations is available, but it can be costly and is not always covered by medical insurance. It is recommended that immediate family members be evaluated for asymptomatic hypercalcemia, and those with testing consistent with familial hypocalciuric hypercalcemia should be reassured.

There is no suggestion of malignancy in this patient's clinical history given the longstanding hypercalcemia and the fact that her intact PTH level is not suppressed. Thus, her hypercalcemia is unlikely to be due to malignancy from PTHrP secretion or multiple myeloma. Therefore, measuring PTHrP (Answer C) or ordering urine protein electrophoresis (Answer D) is incorrect. FNAB of a suspected parathyroid lesion (Answer E) is rarely needed and typically inadvisable because FNAB can distort the parathyroid microarchitecture and lead to difficulty interpreting findings on pathologic review if a biopsied parathyroid is resected.

Educational Objective
Counsel patients that familial hypocalciuric hypercalcemia does not require treatment beyond education and reassurance.

UpToDate Review(s)
Disorders of the calcium-sensing receptor: Familial hypocalciuric hypercalcemia and autosomal dominant hypocalcemia

Reference(s)

Bilezikian JP, Brandi ML, Eastell R, et al. *J Clin Endocrinol Metab.* 2014;99(10):3561-3569. PMID: 25162665

Shinall MC Jr, Dahir KM, Broome JT. Differentiating familial hypocalciuric hypercalcemia from primary hyperparathyroidism. *Endocr Pract.* 2013;19(4):697-702. PMID: 23425644

86 ANSWER: D) Right lobectomy

There are 2 main considerations regarding this patient's right-sided nodule: (1) the nodule is large and the patient is young and (2) the cytology has Hurthle-cell features. Several diagnostic tools provide excellent information about the likelihood of malignancy within a nodule. These include cytologic features and ultrasound characteristics and patterns of the nodule. Although there does not seem to be a clear association with increasing nodule size within the range of 1 to 4 cm, some mixed data suggest that there is a relatively high risk of cancer in nodules greater than 4 cm in dimensions. For example, in one 2009 study in which some of the nodules larger than 4 cm underwent FNAB using palpation guidance, 11 of 96 nodules with either benign, inconclusive, or nondiagnostic cytologic characteristics were found to have cancer within the nodule at the time of surgery, leading to a malignancy rate of 11%. In a more recent study in which the nodules were subject to ultrasound-guided FNAB before surgery, there was a malignancy rate of 10% in nodules that were benign according to FNAB cytology and a malignancy rate of 29% in nodules with indeterminate cytology. These data have led some to recommend lobectomy for cytologically benign nodules that are greater than 4 cm. However, another study showed lower rates of malignancy of 1.8% in nodules greater than 3 cm with benign cytologic characteristics. However, the malignancy rate was 33% in cytologically indeterminate nodules. Thus, in this patient, it is unclear whether the size of his nodule alone should lead to a recommendation for surgery.

An additional consideration in this patient is the specific cytology of his nodule. Hurthle-cell neoplasia is classified as Bethesda cytologic category IV, but it accounts for only a small percentage of this category (*see table*). One study found that 11 of 43 patients undergoing surgery for nodules with this cytologic category had a diagnosis of malignancy. Older patient age and larger nodule size seem to correlate with malignancy. Although it is appealing to consider molecular markers to help decide on the best course of action in this patient, the assessment of molecular markers is less studied for Hurthle-cell neoplasia. In one recent study of such lesions, the Gene Expression Classifier results were "suspicious" for 43 of 46 lesions, with only 6 being confirmed malignant at the time of surgery. Thus, the positive predictive value is low and there is a high rate of false-positive results with this particular cytology. The Gene Expression Classifier (Answer B) would therefore add little additional information. Although not given as an option in this vignette, a 7-gene molecular panel could be considered for obtaining additional information about this nodule. The caveat, however, is that many Hurthle-cell cancers do not have mutations such as *BRAF*, *PET/PTC*, *RAS*, and *PAX8/PPARG*, which are among the mutations included in this gene panel. The performance of such molecular panels in this specific tumor subtype has not been well documented.

Categories	Description	Approximate Frequency	Risk of Malignancy
I	Unsatisfactory	5%-10%	N/A
II	Benign	60%-70%	0%-3%
III	Atypia of undetermined significance or follicular lesion of undetermined significance	15%-20%	5%-15%
IV	Follicular neoplasm or suspicious for follicular neoplasm (includes Hurthle-cell neoplasm or suspicious for Hurthle cell neoplasm)		15%-30%
V	Suspicious for malignancy		60%-75%
VI	Malignant	7%-8%	97%-99%

This patient's 0.7-cm nodule has a low risk of malignancy because it is isoechoic and does not contain intranodular calcifications. It does not require biopsy (Answer E) on the basis of current guidelines.

Thus, although the size of the nodule alone may not be a sufficient indication for surgery, the size combined with the Hurthle-cell neoplasm cytologic characteristics makes surgery the wisest choice and a diagnostic lobectomy (Answer D) is indicated. Follow-up ultrasonography without other action (Answer A) is not the best option given the combination of nodule size and cytology and the patient's young age. Ethanol ablation (Answer C) is most appropriate for cystic nodules, which usually have a very low risk of malignancy.

Educational Objective
Determine whether surgery is indicated for thyroid nodules larger than 4 cm on the basis of their cytologic characteristics.

UpToDate Topic Review(s)
Diagnostic approach to and treatment of thyroid nodules

Reference(s)
Brauner E, Holmes BJ, Krane JF, et al. Performance of the Afirma Gene Expression Classifier in Hurthle cell thyroid nodules differs from other indeterminate thyroid nodules. *Thyroid.* 2015;25(7):789-796. PMID: 25962906

Haugen BR, Alexander EK, Bible KC, et al. 2015 American Thyroid Association Management Guidelines for Adult Patients with Thyroid Nodules and Differentiated Thyroid Cancer: The American Thyroid Association Guidelines Task Force on Thyroid Nodules and Differentiated Thyroid Cancer. *Thyroid.* 2016;26(1):1-133. PMID: 26462967

Lee KH, Shin JH, Ko ES, et al. Predictive factors of malignancy in patients with cytologically suspicious for Hurthle cell neoplasm of thyroid nodules. *Int J Surg.* 2013;11(9):898-902. PMID: 23916366

Wharry LI, McCoy KL, Stang MT, et al. Thyroid nodules (≥4 cm): can ultrasound and cytology reliably exclude cancer? *World J Surg.* 2014;38(3):614-621. PMID: 24081539

87 ANSWER: D) Trial of a statin at a lower dosage

Rheumatoid arthritis is associated with increased cardiovascular morbidity and mortality. Unlike the general population in which hyperlipidemia is strongly associated with adverse cardiovascular outcomes, the link between lipids and cardiovascular risk in persons with rheumatoid arthritis is more complex because of the interplay between metabolic factors, inflammation, antirheumatic treatments, and genetic factors. In active rheumatoid arthritis, in the context of increased inflammation, reductions in total cholesterol levels, as well as HDL- and LDL-cholesterol levels have been seen; this phenomenon is referred to as the "lipid paradox." The increase in inflammation is believed to be the driver of increased cardiovascular risk in these individuals. Observational data suggest this risk might be attenuated by the use of conventional disease-modifying drugs or biologic therapy. Anti-inflammatory therapy increases lipid levels, but whether these therapies favorably alter cardiovascular risk in these patients is not yet known.

While the cardiovascular risk calculator that is available as part of the widely used American College of Cardiology/American Heart Association guidelines for treatment of blood cholesterol includes various nonmodifiable and modifiable variables, it does not address the presence of inflammatory joint disease as a risk factor for cardiovascular disease. Interestingly, the QRISK2 cardiovascular disease risk score developed for use in the United Kingdom takes a different approach and enables the categorical factoring of the presence of rheumatoid arthritis as an additional risk factor. The key is to recognize rheumatoid arthritis as a risk factor for accelerated cardiovascular risk.

Because of significant variability of lipid levels with changes in inflammatory status in rheumatoid arthritis, recommendations from several rheumatology organizations and the National Lipid Association suggest assessing lipid levels when disease activity is stable. It is reasonable to suggest that sustained elevations in LDL cholesterol during remission and/or stable rheumatoid arthritis disease activity (but not during the medication adjustment phase/active uncontrolled rheumatoid arthritis) require treatment with a statin as a first-line lipid-lowering medication. Nevertheless, although the use of statins in rheumatoid arthritis is recommended, thresholds for statin initiation and treatment goals are not known. This patient has stable joint disease while on treatment. Thus, it is reasonable to consider statin therapy for LDL-cholesterol levels greater than 160 mg/dL (>4.14 mmol/L). While this patient has tried high-intensity statin therapy in the past, a lower statin dosage has not been attempted (thus, Answer D is correct and Answer A is incorrect).

Colesevelam (Answer B) is a bile acid sequestrant that can provide modest reductions in LDL cholesterol. Colesevelam also has a modest benefit in hemoglobin A_{1c} reduction. This patient has prediabetes, and hemoglobin

A_{1c} reduction would most likely be beneficial; however, evidence for primary cardiovascular risk reduction with colesevelam is lacking.

Ezetimibe (Answer C), the intestinal cholesterol absorption inhibitor, has modest LDL-cholesterol–lowering effects as a single agent. Current evidence suggests some benefit for secondary prevention of cardiovascular disease in individuals at high risk, but there is no evidence of benefit in primary cardiovascular disease prevention, let alone in patients with inflammatory joint disease.

Proprotein convertase subtilisin/kexin type 9 (PCSK9) inhibitors (Answer E) are antibodies that lower LDL cholesterol in specific patient groups, namely those with genetic hypercholesterolemia or in individuals at high risk when LDL-cholesterol lowering is inadequate on maximum tolerated statin dosages. Because a lower statin dosage has not yet been attempted in this patient, there is currently no immediate indication for injectable therapy.

Educational Objective
Manage increased cardiovascular disease risk in a patient with dyslipidemia and inflammatory joint disease/ rheumatoid arthritis.

UpToDate Topic Review(s)
Coronary artery disease in rheumatoid arthritis: Implications for prevention and management

Reference(s)

Myasoedova E. Lipids and lipid changes with synthetic and biologic disease-modifying antirheumatic drug therapy in rheumatoid arthritis: implications for cardiovascular risk. *Curr Opin Rheumatol.* 2017;29(3):277-284. PMID: 28207495

Choy E, Ganeshalingam K, Semb AG, Szekanecz Z, Nurmohamed M. Cardiovascular risk in rheumatoid arthritis: recent advances in the understanding of the pivotal role of inflammation, risk predictors and the impact of treatment. *Rheumatology (Oxford).* 2014;53(12):2143-2154. PMID: 24907149

88 ANSWER: A) Target hemoglobin A_{1c} value 6.0%-6.5% (42-48 mmol/mol)

In women with diabetes mellitus, the aim of interventions in the preconception period is to reduce complications for both the mother and the fetus. Infants of mothers with pregestational diabetes are at increased risk for congenital malformations, compared with the 2% risk for malformations in mothers without diabetes (*see table*):

Hemoglobin A_{1c}	Risk for Congenital Malformations
<7.0% (<53 mmol/mol)	No increased risk
7.0%-10.0% (53-86 mmol/mol)	3%-7%
10.0%-11.0% (86-97 mmol/mol)	8%-10%
≥11.0% (≥97 mmol/mol)	10%-20% or more

During preconception counseling, the patient should be informed of these risks and the importance of achieving tight glycemic control before pregnancy. In this patient, the appropriate next step would be to initiate basal and bolus insulin therapy with the goals of (1) maintaining her fasting glucose concentration less than 95 mg/dL (<5.3 mmol/L); (2) maintaining her 2-hour postprandial glucose concentration at 120 mg/dL or less (≤6.7 mmol/L); and (3) achieving a hemoglobin A_{1c} level of 6.0% to 6.5% (42-48 mmol/mol) before conception (Answer A). The use of metformin in pregnancy is controversial.

None of the other answers is as important as preconception blood glucose control. Weight loss by lifestyle change (Answer B) would reduce her insulin requirements, but it is of secondary importance compared with glucose control. Blood pressure targets for pregnant women with diabetes and hypertension are 120-160 mm Hg/80-105 mmHg, not less than 120/80 mm Hg (Answer C). This patient has nonproliferative retinopathy, which does not require retinal laser therapy (Answer D) before conception. Hypertriglyceridemia requires follow-up, as triglyceride levels increase during pregnancy, but it does not require immediate therapy in this patient's case (Answer E).

Educational Objective

Provide preconception counseling to women with pregestational diabetes mellitus on how to reduce the risk of maternal and fetal complications.

UpToDate Topic Review(s)

Pregestational diabetes: preconception counseling, evaluation, and management

Reference(s)

Mackeen AD, Trauffer PML. Pregestational diabetes. In: Berghella V, ed. *Maternal-Fetal Evidence Based Guidelines*. 2nd ed. New York, NY: Informa Healthcare; 2012:39-46.

Management of diabetes in pregnancy. 13. American Diabetes Association. *Diabetes Care*. 2017;40(Suppl 1):S114-S119. PMID: 27979900

89 ANSWER: A) Hypophysitis

Checkpoint inhibitors are newly developed immunomodulatory antibodies that aim to augment the immune system. Their use (such as in this vignette) has substantially improved the prognosis for patients with advanced melanoma and they are likely to significantly improve the treatment of advanced disease in a number of other malignancies. The primary targets for checkpoint inhibition include the cytotoxic T-lymphocyte–associated antigen 4 (CTLA-4) and programmed cell death-1 (PD-1) receptor.

Ipilimumab, a CTLA-4 antibody, is approved for use in patients with advanced melanoma on the basis of significant improvement in overall survival. Another CTLA-4 antibody (tremelimumab) is in development. Multiple antibodies against PD-1 and its ligand (PD-L1) are in development and have shown great promise in melanoma, non–small cell lung cancer, and other malignancies. Examples include nivolumab and pembrolizumab, both of which have been approved to treat melanoma. Other agents targeting PD-1 and PD-L1 are under development.

The use of such agents will most likely be more widespread in the near future and it is important to recognize that endocrine dysfunction is thought to occur (albeit with varying severity) in up to 10% of patients treated with CTLA-4 antibodies. This patient presents acutely with headache, vomiting, evidence of thyroid and adrenal insufficiency, and a uniformly enhancing pituitary mass. She has an underlying malignancy and is treated with the CTLA-4 antibody ipilimumab. The pituitary MRI demonstrates a symmetrically enlarged pituitary gland and stalk thickening with generalized enhancement with contrast. The clinical and radiologic picture is consistent with inflammation of the pituitary gland (hypophysitis [Answer A]). This is an increasingly recognized complication of ipilimumab therapy, although the exact incidence remains unclear. If hypophysitis is suspected, glucocorticoid replacement therapy should be commenced immediately. Previously, a course of high-dosage corticosteroids (1 mg/kg of prednisone daily) was recommended, but more recent experience suggests that only physiologic replacement doses of corticosteroids are required and this should reduce the risk of steroid-related side effects.

Pituitary hemorrhage (Answer B) (usually into an underlying tumor) could present in this way, although there is often vision disturbance (diplopia or reduced visual acuity). Moreover, the MRI findings are not consistent with hemorrhage, which usually appears as a hyperintense mass on T1 imaging and demonstrates varying degrees of enhancement.

Pituitary abscess (Answer C) is a rare disorder, with only a few cases (approximately 200) described in the medical literature, and it is estimated to represent less than 1% of all cases of pituitary disorders referred for specialist endocrine opinion. Headache and endocrine dysfunction (especially diabetes insipidus, found in 40%-70% of cases) are the most common presenting features. Evidence of sepsis is not always apparent and, indeed, most pituitary abscesses are diagnosed perioperatively. In this patient, the borderline temperature and mildly elevated white blood cell count and C-reactive protein are relatively nonspecific. A proportion of patients present with vision symptoms (visual field or extraocular movement abnormalities), but neurologic long tract signs are uncommon. The major risk factor for the development of a pituitary abscess is previous pituitary surgery, but in many patients no risk factor is apparent. Typical MRI findings include a cystic sellar mass that demonstrates variable enhancement with gadolinium contrast—such findings are not evident here.

The pituitary gland is an uncommon site for metastases (Answer D), and metastatic disease accounts for only 1% to 2% of sellar masses. Although neoplasms from almost every tissue (including melanoma) have been reported to metastasize to the pituitary, the most common primary tumors are associated with breast or lung cancers. Metastatic deposits demonstrate a predilection for the posterior lobe of the pituitary; the anterior lobe being solely involved in only 15% of cases. Unlike this case, pituitary metastases are often asymptomatic. In one review, only

40 of 200 patients (20%) were symptomatic, and, of these, diabetes insipidus was documented in 28 patients (70%) while only 6 patients (15%) had 1 or more anterior pituitary deficiencies. The presence of obvious symptoms and anterior pituitary dysfunction in this case make hypophysitis a more likely diagnosis.

A pituitary adenoma (Answer E) can cause pituitary dysfunction as described here, as well as hormonal excess syndromes. However, the MRI appearance in such cases is usually of a discrete, low attenuation lesion that enhances with contrast; the generalized pituitary enlargement and enhancement shown in the MRI in this vignette are not typical of a simple pituitary adenoma.

Educational Objective
Identify the clinical and radiologic features of hypophysitis and explain the potential endocrine complications of immunotherapy for malignancy.

UpToDate Topic Review(s)
Toxicities associated with checkpoint inhibitor immunotherapy

Reference(s)

Faje A. Immunotherapy and hypophysitis: clinical presentation, treatment, and biologic insights. *Pituitary*. 2016;19(1):82-92. PMID: 26186958

Faje AT, Sullivan R, Lawrence D, et al. Ipilimumab-induced hypophysitis: a detailed longitudinal analysis in a large cohort of patients with metastatic melanoma. *J Clin Endocrinol Metab*. 2014;99(11):4078-4085. PMID: 25078147

90   ANSWER: A) Combination hormonal contraception

This patient has hirsutism and irregular menstrual cycles. The treatment of choice for both symptoms is combination hormonal contraception (Answer A). Combination hormonal contraception (ethinyl estradiol and a progestin) has been demonstrated to improve hirsutism and acne in women with hyperandrogenism. It works by suppressing LH and theca-cell androgen production as a consequence. It also increases sex hormone–binding globulin, which decreases free androgen hormone.

Spironolactone (Answer C) could be added to block testosterone at the level of the androgen receptor if hirsutism is not controlled after 6 months on hormonal contraception, the timeframe needed for turnover of hair follicles. Importantly, spironolactone should not be used alone (without birth control) in women of reproductive age because of the concern for abnormal genital development in a male fetus. A levonorgestrel-coated intrauterine device (Answer B) would be an acceptable alternative to protect the uterus from unopposed estrogen exposure in a woman with polycystic ovary syndrome and irregular menstrual cycles, but it does not address the cosmetic concern of hirsutism. Metformin (Answer E) can increase the number of ovulatory menstrual cycles in women with polycystic ovary syndrome, but it does not effectively treat hirsutism or acne. Dexamethasone (Answer D) is not an acceptable treatment for polycystic ovary syndrome, even when adrenal androgens are elevated.

Educational Objective
Recommend how to treat women with polycystic ovary syndrome and predominantly adrenal hyperandrogenism.

UpToDate Topic Review(s)
Treatment of polycystic ovary syndrome in adults

Reference(s)

Legro RS, Arslanian SA, Ehrmann DA, et al; Endocrine Society. Diagnosis and treatment of polycystic ovary syndrome: an Endocrine Society clinical practice guideline. *J Clin Endocrinol Metab*. 2013;98(12):4565-4592. PMID: 24151290

Martin KA, Chang RJ, Ehrmann DA, et al. Evaluation and treatment of hirsutism in premenopausal women: an Endocrine Society clinical practice guideline. *J Clin Endocrinol Metab*. 2008;93(4):1105-1120. PMID: 18252793

91 ANSWER: A) Perform a pituitary biopsy

Pituitary pathologic processes are not limited to adenomas, but include a vast range of neoplastic, inflammatory, infiltrative, infectious, and vascular diseases. The presence of diabetes insipidus rules out a pituitary adenoma, which is almost never seen in the setting of non-operated adenomas.

In a young woman who presents with pituitary enlargement and diabetes insipidus, lymphocytic hypophysitis is certainly to be included in the differential diagnosis. This was initially considered the most likely diagnosis in this patient, thus prompting initiation of glucocorticoid therapy. Mass shrinkage with glucocorticoids would not have been pathognomonic of lymphocytic hypophysitis, as other pathologies (eg, sarcoidosis) would most likely respond to such therapy. However, the lack of response and, in fact, the progression of disease despite glucocorticoid therapy raises the suspicion for infectious, infiltrative, or neoplastic disease. Therefore, a diagnostic procedure that provides a final diagnosis is mandatory. Of the listed answer options, the only one that fits in this category is pituitary biopsy (Answer A).

This patient had a pituitary abscess, which required a long course of intravenous and oral antibiotics. Pituitary abscesses are rare, and they can appear de novo or in glands that have been operated or harbor a previous pathologic process. Spread from sinus infection can be seen, but usually no obvious cause is identified. Although abscesses typically appear as cystic lesions on MRI, their appearance may vary.

Measuring angiotensin-converting enzyme (Answer D) would not help even if the value were abnormal, as this test is not sensitive or specific for sarcoidosis. Furthermore, in the case of sarcoidosis, the mass would have most likely shrunk with glucocorticoid therapy. Although pituitary tuberculosis was in the differential diagnosis, a positive tuberculin skin test (Answer B) would not be diagnostic of pituitary tuberculosis. While hemochromatosis (Answer C) can cause hypopituitarism, effects of this condition are rare in women and would not cause pituitary enlargement, headaches, and diabetes insipidus. Pituitary antibody testing (Answer E) is not yet routinely used, and these antibodies may be present in several pituitary diseases. Furthermore, even if positive, the diagnosis of lymphocytic hypophysitis would be unlikely given worsening of mass effect while on glucocorticoid therapy.

Educational Objective
Determine the need for tissue diagnosis in patients with enlarging sellar masses.

UpToDate Topic Review(s)
Causes, presentation, and evaluation of sellar masses

Reference(s)

Carpinteri R, Patelli I, Casanueva FF, Giustina A. Pituitary tumours: inflammatory and granulomatous expansive lesions of the pituitary. *Best Pract Res Clin Endocrinol Metab*. 2009;23(5):639-550. PMID: 25732650

Fukuoka H. Hypophysitis. *Endocrinol Metab Clin North Am*. 2015;44(1):143-149. PMID: 25732650

Karagiannis AK, Dimitropoulou F, Papatheodorou A, Lyra S, Seretis A, Vryonidou A. Pituitary abscess: a case report and review of the literature. *Endocrinol Diabetes Metab Case Rep*. 2016;2016:160014. PMID: 27274845

Chaichana K, Larman T, Salvatori R. Pituitary abscess with unusual MRI appearance. *Endocrine*. 2016;54(3):837-848. PMID: 27655290

92 ANSWER: B) Genetic counseling and genetic testing

The median survival of men with cystic fibrosis (CF) has dramatically increased over the last half century, with many men living into their 30s and 40s. From a reproductive standpoint, more than 95% of men with CF have congenital bilateral absence of the vas deferens, which results in obstructive azoospermia. In addition to the azoospermia, the ejaculate of these men shows a low volume and low pH. Men with CF usually have sperm in the testes and epididymides that can potentially be retrieved for use in assisted reproductive techniques such as intracytoplasmic sperm injection.

The next step for a man with CF contemplating fertility is a referral for the couple for genetic counseling and genetic testing (Answer B) as 1 in 25 white persons is a CF carrier. If his partner has negative CF screening, the risk of having a child with CF is as low as 1 in 400. While genetic testing can detect most carriers, there are more than 1900 described mutations in the *CFTR* gene and most screening panels detect only the most common mutations. In addition to genetic testing, couples should have an honest discussion with a genetic counselor regarding other potential risks for a child, including losing his or her father at a young age.

Referral to an adoption agency at this point (Answer A) is incorrect as this man inquired about his own fertility potential and because men with CF need to be aware of their reproductive options to make an informed decision. Obtaining a semen analysis (Answer C) would not be helpful because it would most likely show no sperm (in almost all men with CF). Proceeding to harvest sperm from either the epididymis or testis (Answers D and E) is incorrect without knowing the CF carrier status of his partner. If the couple decides to pursue pregnancy, Answers D and E could be options.

Educational Objective
Recommend genetic counseling and genetic testing to men with cystic fibrosis who desire fertility.

UpToDate Topic Review(s)
Cystic fibrosis: Clinical manifestations and diagnosis

Reference(s)

Ahmad A, Ahmed A, Patrizio P. Cystic fibrosis and fertility. *Curr Opin Obstet Gynecol.* 2013;25(3):167-172. PMID: 23429570

Popli K, Stewart J. Infertility and its management in men with cystic fibrosis: review of literature and clinical practices in the UK. *Hum Fertil (Camb).* 2007;10(4):217-221. PMID: 18049957

93 ANSWER: D) Bilateral macronodular adrenal hyperplasia

This middle-aged woman has features of cortisol excess, including weight gain, hypertension, and glucose intolerance. The biochemical findings suggest ACTH-independent cortisol excess with a low morning plasma ACTH level and inadequate suppression of plasma cortisol on overnight dexamethasone suppression testing. The unenhanced CT scan demonstrates bilateral adrenal macronodular hyperplasia (BMAH) (Answer D).

BMAH results in hypercortisolism through a number of mechanisms. In most patients with BMAH, cortisol is regulated by a variety of aberrant G-protein–coupled hormone receptors and by locally produced ACTH. The most commonly described aberrant receptors include vasopressin, serotonin 5-hydroxytryptamine 4, gastric inhibitory polypeptide, β-adrenergic, LH/hCG, and others. Recent advances in understanding the molecular basis of BMAH have determined that up to 50% of persons with this condition have a germline mutation in the *ARMC5* gene (armadillo repeat containing 5 gene). Thus, while most cases of BMAH are sporadic, this may be a familial condition with an autosomal dominant mode of transmission in some patients.

BMAH typically presents in the fourth to sixth decade of life and may only demonstrate subtle clinical features of cortisol excess. The biochemical findings are similar to those seen in any other cause of ACTH-independent Cushing syndrome: low or undetectable ACTH in the context of plasma and/or urinary cortisol excess. Imaging findings can be variable and range from apparent unilateral nodules to massive bilateral adrenal enlargement. Typically (as is seen here), there are multiple nonpigmented nodules larger than 10 mm in diameter in both adrenals. However, in some cases, diffuse enlargement of both adrenals occurs without distinct nodules.

Primary pigmented nodular adrenal hyperplasia (PPNAD) (Answer B) also presents with ACTH-independent Cushing syndrome. However, the key difference between PPNAD and BMAH is in adrenal imaging. In PPNAD, the adrenal nodules are so small that they can be missed on conventional CT or MRI or the adrenals may be reportedly normal. Classically in PPNAD, the adrenal glands are often not enlarged, but instead they are occupied by several small black or brown nodules spread in an otherwise atrophic cortex; this can be seen as a string of beads on thin-section high-resolution CT. The CT in this vignette shows obvious adrenal hyperplasia, so PPNAD is incorrect.

Carney complex (Answer A) is a rare, autosomal dominant, multiple neoplasia syndrome that is characterized by skin pigmentation, endocrine tumors, and nonendocrine tumors such as cutaneous and atrial myxomas. The most common endocrine tumor is PPNAD. As already discussed, this patient does not have imaging characteristics typical of PPNAD. Moreover, she has no other diagnostic criteria required to diagnose Carney complex. While multiple areas of skin pigmentation (eg, lentigines and blue nevi) are very common, these are usually found on mucosal surfaces and not simply confined to the shoulders.

This patient has no clinical features consistent with pheochromocytoma (Answer C). Moreover, pheochromocytomas are heterogenous and often highly vascular adrenal lesions with high attenuation and do not resemble the low-attenuation nodular adrenals demonstrated in this patient's CT. Therefore, the elevated plasma normetanephrine represents a false-positive result. In this scenario, it is prudent to look at the patient's medication history, as medications may account for up to 20% of false-positive results in such circumstances. The most likely interfering drug in this case is the tricyclic antidepressant amitriptyline. This medication blocks neuronal reuptake of norepinephrine, thus increasing its major metabolite, normetanephrine. Plasma epinephrine and metanephrine levels are not as significantly affected.

The enlarged adrenals and high-normal 17α-hydroxyprogesterone level could be suggestive of nonclassic (late-onset) congenital adrenal hyperplasia (Answer E). However, such patients do not present with cortisol excess, but rather most often have a clinical phenotype similar to that of polycystic ovary syndrome with menstrual disorder, mild androgen excess, and subfertility. In many cases, the clinical phenotype is so subtle that is goes undiagnosed. Nonclassic congenital adrenal hyperplasia is due to a partial defect in the 21-hydroxylase enzyme, and the subsequent mild ACTH excess leads to adrenal androgen excess. The high-normal 17α-hydroxyprogesterone in this case is due to inefficient steroid biosynthesis, which can be a common consequence of BMAH.

Educational Objective
Construct a differential diagnosis of bilateral adrenal abnormalities on the basis of imaging and biochemical findings.

UpToDate Topic Review(s)
Cushing's syndrome due to primary bilateral macronodular adrenal hyperplasia

Reference(s)

Assié G, Libé R, Espiard S, Rizk-Rabin M, et al. ARMC5 mutations in macronodular adrenal hyperplasia with Cushing's syndrome. *N Engl J Med.* 2013;369(22):2105-2114. PMID: 24283224

Libé R, Coste J, Guignat L, et al. Aberrant cortisol regulations in bilateral macronodular adrenal hyperplasia: a frequent finding in a prospective study of 32 patients with overt or subclinical Cushing's syndrome. *Eur J Endocrinol.* 2010;163(1):129-138. PMID: 20378721

94   ANSWER: B) Stop metformin and continue with diet treatment

Maturity-onset diabetes of the young (MODY) is a heterogeneous disorder of glucose metabolism that comprises approximately 2% of all diabetes cases. This nonketotic monogenic form of diabetes is characterized by absence of autoimmune antibodies and measurable C-peptide levels. Patients with MODY are typically diagnosed with diabetes in the second or third decade of life, and there is an autosomal dominant form of inheritance. The syndrome is characterized by single-gene mutations, each of which leads to a characteristic type of diabetes that may involve abnormal β-cell development, regulation, or function. Mutations can also occur in the insulin gene itself. The course of the disease, microvascular complications, and associated non-pancreatic manifestations are dependent on the molecular defect in each subtype of monogenic diabetes. The disease is often misclassified as either type 1 or type 2 diabetes, which can lead to inappropriate treatment as is the case in this vignette.

There are at least 11 monogenic forms of diabetes. The prevalence of each subtype varies depending on ethnicity. The most common MODY subtype is due to one of several mutations in the hepatic nuclear factor 1α (*HNF1A*; MODY3), which leads to a defect in insulin secretion. There is also a lower renal threshold for glycosuria, and these patients have lifelong glycosuria that is often first detected in childhood. Patients with MODY3 are extremely sensitive to sulfonylureas and account for 52% to 65% of all cases of MODY.

Glucokinase acts as the glucose sensor for the β cell and catalyzes the transfer of phosphate from ATP to glucose. Glucokinase is the rate-limiting step in glycolysis and glycogen storage. Patients who have one of the numerous mutations in the *GCK* gene have MODY 2, which is characterized by a higher threshold for glucose-stimulated insulin secretion. The resultant hyperglycemia is usually mild and stable. The fasting glucose is typically in the range of 90 to 104 mg/dL (5.0-5.8 mmol/L). Patients with *GCK* mutations account for 15% to 31% of all cases of MODY. Affected patients do not typically develop microangiopathic complications. Diet therapy alone is the treatment of choice in almost all cases of MODY2 as long as the patient maintains a normal body weight. The exception is during pregnancy when women may need insulin therapy.

The patient in this vignette has a sibling who was found to have a *GCK* mutation. All affected members of the immediate family with diabetes are assumed to have the same defect in β-cell function. The correct treatment for this patient's hyperglycemia is diet therapy alone (Answer B).

Because this patient was having gastrointestinal adverse effects that may be attributable to metformin, the drug should be stopped (thus, Answer A is incorrect). Furthermore, metformin does not address the defect in

GCK function and is largely ineffective in the treatment of this patient's mild diabetes. Pharmacologic treatment of the hyperglycemia with a sulfonylurea (Answer C), sodium-glucose cotransporter 2 inhibitor (Answer D), or a glucagonlike peptide 1 analogue (Answer E) is not needed. Additionally, use of a sulfonylurea could potentially cause hypoglycemia in this setting.

Educational Objective
Manage monogenic diabetes due to a mutation in the glucokinase gene.

UpToDate Topic Review(s)
Classification of diabetes mellitus and genetic diabetic syndromes

Reference(s)

Fajans SS, Bell GI, Polonsky KS. Molecular mechanisms and clinical pathophysiology of maturity-onset diabetes of the young. *N Engl J Med.* 2001;345(13):971-980. PMID: 11575290

Thanabalasingham G, Owen KR. Diagnosis and management of maturity onset diabetes of the young (MODY). *BMJ.* 2011;343:d6044. PMID: 22012810

Naylor R, Philipson LH. Who should have genetic testing for maturity-onset diabetes of the young? *Clin Endocrinol.* 2011;75(4):422-426. PMID: 21521318

Steele AM, Shields BM, Wensley KJ, Colclough K, Ellard S, Hattersley AT. Prevalence of vascular complications among patients with glucokinase mutations and prolonged, mild hyperglycemia. *JAMA.* 2014;311(3):279-286. PMID: 24430320

95 ANSWER: E) Levothyroxine therapy is not indicated

Subclinical hypothyroidism is an early condition of mild thyroid hormone deficiency, characterized by above-normal serum TSH and normal free T_4 and free T_3. A further distinction is usually made between mildly elevated TSH (4.0-10.0 mIU/L) and more markedly elevated TSH (>10 mIU/L). Subclinical hypothyroidism is reported in 4% to 20% of adults, and this wide range reflects important differences among the populations studied in terms of race and dietary iodine intake, the dissimilar characteristics (age, sex, and BMI) among the patients evaluated, and the different methods of TSH assessment. Generally, the condition is more common in women, in older persons, in white populations, and in areas of iodine sufficiency. Etiologically, most cases of persistent subclinical hypothyroidism are due to autoimmune (Hashimoto) thyroiditis; however, germline loss-of-function mutations in the TSH receptor gene account for a small proportion of cases. In addition, transient TSH elevations may occur in numerous circumstances, such as recovery from subacute or painless thyroiditis, following withdrawal of levothyroxine, during recovery from significant nonthyroidal illness, and during treatment with various drugs (eg, lithium, amiodarone). Furthermore, there is a widening of the reference range for serum TSH with increasing age, such that a mild TSH elevation (4.0-7.0 mIU/L) in persons older than 80 years should be considered a physiologic adaptation to aging.

Measurement of serum thyroid autoantibodies (TPO antibodies and/or thyroglobulin antibodies) establishes a firm etiologic diagnosis of autoimmune thyroiditis. Measurement of TPO antibodies represents the most sensitive serologic test for thyroid autoimmunity in subclinical hypothyroidism and provides valuable information regarding the rate of progression to overt hypothyroidism, which occurs most rapidly in patients with positive TPO antibodies (4.3% per year) as compared with those with negative TPO antibodies (2.6% per year). An initially elevated serum TSH, with free T_4 in reference range, should be investigated with repeated measurement of both serum TSH and free T_4 along with TPO antibodies, preferably after a 2- to 3-month interval.

There is ongoing controversy regarding the effects of subclinical hypothyroidism on mood disturbance, lipid profiles, long-term cardiovascular risk and the need for treatment. Most patients with subclinical hypothyroidism do not have significant symptoms, and current guidelines do not recommend treatment in asymptomatic patients with very mildly elevated serum TSH concentrations. Treatment should be considered if the serum TSH level is greater than 10 mIU/L, even in asymptomatic patients, because of long-term risks of cardiovascular disease. In addition, a trial of levothyroxine may be warranted in patients younger than 65 years who have a serum TSH level between 5 and 10 mIU/L if they have significant symptoms. The patient in this vignette has very mild symptoms (fatigue and minimal weight gain) and while some physicians may consider levothyroxine replacement for the minimally raised serum TSH concentration, it is notable that the TSH measurement has not changed for at least 5 years. Expert opinion documented in current clinical practice guidelines does not recommend levothyroxine therapy for the patient described in this vignette (thus, Answer E is correct).

Subclinical hypothyroidism has been linked to heart failure and increased coronary heart disease morbidity and mortality. Despite some heterogeneity in the literature regarding the relationship between subclinical hypothyroidism and cardiovascular disease, the available data suggest that the dominant risk of mild serum TSH elevations (<10 mIU/L) is in patients younger than 65 years, although most data are derived from observational studies and not from large randomized controlled trials. While evidence of significant cardiac disease may influence treatment decisions, the finding of hypertension alone (Answer B) is insufficient to warrant levothyroxine replacement.

The measurement of serum total or free T_3 is generally unhelpful in the management of patients with subclinical or overt hypothyroidism. The clinical significance of perturbations in serum free T_3 concentrations within the reference range, as well as below-normal serum T_3 concentrations (Answer A), is unknown, and treatment decisions should not be based on the finding of a slightly reduced free T_3 value. Patients with subclinical hypothyroidism may have a hypoechoic or inhomogeneous thyroid echo pattern on ultrasonography and this may be present before circulating autoantibodies become detectable, thereby providing early evidence for thyroid autoimmunity. However, guidelines do not recommend routine evaluation with thyroid ultrasonography in patients with subclinical hypothyroidism, and findings consistent with thyroiditis on sonography (Answer D) generally do not influence decisions regarding the need for treatment.

Several observational studies have investigated the relationship between subclinical hypothyroidism and dyslipidemia with heterogeneous results, and various observational studies and small randomized controlled trials have indicated reductions in total and LDL-cholesterol concentrations in patients with subclinical hypothyroidism treated with levothyroxine. Normalization of serum lipids, however, is rarely achieved and most of the beneficial effects are observed in patients with a serum TSH level greater than 10 mIU/L. Current guidelines do not recommend levothyroxine replacement on the basis of serum cholesterol concentrations (Answer C).

Educational Objective
Manage subclinical hypothyroidism.

UpToDate Topic Review(s)
Subclinical hypothyroidism in nonpregnant adults

Reference(s)

Pearce S, Brabant G, Duntas L, et al. 2013 ETA guideline: management of subclinical hypothyroidism. *Eur Thyroid J*. 2013;2(4):215-228. PMID: 24783053

Jonklaas J, Bianco AC, Bauer AJ, et al; American Thyroid Association Task Force on Thyroid Hormone Replacement. Guidelines for the management of hypothyroidism: prepared by the American Thyroid Association Task Force on Thyroid Hormone Replacement. *Thyroid*. 2014;24(12):1670-1751. PMID: 25266247

Garber JR, Cobin RH, Gharib H, et al; American Association of Clinical Endocrinologists and American Thyroid Association Taskforce on Hypothyroidism in Adults. Clinical practice guidelines for hypothyroidism in adults: cosponsored by the American Association of Clinical Endocrinologists and the American Thyroid Association [published corrections appear in *Thyroid*. 2013;23(2):251 and *Thyroid*. 2013;23(1):129]. *Thyroid*. 2012;22(12):1200-1235. PMID: 22954017

96 ANSWER: B) Fibroblast growth factor 23 measurement

This patient presents with progressive weakness and bone pain associated with severe hypophosphatemia, elevated alkaline phosphatase, and inappropriately low calcitriol. This is suspicious for tumor-induced osteomalacia (TIO) or oncogenic osteomalacia, a paraneoplastic syndrome associated with tumors of mesenchymal origin (eg, sclerosing angioma, benign angiofibroma, hemangiopericytoma, chondrosarcoma). The radiologic imaging shows bilateral rib fractures with no trauma history. Typically, tumors associated with TIO are slow growing, small, and very difficult to localize, which can delay diagnosis of the underlying etiology of osteomalacia.

Tumors associated with TIO overproduce fibroblast growth factor 23 (Answer B), which causes renal tubular loss of phosphate and inhibits 1α-hydroxylase, thus lowering the 1,25-dihydroxyvitamin D level and perpetuating hypophosphatemia. In normal physiology, a low serum phosphate level should activate the 1α-hydroxylase enzyme and cause 1,25-dihydroxyvitamin D to rise to stimulate more intestinal absorption of both phosphate and calcium; this is inhibited by fibroblast growth factor 23 in TIO. In the workup of this disorder, a ratio of tubular maximum reabsorption of phosphate to glomerular filtration rate will be lower than expected for the degree of hypophosphatemia. TIO may be difficult to distinguish from inherited forms of hypophosphatemic rickets

(X-linked and autosomal dominant, which are caused by mutations in the *PHEX* and *FGF23* genes, respectively). However, a careful evaluation of the family history can exclude a genetic cause of osteomalacia.

Bone turnover markers can be quite elevated in these patients, but documenting their levels (Answers C and E) will not establish a diagnosis. Multiple myeloma could lead to bone pain and fractures, but with normal renal function and normal complete blood cell count, it is less likely in this case. Thus, performing serum electrophoresis (Answer A) is incorrect. With TIO, the bone density reflects low mineralization and bone mass; however, assessing bone mineral density (Answer D) will not be informative as to the etiology.

Definitive treatment of TIO involves localizing the underlying tumor and treating it, most often by surgery or radiation. As the localization of these small tumors can be challenging, immediate medical therapy should include both calcitriol (to increase intestinal absorption of phosphate and calcium) and potassium phosphate, with the goal of alleviating bone pain.

Educational Objective
Diagnose tumor-induced osteomalacia, a paraneoplastic syndrome, due to overproduction of fibroblast growth factor 23 by the tumor.

UpToDate Topic Review(s)
Hereditary hypophosphatemic rickets and tumor-induced osteomalacia

Reference(s)

Jan de Beur SM. Tumor-induced osteomalacia. In: Favus MJ, ed. *Primer on the Metabolic Bone Diseases and Disorders of Mineral Metabolism*. 6th ed. American Society for Bone and Mineral Research. 2006:345-351.

Jonsson KB, Zahradnik R, Larsson T, et al. Fibroblast growth factor 23 in oncogenic osteomalacia and X-linked hypophosphatemia. *N Engl J Med*. 2003:348(17):1656-1663. PMID: 12711740

97 ANSWER: B) "False-positive" results related to venlafaxine use

Pheochromocytomas are neuroendocrine tumors of the adrenal medulla that are capable of synthesizing and secreting dopamine, norepinephrine, and epinephrine. Paragangliomas are neuroendocrine tumors that usually arise from chromaffin cells of the autonomic nervous system and are capable of synthesizing and secreting dopamine and norepinephrine, but not epinephrine. Therefore, elevations in plasma normetanephrine (the metabolite of norepinephrine) may indicate either a functional pheochromocytoma or paraganglioma, whereas elevations in plasma metanephrine are associated with pheochromocytomas. Importantly, symptomatic pheochromocytomas and paragangliomas that induce a syndrome of catecholamine excess typically have substantial elevations in plasma metanephrines—usually at least 4-fold above the upper limit of the reference range, but almost always greater than 2-fold. In this case, the 1.5-fold elevations above the upper normal limit (both normetanephrine and metanephrine) are inconsistent with symptomatic pheochromocytoma or paraganglioma (thus, Answers D and E are incorrect).

An increasingly common cause of false-positive test results in this setting is the use of medications such as tricyclic antidepressants, serotonin reuptake inhibitors, and norepinephrine and/or epinephrine reuptake inhibitors. These medications (such as venlafaxine [Answer B]) can induce mild elevations in plasma normetanephrine and metanephrine that are usually less than 2-fold greater than the upper limit of the reference range; however, in rare cases these medications can induce greater than 2-fold elevations in metanephrines. This suspicion is difficult to confirm since stopping the medication may not be safe from a psychiatric view point and it can take 6 to 8 weeks after medication cessation for metanephrines to normalize. A clonidine suppression test may eliminate the source of sympathetic nervous system false-positive results, but it is rarely used in clinical practice. Therefore, one must often rely on clinical judgment and close monitoring to assess for progressive symptoms.

Another cause of increased sympathoadrenergic tone is anxiety (Answer A). Increased sympathetic nervous system activity with anxiety, or even seated or upright posture, can mildly increase plasma normetanephrine levels. However, these elevations are typically much less than 2-fold greater than the upper limit of the reference range, and anxiety is less likely than antidepressants to induce such elevations.

Alprazolam (Answer C) does not induce elevations in plasma metanephrines.

Educational Objective
Interpret laboratory measurement of metanephrines when evaluating for a catecholamine-secreting tumor and identify potential causes of false-positive results.

UpToDate Topic Review(s)
Clinical presentation and diagnosis of pheochromocytoma

Reference(s)

Lenders JW, Duh QY, Eisenhofer G, et al; Endocrine Society. Pheochromocytoma and paraganglioma: an Endocrine Society Clinical Practice Guideline. *J Clin Endocrinol Metab.* 2014;99(6):1915-1942. PMID: 24893135

Neary NM, King KS, Pacak K. Drugs and pheochromocytoma--don't be fooled by every elevated metanephrine. *N Engl J Med.* 2011;364(23):2268-2270. PMID: 21651412

98 ANSWER: C) Measure serum calcitonin and perform neck ultrasonography

The progression of medullary thyroid cancer is strongly influenced by the *RET* genotype. Mutations in codon 918 carry the highest risk, with the median age of medullary thyroid cancer diagnosis without the presence of lymph node metastases being 3 years. Mutations in codons 922 and 883 carry a similarly very high risk of early-onset malignancy. Mutations in codons 609, 611, 618, 620, 630, and 634 are also characterized by early progression from C-cell hyperplasia to medullary thyroid cancer. C-cell hyperplasia develops between age 8 and 20 years, whereas medullary thyroid cancer itself develops between age 10 and 43 years. The mutation described in this question (Leu790Phe) is one of several mutations (including others in codons 768, 791, 804, and 891) that are characterized by progression to C-cell hyperplasia at age 7 to 29 years and progression to medullary thyroid cancer at age 30 to 47 years. The earliest age of medullary thyroid cancer diagnosis is 9 months for a codon 918 mutation, 7 years for a codon 711 mutation, and 12 years for a codon 790 mutation.

Because of these different risks, recommendations regarding the timing of prophylactic thyroidectomy differ depending on the mutation. Thyroidectomy is recommended within the first month to first year of life for infants who have a mutation in codon 918, 922, or 883. The suggested timing for thyroidectomy for children with a mutation in codon 609, 611, 618, 620, 630, or 634 is generally before age 5 years. For the lowest-risk mutations, thyroidectomy is suggested between age 5 and 10 years. For persons with a mutation in codon 790, it has been suggested that thyroidectomy can even be deferred longer if calcitonin levels are normal, cervical ultrasonography is normal, and there is no family history of aggressive medullary thyroid cancer.

In determining the appropriate plan for this patient, one consideration is that although this mutation is characteristically less aggressive, there does appear to be a history of aggressive medullary thyroid cancer in this particular kindred. Waiting until age 30 years before considering evaluation directed at the disease risks conferred by his mutation (Answer E) would be inappropriate. In the setting of an identified mutation and a kindred with aggressively behaving disease, a serum calcitonin level alone would also be inadequate.

Codon 790 is located in exon 13 in the intracellular domain of the RET tyrosine kinase receptor. Mutations in codon 790 are typically associated with familial medullary thyroid cancer, rather than multiple endocrine neoplasia. The frequency of hyperparathyroidism is very low with this mutation, as is the case for other *RET* mutations involving the intracellular domain. Although pheochromocytoma is generally not seen with codon 790 mutations, it has been reported and biochemical screening therefore would be prudent. The history of a hypertensive crisis during thyroidectomy in the patient's uncle could be suggestive of a pheochromocytoma. Thus, one must always keep in mind the patient's family history in the setting of a genetic syndrome. Therefore, screening for pheochromocytoma in this patient is clearly indicated. The best approach is to additionally measure his serum calcitonin levels and perform neck ultrasonography (Answer C). If results of serum calcitonin measurement and neck ultrasonography are suggestive of C-cell hyperplasia or medullary thyroid cancer, proceeding to thyroidectomy in a timely manner would be advisable. If results from these evaluations are normal, a full discussion between the patient and his health care team could help decide on the most appropriate timing of potential thyroidectomy. If the only abnormal result were 24-hour urinary catecholamine excretion, completion of evaluation for a pheochromocytoma, and adrenalectomy if the diagnosis were confirmed, would be wise. This would then allow for thyroidectomy to proceed whenever it is deemed appropriate.

Immediate thyroidectomy (Answer D) would be unwise without a serum calcitonin measurement to help assess whether medullary thyroid cancer is present (and might even have metastasized) and before evaluation for cervical lymph node involvement. Pituitary adenomas, including prolactinomas, and duodenopancreatic neuroendocrine tumors, including gastrinomas, are features of multiple endocrine neoplasia type 1, rather than multiple endocrine neoplasia type 2, which is associated with *RET* mutations (thus, Answers A and B are incorrect).

Educational Objective

Use genotype-phenotype correlations to recommend management for patients at risk of familial medullary thyroid cancer who carry a *RET* proto-oncogene mutation.

UpToDate Topic Review(s)

Medullary thyroid cancer: Clinical manifestations, diagnosis, and staging

References

Machens A, Dralle H. Genotype-phenotype based surgical concept of hereditary medullary thyroid carcinoma. *World J Surg*. 2007;31(5):957-968. PMID: 17453286

Machens A. Early malignant progression of hereditary medullary thyroid cancer. *N Engl J Med*. 2004;350(9):943. PMID: 14985494

Wells SA Jr, Pacini F, Robinson BG, Santoro M. Multiple endocrine neoplasia type 2 and familial medullary thyroid carcinoma: an update. *J Clin Endocrinol Metab*. 2013;98(8):3149-3164. PMID: 23744408

99 ANSWER: E) Recommend intensive lifestyle modifications

Categories of increased risk for diabetes (prediabetes) include impaired fasting glucose (fasting glucose between 100 and 125 mg/dL [5.6-6.9 mmol/L]) and impaired glucose tolerance (2-hour glucose between 140 and 199 mg/dL [7.8-11.0 mmol/L] during a 2-hour 75-g oral glucose tolerance test). In addition, patients in whom hemoglobin A_{1c} is between 5.7% and 6.4% also have an increased risk of developing diabetes. Testing for prediabetes or diabetes should be considered in patients who are overweight or obese and have 1 or more of the following risk factors: a first-degree relative with diabetes, history of hypertension or cardiovascular disease, low HDL-cholesterol level and/or a high triglyceride level, sedentary lifestyle, history of gestational diabetes and/or polycystic ovary syndrome, nonwhite ethnicity, or the presence of clinical features associated with insulin resistance such as acanthosis nigricans. Testing should start at age 45 years.

The patient in this vignette has had 2 elevated fasting glucose measurements in the last 6 months and has an elevated hemoglobin A_{1c} value; she therefore has prediabetes. Her risk factors include a sedentary lifestyle, dyslipidemia, hypertension, and coronary artery disease. Strategies to delay or prevent progression to diabetes are warranted. Several large randomized controlled trials have demonstrated that diet, weight loss, and exercise can delay or prevent progression of impaired fasting glucose and or impaired glucose tolerance to diabetes. The Finnish Diabetes Prevention Study evaluated 522 middle-aged overweight patients with impaired glucose tolerance and found that weight loss, increased fiber intake, and regular physical activity reduced the risk of developing diabetes by 58% after 3.2 years. The Diabetes Prevention Program was a larger study conducted in the United States that enrolled more than 3200 patients who had impaired glucose tolerance, impaired fasting glucose, or both. Patients were randomly assigned to intensive lifestyle modification with diet, exercise with a goal of 150 or more minutes per week, and a weight reduction goal of 7% of body weight vs a metformin and placebo arm. After 2.8 years, the individuals in the intensive lifestyle arm had a 58% reduction in the development of diabetes compared with that observed in the placebo group. The group treated with metformin had a 31% reduction in risk of progressing to diabetes. The salutary effects of intensive lifestyle were most pronounced in older and leaner individuals. Other lifestyle modification studies conducted in China and India have demonstrated similar findings in the prevention of diabetes.

Intensive lifestyle modification is the best treatment for this patient given her age and the fact that she is overweight (Answer E). She should be referred to a dietician to modify her diet and should be advised to exercise more than 150 minutes per week (with a goal of losing 5% to 7% of her body weight).

Metformin (Answer C) would not be expected to be as effective in reducing the risk of diabetes in this case. If she fails to exercise and lose weight, treatment with metformin could be considered at a later date. The cost of sitagliptin (Answer D) is high for the prevention of diabetes and it is not the treatment of choice in this case.

Several large trials have demonstrated that high-potency statins (eg, atorvastatin and rosuvastatin) increase the risk of developing diabetes. A primary cardiovascular prevention trial (JUPITER trial) of more than 17,000 patients without diabetes treated with rosuvastatin or placebo demonstrated that the risk of diabetes increased by 28% in patients treated with the statin (hazard ratio, 1.28; 95% confidence interval, 1.07 to 1.54; $P=.01$). A meta-analysis of 13 statin trials with more than 91,000 participants reported that statin use led to an 8% increased risk of developing diabetes during a mean treatment period of 4 years (odds ratio, 1.09; 95% confidence interval, 1.02 to 1.17). A meta-analysis of 5 studies with more than 32,000 patients without diabetes at baseline compared moderate-potency statins (eg, simvastatin) with high-potency statins and demonstrated a slightly higher risk of developing diabetes in the group treated with high-potency statins (odds ratio, 1.12; 95% confidence interval, 1.04 to 1.22).

The beneficial effects of statins in lowering cardiovascular events greatly outweigh the slightly increased risk of developing diabetes. In addition, most of the patients in the large statin trials had multiple risk factors for the development of diabetes. Lowering the atorvastatin dosage (Answer A) or stopping the medication (Answer B) in this patient with documented coronary artery disease would be counterproductive and potentially risky. She should continue on the same atorvastatin dosage.

Educational Objective
Recommend appropriate treatment of impaired fasting glucose or prediabetes, taking into account the patient's history, age, and body mass index.

UpToDate Topic Review(s)
Prevention of type 2 diabetes mellitus

Reference(s)

American Diabetes Association. 2. Classification and diagnosis of diabetes. *Diabetes Care.* 2016;39(Suppl 1):S13-S22. PMID: 26696675

Tuomilehto J, Lindstrom J, Eriksson JG, et al; Finnish Diabetes Prevention Study Group. Prevention of type 2 diabetes mellitus by changes in lifestyle among subjects with impaired glucose tolerance. *N Engl J Med.* 2001;344(18):1343-1350. PMID: 11333990

Knowler WC, Barrett-Connor E, Fowler SE, et al; Diabetes Prevention Program Research Group. Reduction in the incidence of type 2 diabetes mellitus with lifestyle intervention or metformin. *N Engl J Med.* 2002;346(6):393-403. PMID: 11832527

Ridker PM, Pradhan A, MacFadyen JG, Libby P, Glynn RJ. Cardiovascular benefits and diabetes risk of statin therapy in primary prevention: an analysis from the JUPITER trial. *Lancet.* 2012;380(9841):565-571. PMID: 22883507

Sattar N, Preiss D, Murray HM, et al. Statins and risk of incident diabetes: a collaborative meta-analysis of randomized statin trials. *Lancet.* 2010;375(9716):735-742. PMID: 20167359

Preiss D, Seshasai SR, Welsh P, et al. Risk of incident diabetes with intensive-dose compared with moderate-dose statin therapy: a meta-analysis. *JAMA.* 2011;305(24):2556-2564. PMID: 21693744

100 ANSWER: C) Methadone use

Naltrexone sustained release/bupropion sustained release is a weight-loss medication approved by the US FDA in 2014. Naltrexone is a competitive opioid antagonist and bupropion is a norepinephrine and dopamine reuptake inhibitor. Phase 3 clinical trials showed 5.0% to 9.3% weight loss in the treatment group compared with a 1.2% to 5.1% weight loss in the placebo group after 56 weeks. The most frequent adverse effects include nausea, constipation, headache, vomiting, dizziness, insomnia, dry mouth, and diarrhea.

Chronic opioid use (Answer C) is a contraindication to use of naltrexone/bupropion, as naltrexone blocks the opioid's effect. Additional contraindications are uncontrolled hypertension (thus, Answer B is incorrect as he has controlled hypertension); seizure disorders; anorexia nervosa or bulimia; pregnancy; concomitant use of a monoamine oxidase inhibitor; or abrupt discontinuation of alcohol, benzodiazepines, barbiturates, and anticonvulsant agents. The naltrexone/bupropion dosage must be adjusted depending on the patient's kidney function. This patient's current glomerular filtration rate (Answer D) is not a contraindication to use of naltrexone/bupropion, although the medication is not recommended for patients with end-stage renal disease. Nephrolithiasis (Answer E) and cholelithiasis (Answer A) are also not contraindications.

Antiobesity drugs that could be considered for this patient include liraglutide or lorcaserin.

Educational Objective
Counsel patients regarding contraindications to weight-loss medications.

Reference(s)

US Food and Drug Administration. FDA approves weight-management drug Contrave. Available at: http://www.fda.gov/newsevents/newsroom/
    pressannouncements/ucm413896.htm. September 10, 2014.

Contrave [package insert]. Deerfield, IL: Takeda Pharmaceuticals America, Inc; 2014.

Ali KF, Shukla AP, Aronne LJ. Bupropion-SR plus naltrexone-SR for the treatment of mild-to-moderate obesity. *Expert Rev Clin Pharmacol.* 2016;9(1):27-34.
    PMID: 26512740

101

ANSWER: D) Intravenous zoledronic acid

Paget disease of bone is a derangement in bone metabolism caused by increased bone resorption due to abnormal osteoclast physiology. Osteoclasts in pagetic bone are abnormal, with a bizarre appearance. They are multinucleated and are present in excessive numbers. This is a fairly common finding and is seen at a prevalence of 2% to 9% in some populations. The average age at diagnosis is in the fifth decade of life with a slight predilection for men. Paget disease is rarely seen in persons younger than 40 years. Most patients with Paget disease are asymptomatic and the diagnosis is made after an elevated alkaline phosphatase concentration is detected on routine laboratory evaluation or abnormalities are noted on radiographs. Paget disease can affect any bone, but it is most typically seen in the skull, spine, pelvis, and long bones. More significant clinical manifestations include pain, deformity, fractures, increased predisposition to development of bone tumors, abnormalities in calcium and phosphate metabolism (especially when immobilized), and hypervascularity of lesions, as seen in this patient, which can increase the risk of bleeding complications with orthopedic surgery.

The mainstay of pharmacotherapy for Paget disease is antiresorptive medications, including bisphosphonates and calcitonin. The more potent bisphosphonates—alendronate, risedronate, and zoledronic acid (Answer D)—can induce biochemical remissions in most patients. Zoledronic acid is the most likely agent to produce a long remission. Treatment with antiresorptive therapy *before* orthopedic surgery is indicated to diminish the vascularity of the bone and surrounding soft tissue and should reduce perioperative bleeding (thus, Answer C is incorrect). Additionally, treatment of asymptomatic Paget disease may be indicated depending on the location and activity of the disease. Disease sites at high risk of complications include weight-bearing bones, skull, spine, and a bone contiguous with a joint. It is reasonable to initiate pharmacotherapy if disease is present at other sites when elevations in alkaline phosphatase exceed 2 to 4 times the upper normal limit for the assay. The most potent antiresorptive agent, denosumab (Answer A), has been reported to decrease disease activity in 1 patient with Paget disease, but this has not been studied extensively and it would not be considered first-line therapy.

A rare complication of Paget disease is the transformation of pagetic bone into malignant osteosarcoma. Due to this increased risk of sarcoma, radiation therapy to pagetic bone (Answer B) is not recommended. Likewise, therapy with teriparatide (Answer E) would be contraindicated.

Educational Objective

Recommend preoperative medical treatment to reduce abnormal bone turnover in the setting of Paget disease.

Reference(s)

Ralston SH, Langston AL, Reid IR. Pathogenesis and management of Paget's disease of bone. *Lancet.* 2008;372(9633):155-163. PMID: 18620951

Lyles KW, Siris ES, Singer FR, Meunier PJ. A clinical approach to the diagnosis and management of Paget's disease of bone. *J Bone Miner Res.*
    2001;16(8):1379-1387. PMID: 11499860

Siris ES, Lyles KW, Singer FR, Meunier PJ. Medical management of Paget's disease of bone: indications for treatment and review of current therapies. *J Bone
    Miner Res.* 2006;21(Suppl 2):P94-P98. PMID: 17229018

102

ANSWER: A) *SDHB*

This patient's clinical presentation is concerning for pheochromocytoma, with biochemical evidence to support the presence of a catecholamine-secreting tumor and imaging that demonstrates a lipid-poor adrenal mass in addition to a probable renal cell carcinoma. This combination of pheochromocytoma and renal cell carcinoma should raise the possibility of an inherited tumor predisposition syndrome such as von-Hippel–Lindau syndrome (*VHL* gene), one of the succinate dehydrogenase gene mutation syndromes (*SDHA, SDHB, SDHC, SDHD,* or *SDHAF2*), or a mutation in the *TMEM127* gene. These autosomal dominant syndromes all carry a lifetime risk for developing pheochromocytoma, paraganglioma, and renal cell carcinoma. *VHL* mutations are also associated with many other vascular and nervous system tumors, while *SDHx* mutations can be associated with gastrointestinal stromal tumors (as seen in the patient's brother) and potentially with pancreatic neuroendocrine tumors and pituitary adenomas. Although a pathogenic mutation in either *SDHB* (Answer A) or *SDHAF2* (Answer C) could potentially explain this patient's presentation, an *SDHB* mutation is statistically far more likely because *SDHAF2* mutations are exceedingly rare (only a few cases have been identified).

Mutations in the *RET* proto-oncogene (Answer B), which cause multiple endocrine neoplasia type 2, and mutations in the *NF1* gene (Answer E), which cause neurofibromatosis type 1, increase the risk for pheochromocytoma, but neither syndrome is known to be associated with renal tumors or gastrointestinal stromal tumors. Mutations in the *MEN1* gene (Answer D), which cause multiple endocrine neoplasia type 1, are not associated with pheochromocytoma, renal cell carcinoma, or gastrointestinal stromal tumors.

The prevalence of a germline mutation in patients with pheochromocytoma or paraganglioma is estimated to be 25% to 40%. Many gene mutations are associated not only with pheochromocytoma and paraganglioma, but also with other tumors (eg, renal cell carcinoma, gastrointestinal stromal tumors). Genetic testing should be discussed with every patient, as recommended by the Endocrine Society Clinical Practice Guidelines in 2014. The discovery of a germline mutation has important surveillance implications for affected patients and their family members. Patients with a known mutation can be screened (with imaging) for tumors associated with that specific mutation. Although the exact surveillance recommendations have not been validated with evidence yet, it is generally recommended that patients with a known pheochromocytoma-paraganglioma genetic syndrome undergo longitudinal surveillance with a combination of plasma metanephrine measurement and imaging.

Educational Objective
Differentiate among the inherited pheochromocytoma-paraganglioma syndromes.

UpToDate Topic Review(s)
Pheochromocytoma in genetic disorders

Reference(s)

Lenders JW, Duh QY, Eisenhofer G, et al; Endocrine Society. Pheochromocytoma and paraganglioma: an Endocrine Society Clinical Practice Guideline. *J Clin Endocrinol Metab.* 2014;99(6):1915-1942. PMID: 24893135

Rana HQ, Rainville IR, Vaidya A. Genetic testing in the clinical care of patients with pheochromocytoma and paraganglioma. *Curr Opin Endocrinol Diabetes Obes.* 2014;21(3):166-176. PMID: 24739310

103

ANSWER: C) Ethinyl estradiol, 20 mcg daily, and norethindrone acetate, 1 mg daily

In the absence of medical contraindications, women between the ages of 40 and 50 years are still candidates for oral contraceptive use according to current US FDA guidelines. The lowest dosage of ethinyl estradiol, 20 mcg daily (Answer C), should be used in women older than 40 years. The risk of venous thromboembolism is lower than that associated with 30/35 mcg ethinyl estradiol preparations. In this patient, a low-dosage contraceptive pill could be given cyclically or could be given continuously to avoid the hot flashes that occur during the placebo break. Both regimens protect against pregnancy.

A higher-dosage contraceptive with 35 mcg ethinyl estradiol (Answer A) does not provide additional contraceptive or symptomatic benefit and is therefore not recommended. Continuous, combined hormone replacement therapy with estradiol, 0.025 mg transdermal daily, and micronized progesterone, 100 mg daily (Answer B), or with estradiol, 0.5 mg daily, and medroxyprogesterone, 2.5 mg daily (Answer D), will not provide birth control, and the patient does not want another pregnancy. Similarly, transdermal estradiol and norethindrone acetate (Answer E) will not prevent pregnancy. However, all these hormone replacement regimens would treat the hot flashes that occur in perimenopause.

Educational Objective
Recommend the most appropriate hormone treatment for a perimenopausal woman who does not desire pregnancy.

UpToDate Topic Review(s)
Treatment of menopausal symptoms with hormone therapy

Reference(s)

Martin KA, Manson JE. Approach to the patient with menopausal symptoms. *J Clin Endocrinol Metab*. 2008;93(12):4567-4575. PMID: 19056840

Taylor HS, Manson JE. Update in hormone therapy use in menopause. *J Clin Endocrinol Metab*. 2011;96(2):255-264. PMID: 21296989

Warren MP. Hormone therapy for menopausal symptoms: putting benefits and risks into perspective. *J Fam Pract*. 2010;59(12):E1-E7. PMID: 21135919

104 ANSWER: D) Celiac disease

Children with type 1 diabetes mellitus are at risk for a number of immune-mediated disorders, of which celiac disease and thyroid disease are the most common. In children, celiac disease may present with symptoms such as diarrhea, bloating, and fatigue. Affected children can have short stature and abnormalities of dental enamel, which can range in severity from grade 1 to 4:

- Grade 1—defect in color of enamel, 1 or more areas that are yellow, cream, or brown
- Grade 2—slight structural defects such as rough enamel surface, shallow pits, or horizontal grooves
- Grade 3—evident structural defects, deep horizontal grooves, large vertical pits
- Grade 4—severe structural defects, shape of tooth may be changed

Celiac disease is estimated to be present in 5% of persons with type 1 diabetes. About 85% of those affected are asymptomatic at diagnosis. In this vignette, the child has decreased growth velocity, mild gastrointestinal symptoms (ie, bloating), hypoglycemia, and dental enamel defects, which together make celiac disease (Answer D) the most likely diagnosis.

In children, hypothyroidism (Answer E) can be insidious in onset and is quite common in those with type 1 diabetes. Autoimmune thyroid disease is present in 5% of children with type 1 diabetes, and the incidence is higher in girls and increases with age. Clinical presentation can include fatigue, short stature, cold intolerance, constipation, poor school performance, and hypoglycemia. Signs often include bradycardia and delayed relaxation phase of reflexes. Decreased growth velocity should also raise suspicion for hypothyroidism. In clinical practice, TSH measurement would very likely be part of this child's evaluation. However, the dental enamel abnormalities and the low vitamin D level are more consistent with celiac disease than thyroid dysfunction in this case.

GH deficiency (Answer A) can be congenital or acquired. Congenital forms manifest with growth abnormality by 12 months of age. In the acquired form, children have increased weight-to-height ratios, infantile appearance, "cherubic face," and an underdeveloped nasal bridge. These children have short stature and, in severe cases or in those with ACTH deficiency, they may have hypoglycemia. However, the rest of this patient's presentation is not consistent with GH deficiency.

Gastroparesis (Answer B) is most often observed in those with poor diabetes control. It is associated with bloating and hypoglycemia and often develops more than 5 years following the diagnosis of diabetes. Gastroparesis is observed in those with poor diabetes control. However, in this patient, diabetes was diagnosed only 3 years ago and her glycemic control has been fairly good.

Adrenal insufficiency (Answer C) presents with a constellation of findings such as fatigue, nausea, and abdominal pain. On physical examination, she does not have skin hyperpigmentation, which may be seen in primary adrenal insufficiency. This patient has no headaches or vision changes to make one suspect secondary adrenal insufficiency.

Educational Objective
Assess for autoimmune disorders in patients with type 1 diabetes mellitus.

UpToDate Topic Review(s)

Associated autoimmune diseases in children and adolescents with type 1 diabetes mellitus

Reference(s)

Pham-Short A, Donaghue KC, Ambler G, Phelan H, Twigg S, Craig ME. Screening for celiac disease in type 1 diabetes: a systematic review. *Pediatrics.* 2015;136(1)e170-e176. PMID: 26077482

Hill ID, Dirks MH, Liptak GS, et al; North American Society for Pediatric Gastroenterology. Hepatology and Nutrition. Guideline for the diagnosis and treatment of celiac disease in children: recommendations of the North American Society for Pediatric Gastroenterology, Hepatology and Nutrition. *J Pediatr Gastroenterol Nutr.* 2005;40(1):1-19. PMID: 15625418

Rashid M, Zarkadas M, Anca A, Limeback H. Oral manifestations of celiac disease: a clinical guide for dentists. *J Can Dent Assoc.* 2011;77:b39. PMID: 21507289

105 ANSWER: A) Decrease her methimazole dosage

Both methimazole and propylthiouracil can be detected in the breast milk of lactating women being treated for hyperthyroidism. The amount of propylthiouracil that reaches breast milk is very small (0.007%-0.077% of the ingested dose) and generally does not affect the infant's thyroid function. Proportionally more methimazole or carbimazole is transferred into breast milk (0.1%-0.2% of the administered dose). Nevertheless, infants of mothers being treated with methimazole have been shown to have normal thyroid function. The available follow-up data also suggest that the intellectual development and physical growth of the child are unaffected by previous methimazole treatment of the mother. However, because the number of studied patients is small, the recent American Thyroid Association guidelines for treatment of thyroid disease during pregnancy and the postpartum period recommend that the maximal methimazole dosage used during lactation should be 20 mg daily and the maximal propylthiouracil dosage should be 450 mg daily. The patient described in this vignette required 40 mg daily of methimazole to maintain a normal TSH and slightly high levels of thyroid hormone during pregnancy. Now post partum, her TSH is the middle of the normal range on this same dosage. As the recommendation during lactation is to use the lowest possible effective dosage of methimazole or propylthiouracil, it would be reasonable to see if she could maintain euthyroidism on a lower methimazole dosage (Answer A). After her methimazole dosage is reduced, her thyroid function can be checked to make sure that her hyperthyroidism is still well controlled.

Maintaining the patient's current methimazole dosage (Answers B and C) would not be the best choice as her dosage is above that recommended during lactation and no attempt has yet been made to determine whether a lower dosage will maintain euthyroidism. A normal iodine status is important in lactating women, as iodine within breast milk is the sole source of iodine for breastfed infants. This mother is already taking a multivitamin containing 150 mcg of iodine. The iodine supplementation recommended by the American Thyroid Association during lactation is 150 mcg daily. Thus, this patient is receiving sufficient supplemental iodine and she does not need further supplementation with an additional 400 mcg dose. Indeed, sustained iodine intakes of more than 500 mcg daily are not recommended because of concern for inducing hypothyroidism in the baby.

This mother has some concerns about the quantity of her breast milk. Both hypothyroidism and hyperthyroidism may potentially have an adverse effect on lactation. The data regarding hypothyroidism leading to poor lactation are stronger than the data regarding hyperthyroidism, the latter being based mainly on animal studies. Thus, another consideration in this patient is to avoid any trend towards iatrogenic subclinical hypothyroidism, which might potentially have an adverse effect on milk production and let down. This patient is currently euthyroid, so her thyroid status should not be having a negative effect on milk production. Several galactogogues, including dopamine antagonists such as metoclopramide or domperidone, have occasionally been used to try and enhance lactation in women with poor milk production. However, these should not be considered until nonpharmacologic measures such as proper breastfeeding techniques and stress management have been used. Moreover, the American Academy of Pediatrics considers metoclopramide, a dopamine antagonist (Answer D), to be a medication with unknown side effects for the infant.

There is no compelling reason to switch this patient's regimen from methimazole to propylthiouracil (Answer E) because she is breastfeeding. Each of these medications can be safely used during lactation as long as the lowest effective dosage is used. Disadvantages of switching to propylthiouracil would be the greater risk of hepatotoxicity and the need to take propylthiouracil more than once daily.

Educational Objective
Guide the medical management of hyperthyroidism in lactating women.

UpToDate topic review(s)
Hyperthyroidism during pregnancy: Treatment

Reference(s)

Alexander EK, Pearce EN, Brent GA, et al. 2016 Guidelines of the American Thyroid Association for the Diagnosis and Management of Thyroid Disease during Pregnancy and the Postpartum. *Thyroid.* 2017;27(3):315-389. PMID: 28056690

106 ANSWER: E) Total testosterone, ↑; bioavailable testosterone, ↓; sex hormone–binding globulin, ↑

Most of the total testosterone measured in serum is bound to the carrier protein sex hormone–binding globulin (SHBG). When interpreting total testosterone levels, clinicians should keep in mind the medical conditions that can affect SHBG levels and consequently alter the levels of total testosterone.

SHBG is a glycoprotein produced in the liver under the influence of sex hormones and other nonhormonal factors. SHBG monomers dimerize during synthesis and secretion and contain 2 steroid binding sites. SHBG serves as a reservoir for bound steroids and regulates their bioavailability. SHBG binds various sex hormones with the highest affinity for dihydrotestosterone, followed by testosterone, followed by estradiol. SHBG levels in premenopausal women are greater than 2-fold higher than in men. This is due to estrogen, which increases SHBG levels. In healthy individuals, energy balance and physical activity are important factors in determining SHBG levels.

The man in this vignette has a history of possible hypogonadism and is currently hyperthyroid. Answer E is correct because thyroxine increases SHBG production and total testosterone levels. Bioavailable testosterone would decrease because there is less free and albumin-bound testosterone. None of the other patterns (Answers A, B, C, or D) is correct due to the effects explained above. The evaluation for hypogonadism should be deferred until the patient is euthyroid as a normal total testosterone value could be falsely reassuring in the setting of hyperthyroidism.

In addition to elevated thyroxine, elevated SHBG and total testosterone levels can be seen in men with HIV, acute and chronic hepatitis, cirrhosis, and alcoholism. Medications that induce hepatic enzymes (phenobarbital, phenytoin, and carbamazepine) also increase SHBG. In contrast, decreased SHBG and total testosterone levels can be seen in men with obesity and diabetes mellitus (due to the effects of insulin), nonalcoholic fatty liver disease, and hyperprolactinemia.

Educational Objective
Identify conditions that can alter levels of testosterone and sex hormone–binding globulin.

UpToDate Topic Review(s)
Clinical features and diagnosis of male hypogonadism

Reference(s)

Hammond GL, Wu TS, Simard M. Evolving utility of sex hormone-binding globulin measurements in clinical medicine. *Curr Opin Endocrinol Diabetes Obes.* 2012;19(3):183-189. PMID: 22531107

Thaler MA, Seifert-Klauss V, Luppa PB. The biomarker sex hormone-binding globulin - from established applications to emerging trends in clinical medicine. *Best Pract Res Clin Endocrinol Metab.* 2015;29(5):749-760. PMID: 26522459

107 ANSWER: E) Perform subtotal parathyroidectomy

This patient has secondary hyperparathyroidism from chronic kidney disease and prolonged hyperphosphatemia. Without evidence of hypercalcemia, he does not have tertiary hyperparathyroidism. Metabolic bone disease from secondary hyperparathyroidism (high bone resorption, bone pain and fractures) is seen in 40% to 87% of patients receiving dialysis. Extraskeletal manifestations due to high calcium-phosphate product include soft-tissue and vascular calcification, which increase the risk of cardiovascular disease and mortality. This patient's clinical presentation exemplifies the burden of extraskeletal manifestations of secondary hyperparathyroidism.

Management of secondary hyperparathyroidism is primarily with medical therapies to lower PTH levels (goal intact PTH is 150-300 pg/mL in patients with stage 5 chronic kidney disease), including calcium-free phosphate binders, vitamin D analogues, and a calcimimetic. Despite maximum-dosage treatment with a phosphate binder, this patient still has marked hyperphosphatemia causing secondary hyperparathyroidism. Thus, increasing the dosage of sevelamer (Answer A) is incorrect. Treatment with cinacalcet is the best course of action and is effective, but this patient was not able to tolerate it due to nausea and hypocalcemia, so restarting this medication (Answer B) is not a good option. Restarting calcitriol (Answer C) is not recommended because of the uncontrolled hyperphosphatemia and history of hypercalcemia in this patient. Ergocalciferol (Answer D) will not be fully effective in this severe case and will most likely further increase phosphate levels.

Subtotal parathyroidectomy (Answer E) is the best treatment given the potential for high cardiovascular mortality associated with calciphylaxis seen in this patient with vascular calcifications (throughout vessels seen on lateral spine x-ray) and ectopic calcium deposits subcutaneously (seen on left elbow x-ray). Surgical parathyroidectomy has been reported to improve quality of life and to increase survival rates in patients receiving dialysis.

Educational Objective
Determine when surgery is indicated in a patient with hyperparathyroidism associated with end-stage renal disease.

UpToDate Topic Review(s)
Parathyroidectomy in end-stage renal disease

Reference(s)

Lorenz K, Bartsch DK, Sancho JJ, Guigard S, Triponez F. Surgical management of secondary hyperparathyroidism in chronic kidney disease--a consensus report of the European Society of Endocrine Surgeons. *Langenbecks Arch Surg*. 2015;400(8):907-927. PMID: 26429790

Madorin C, Owen RP, Fraser WD, et al. The surgical management of renal hyperparathyroidism. *Eur Arch Otorhinolaryngol*. 2012;269(6):1565-1576. PMID: 22101574

Rodriquez M, Goodman WG, Liakopoulos V, Messa P, Wiecek A, Cunningham J. The use of calcimimetics for the treatment of secondary hyperparathyroidism: a 10 year evidence review. *Semin Dial*. 2015;28(5):497-507. PMID: 25752650

108

ANSWER: A) Weight ↔/↓; triglycerides ↓; hypoglycemia ↔; creatinine ↔; vitamin B$_{12}$ ↔/↓
The American Diabetes Association recommends metformin as the initial antihyperglycemic agent of choice for most patients with type 2 diabetes. Hemoglobin A$_{1c}$ levels commonly decrease by 1.0% to 1.5% with metformin use through reductions in hepatic gluconeogenesis and improvements in peripheral insulin resistance. The expected pattern of effects on weight, triglycerides, hypoglycemia, creatinine, and vitamin B$_{12}$ 6 months after starting metformin therapy is best characterized in Answer A.

Metformin has either a neutral effect on weight or leads to modest weight loss, and it often blunts weight gain when used in combination with sulfonylureas, insulin, or thiazolidinediones.

Initiation of metformin leads to reductions in triglycerides, more modest reductions in LDL cholesterol, increases in HDL cholesterol, and reductions in several clotting factors. These findings most likely contribute to beneficial cardiovascular effects observed with long-term metformin use. When compared with outcomes with sulfonylurea or insulin therapy in the United Kingdom Prospective Diabetes Study, metformin monotherapy led to reductions in total mortality in obese patients with type 2 diabetes, as well as reductions in myocardial infarction and death of any cause after longer-term follow-up of these study patients. Metformin monotherapy reduced long-term cardiovascular mortality in a meta-analysis of observational studies comparing metformin with sulfonylurea therapy.

Because metformin does not stimulate insulin secretion, it is not usually associated with hypoglycemia unless used in combination with insulin or sulfonylureas.

Given metformin's renal clearance, its use is contraindicated in those with an estimated glomerular filtration rate below 30 mL/min per 1.73 m^2. Its use does not affect renal function or creatinine levels.

In up to 30% of patients, metformin reduces the absorption of vitamin B$_{12}$ in a dosage- and duration-dependent manner. This can lower vitamin B$_{12}$ levels and rarely lead to vitamin B$_{12}$ deficiency, peripheral neuropathy, or megaloblastic anemia. Periodic monitoring of vitamin B$_{12}$ is therefore recommended in patients using metformin.

Adverse effects due to metformin are mostly gastrointestinal in nature and include diarrhea, flatulence, and abdominal pain. These effects are dosage related, often transient, and reduced by administration of the drug with food. Lactic acidosis is an adverse effect seen more commonly with another biguanide (phenformin), and it rarely occurs with metformin (typically only in individuals who have concomitant illnesses associated with lactic acidosis).

Educational Objective
Explain the nonglycemic effects of metformin therapy.

UpToDate Topic Review(s)
Metformin in the treatment of adults with type 2 diabetes mellitus

Reference(s)

Holman RR, Paul SK, Bethel MA, Matthews DR, Neil HA. 10-year follow up of intensive glucose control in type 2 diabetes. *N Engl J Med.* 2008;359(15):1577-1589. PMID: 18784090

Maruthur NM, Tseng E, Hutfless S, et al. Diabetes medications as monotherapy or metformin-based combination therapy for type 2 diabetes: a systematic review and meta-analysis. *Ann Intern Med.* 2016;164(11):740-751. PMID: 27088241

109 ANSWER: A) Elevated titers of TSH receptor antibodies (TRAb) in the mother

TSH receptor antibodies (TRAb) can effectively cross the placenta and can cause fetal hyperthyroidism once the fetal thyroid gland is functional. If the maternal TRAb concentration is high (generally considered >3 times the upper reference for the assay), the fetus should be carefully monitored throughout pregnancy for development of fetal hyperthyroidism. Most commonly, fetal hyperthyroidism caused by passage of TRAb across the placenta occurs at or after 20 to 22 weeks' gestation. When transplacental passage of TRAb occurs in a woman with Graves disease who is being treated with antithyroidal medications, the fetal hyperthyroidism may be ameliorated by the fact that the antithyroidal medication is also crossing the placenta and is reaching the fetus. Following delivery, the antithyroidal drug is cleared by the fetus more rapidly than TRAb and the neonate's degree of hyperthyroidism will worsen.

The 2011 American Thyroid Association Guidelines for Managing Hyperthyroidism During Pregnancy recommend checking TRAb levels at 20 to 24 weeks' gestation. The current American Thyroid Association Guidelines for Managing Hyperthyroidism During Pregnancy and Post Partum recommend checking TRAb in early pregnancy when thyroid function is first assessed. If the TRAb titer is high in early pregnancy, repeated testing at 18 to 22 weeks' gestation is recommended. If TRAb is elevated at 18 to 22 weeks, additional TRAb testing at 30 to 34 weeks is recommended to help guide postnatal monitoring.

Importantly, TRAb may also persist in women who have received definitive therapy for hyperthyroidism. These antibodies trend down after definitive therapy, but may persist in some patients. Generally, persistence is seen more often if the therapy used was radioiodine therapy. A history of Graves disease previously treated with radioactive iodine or thyroidectomy is an indication to check TRAb during pregnancy. In this situation, the mother may be euthyroid while receiving levothyroxine therapy, but the fetus, nevertheless, becomes hyperthyroid due to TRAb crossing the placenta from the mother. Typically, such hyperthyroidism occurs after 20 to 22 weeks' gestation. However, fetal hyperthyroidism due to transplacental TRAb passage has also been reported as early as week 18. Fetal hyperthyroidism, due to maternal TRAb in a woman who requires levothyroxine after definitive treatment of Graves disease, is one of the few potential indications for "block and replace therapy." In this situation, the antithyroidal drug, given to the mother, crosses the placenta and treats the fetal hyperthyroidism, while the levothyroxine, which crosses the placenta less effectively than antithyroidal drugs, treats the mother's hypothyroidism.

Consequences of fetal hyperthyroidism include fetal tachycardia, intrauterine growth restriction, fetal goiter, accelerated bone maturation, congestive heart failure, and fetal hydrops. In the patient described in this vignette, there are indications that fetal hyperthyroidism occurred during her previous pregnancy, in addition to the current one. The best explanation for this is a high titer of TRAb (Answer A), and these antibodies should be checked. In this particular situation, the thyroid status of the mother (euthyroid) does not reflect the thyroid status of the fetus (hyperthyroid). Therefore, the mother's free T_4 and total T_3 would be expected to be normal, as indicated by her serum TSH level (thus, Answers B and C are incorrect). The fetus would be expected to have a goiter and high thyroid hormone levels due to the action of TRAb. The fetus should have a low TSH level and therefore umbilical cord blood TSH levels should also be low (thus, Answer E is incorrect). Fetal hyperthyroidism is associated with accelerated bone maturation, not delayed maturation (thus, Answer D is incorrect). Close collaboration with the patient's obstetrician and the neonate's pediatrician is essential for successful management of a case such as this.

Educational Objective
Explain that neonatal Graves disease can occur in an athyreotic patient with Graves disease due to thyroid-stimulating antibodies and that this can occur earlier than 22 weeks' gestation.

UpToDate Topic Review(s)
Evaluation and management of neonatal Graves disease

Reference(s)

Alexander EK, Pearce EN, Brent GA, et al. 2017 Guidelines of the American Thyroid Association for the Diagnosis and Management of Thyroid Disease during Pregnancy and the Postpartum. *Thyroid.* 2017;27(3):315-389. PMID: 28056690

Dierickx I, Decallonne B, Billen J, et al. Severe fetal and neonatal hyperthyroidism years after surgical treatment of maternal Graves' disease. *J Obstet Gynaecol.* 2014;34(2):117-122. PMID: 24456429

Donnelly MA, Wood C, Casey B, Hobbins J, Barbour LA. Early severe fetal Graves disease in a mother after thyroid ablation and thyroidectomy. *Obstet Gynecol.* 2015;125(5):1059-1062. PMID: 25710616

Laurberg P, Nygaard B, Glinoer D, Grussendorf M, Orgiazzi J. Guidelines for TSH-receptor antibody measurements in pregnancy: results of an evidence-based symposium organized by the European Thyroid Association. *Eur J Endocrinol.* 1998;139(6):584-586. PMID: 9916861

Laurberg P, Wallin G, Tallstedt L, Abraham-Nordling M, Lundell G, Torring O. TSH-receptor autoimmunity in Graves' disease after therapy with anti-thyroid drugs, surgery, or radioiodine: a 5-year prospective randomized study. *Eur J Endocrinol.* 2008;158(1):69-75. PMID: 18166819

110 ANSWER: B) ACTH stimulation test
Based on the presence of 21-hydroxylase antibodies, this patient has autoimmune primary ovarian insufficiency. In virtually all cases in which the precursor to autoimmune ovarian insufficiency can be demonstrated (ie, autoimmune oophoritis), primary ovarian insufficiency is associated with adrenal autoimmunity or adrenal insufficiency. Therefore, autoimmune ovarian insufficiency is most accurately diagnosed with antiadrenal or 21-hydroxylase antibodies because these antibodies are directed at steroid enzymes that are present in both the ovary and adrenal or adrenal cells secreting steroids common to the ovary and adrenal. Ovarian antibodies (Answer A) are not specific and should therefore not be used in the assessment of autoimmune ovarian insufficiency. The presence of adrenal antibodies is associated with development of adrenal failure in 50% of adults. Thus, in a woman with suspected autoimmune ovarian insufficiency and adrenal autoimmunity, a morning cortisol level should be assessed and/or an ACTH stimulation test should be performed (Answer B) if the morning cortisol concentration is less than 18 µg/dL (<496.6 nmol/L).

Women with autoimmune ovarian insufficiency and adrenal autoimmunity have autoimmune polyglandular syndrome type II, characterized by primary adrenal insufficiency and an additional autoimmune disease. Autoimmune thyroid disease is common in women with primary ovarian insufficiency. However, TSH is normal in the patient in this vignette and measurement of TPO antibodies (Answer D) is not the most important next test. Other autoimmune associations include diabetes mellitus, pernicious anemia, rheumatoid arthritis, systemic lupus erythematosus, myasthenia gravis, vitiligo, and premature gray hair. However, without symptoms, measurement of hemoglobin A_{1c} to assess for diabetes (Answer E) is also not the next best test. Finally, antimullerian hormone levels (Answer C) correlate with the number of small antral follicles in the ovary. In a patient with a high FSH level in the postmenopausal range, antimullerian hormone levels will be low and would not provide additional diagnostic information (Answer C).

Educational Objective
Determine the most important tests to order in a patient with polyglandular autoimmune syndrome type II.

UpToDate Topic Review(s)
Clinical features and diagnosis of autoimmune primary ovarian insufficiency (premature ovarian failure)

Reference(s)

Abraham SB, Abel BS, Sinaii N, Saverino E, Wade M, Nieman LK. Primary vs secondary adrenal insufficiency: ACTH-stimulated aldosterone diagnostic cut-off values by tandem mass spectrometry. *Clin Endocrinol (Oxf)*. 2015;83(3):308-314. PMID: 25620457

Hoek A, Schoemaker J, Drexhage HA. Premature ovarian failure and ovarian autoimmunity. *Endocr Rev*. 1997;18(1):107-134. PMID: 9034788

111 ANSWER: D) Change to insulin glargine, 150 units, and insulin aspart, 50 units, with meals + correction dosing—total daily dose 300 units

The scenario in this vignette is becoming more common with the obesity epidemic and the increasing use of U500 insulin. While there are very few prospective data on U500 insulin use, a number of retrospective studies have demonstrated the utility of this concentrated insulin in treating individuals with marked insulin resistance. Many clinicians consider U500 insulin use in patients requiring more than 200 units of insulin daily, or more than 2 units/kg per day. In outpatient use, U500 insulin has been reported to lead to improved glycemic control and improved patient satisfaction, most likely because of smaller injection volumes facilitating the administration of large insulin doses. In the United States, a U500 insulin pen and syringe were recently released in which the administration of the insulin dose is indicated by units (in 5-unit increments). However, many U500 insulin users still administer it by syringe, and thus prescriptions should clarify dosing by both volume (in mL) or insulin syringe units and specify total insulin (U100 insulin) units.

When a patient on a U500 insulin regimen is admitted to hospital, diabetes management can be challenging. Many hospitals do not use U500 insulin in inpatients because of concerns about dosing errors between U100 and U500 insulin administration orders, particularly the increased risk of hypoglycemia. Furthermore, many patients with diabetes have decreased insulin needs during their hospital stay. Previous studies of glucose control in patients in general wards (excluding intensive care units) have indicated that severe hypoglycemia occurs in up to 8% of patients with diabetes, and hypoglycemic events during admissions are associated with increased inpatient mortality and length of stay. While tight glycemic control during inpatient admissions has demonstrated benefits in critically ill patients, there is no evidence to support tight glycemic control in patients admitted to general wards and avoidance of severe hypoglycemia may be the first priority.

Very few data are available regarding the use of U500 insulin in hospitalized patients. One single-center retrospective study compared 41 U500 users who were maintained on U500 during admission with 20 U500 users whose regimens were converted to U100 insulin during admission. The group maintained on U500 had higher home insulin doses and an average reduction in total daily dose of 15%, whereas the group converted to U100 insulin had lower home insulin doses but a larger drop in inpatient insulin dose (decreased by 65%). However, the glucose levels were not significantly different between the groups. The group maintained on U500 insulin had more days with hypoglycemia but a shorter length of stay than the group converted to U100 insulin, and the authors concluded that use of U500 insulin during admission may be appropriate for some patients. Another single-center retrospective study compared inpatient insulin doses with home insulin doses for U500 insulin users (all patients' regimens were converted to U100 insulin during admission) and reported that the average inpatient insulin dose was only 22.6% of the usual home dose. Patients were stratified into 3 groups based on their preadmission hemoglobin A_{1c} level (<8%, 8%-9%, >9% [<64, 64-75, >75 mmol/mol]). All 3 groups had dose reductions of 75% to 80% compared with the home insulin dose, yet hypoglycemia was present in 2% to 4% of point-of-care blood glucose readings. The group with the highest preadmission hemoglobin A_{1c} value had the most hyperglycemia during inpatient admissions. A notable difference between the 2 studies is the home total daily insulin use: the first study (Tripathy et al) had home insulin doses of 200 U100 units daily, whereas the second study (Palladino et al) reported home insulin doses of 300 to 500 U100 units daily.

For the patient in this vignette, use of U500 insulin during the inpatient stay at either the usual home dose (Answer A) or 90% of the usual home dose (Answer B) could put him at high risk for hypoglycemia. He admits to poor dietary adherence at home, and although his current illness could be expected to increase insulin resistance, the effect of decreased caloric and carbohydrate intake from his diabetes diet in the hospital is likely to dominate his inpatient insulin needs. Furthermore, the long half-life of U500 insulin is less desirable in inpatients in whom nothing-by-mouth status can change suddenly. Thus, use of U500 insulin during his admission is not the best answer. While conversion of his home insulin dose to U100 insulin (Answer C) is an option, his most likely decreased inpatient caloric intake raises the concern for hypoglycemia. Use of basal-bolus U100 insulin during hospital admission with a dose reduction of at least 50% (Answer D) is appropriate to decrease the risk of hypoglycemia. Daily follow-up and titration of the dose can reduce his risk of uncontrolled hyperglycemia. Although use of intravenous insulin (Answer E) has been well validated in critically ill patients, it is often not practical on general wards and is very difficult to manage in patients who are eating.

Educational Objective
Manage the insulin regimen of an inpatient whose home regimen consists of U500 insulin.

UpToDate Topic Review(s)
Management of diabetes mellitus in hospitalized patients

Reference(s)

Palladino CE, Eberly ME, Emmons JT, Tannock LR. Management of U-500 insulin users during inpatient admissions within a Veterans Affairs Medical Center. *Diabetes Res Clin Pract.* 2016;114:32-36. PMID: 27103366

Tripathy PR, Lansang MC. U-500 regular insulin use in hospitalized patients. *Endocr Pract.* 2015;21(1):54-58. PMID: 25628119

Turchin A, Matheny ME, Shubina M, Scanlon JV, Greenwood B, Pendergrass ML. Hypoglycemia and clinical outcomes in patients with diabetes hospitalized in the general ward. *Diabetes Care.* 2009;32(7):1153-1157. PMID: 19564471

112 ANSWER: C) Ultrasound-guided FNAB of the left-sided thyroid nodule

This patient has mild subclinical hyperthyroidism and a palpable thyroid nodule. A technetium scan has been performed to investigate the underlying etiology of his mild thyrotoxicosis. Because there is significant tracer uptake on this scan, a diagnosis of thyroiditis is unlikely and the differential diagnosis is Graves disease or toxic nodular hyperthyroidism. On physical examination, only 1 right-sided nodule is detected, but on ultrasonography, a left-sided nodule is also present. To evaluate which of the thyroid nodules is functioning, careful comparison of the isotope and ultrasound imaging is required.

The technetium scan indicates significant tracer uptake in the lowest portion of the right thyroid lobe corresponding to the palpable thyroid abnormality with reduced uptake in the upper part of the right lobe consistent with the presence of a right-sided autonomous nodule as the cause of subclinical hyperthyroidism. This nodule corresponds to a benign-appearing mixed cystic/solid nodule. Careful inspection of the technetium scan also indicates a markedly photopenic area, lacking all pixels, in the left thyroid lobe representing a "cold," nonfunctioning nodule. This corresponds to an isoechoic solid thyroid nodule without calcification on ultrasonography, and current American Thyroid Association guidelines classify this as a nodule with low suspicion of malignancy. The risk of malignancy in such nodules is estimated to be 5% to 10%. FNAB is recommended in low-suspicion nodules that are 1.5 cm or larger in maximum diameter. On the basis of size criteria, a decision to proceed with FNAB is debatable. However, the complete absence of isotope uptake should raise suspicion that thyroid cancer may be present, and the most appropriate action is to perform ultrasound-guided FNAB of the left-sided cold nodule (Answer C). If the cytologic findings are benign, then radioactive iodine to treat subclinical hyperthyroidism is warranted because the serum TSH concentration is less than 0.1 mIU/L. However, if cytologic findings are indeterminate or suspicious, then surgery is the most appropriate treatment option.

FNAB of functioning nodules (the right-sided nodule) (Answers A and B) is not recommended since the risk of malignancy is very low. Measurement of serum thyroid-stimulating immunoglobulin (Answer E) may be useful in determining the etiology of hyperthyroidism, but because the presence of an autonomous nodule has already been confirmed this is not the best option. Measurement of serum thyroglobulin (Answer D) is useful in the follow-up of patients with thyroid cancer who have undergone a total thyroidectomy, but it does not help establish the etiology of hyperthyroidism, nor does it predict the malignancy risk in thyroid nodules.

Educational Objective
Combine thyroid ultrasonography and scintigraphy findings to guide the investigation of functioning and nonfunctioning thyroid nodules.

UpToDate Topic Review(s)
Diagnostic approach to and treatment of thyroid nodules

Ross DS, Burch HB, Cooper DS, et al. 2016 American Thyroid Association guidelines for diagnosis and management of hyperthyroidism and other causes of thyrotoxicosis. *Thyroid.* 2016;26(10):1343-1420. PMID: 27521067

Haugen BR, Alexander EK, Bible KC, et al. 2015 American Thyroid Association management guidelines for adult patients with thyroid nodules and differentiated thyroid cancer: The American Thyroid Association Guidelines Task Force on Thyroid Nodules and Differentiated Thyroid Cancer. *Thyroid.* 2016;26(1):1-133. PMID: 26462967

113 ANSWER: A) Add insulin

Diabetic proximal neuropathy, also called diabetic amyotrophy, diabetic lumbosacral radiculopathy, or Bruns-Garland syndrome, is an uncommon form of mixed sensory-motor dysfunction that is most commonly found in middle-aged or elderly men who have type 2 diabetes. Diabetic amyotrophy is almost always associated with coexisting peripheral neuropathy. The etiology of the syndrome is unknown, but it has been attributed to metabolic derangements, inflammatory factors, and ischemia. A prospective study of 33 patients with diabetic proximal neuropathy who underwent sural or superficial peroneal nerve biopsy demonstrated evidence of ischemic injury (which included findings of axonal degeneration, multifocal fiber loss, focal perineural necrosis, and neovascularization) compared with findings in healthy control patients. The proposed cause of the ischemia was microscopic vasculitis. Electromyography and nerve conduction studies demonstrate slowed conduction time and velocity in both motor and sensory nerves. There is evidence of denervation of the involved proximal muscle groups.

Patients with diabetic amyotrophy usually present with unilateral thigh pain followed by weakness in the proximal muscles of the lower extremities. In most patients, the symptoms progress to involve both thighs and obturator muscles. Distal muscle involvement may develop later. Some patients present with bilateral lower-extremity pain. Weight loss is common and some patients have cachexia. The typical course is progression of symptoms over 6 to 12 months. This is followed by partial to full recovery in most patients over a period of months to years. However, some patients do not fully recover muscle function and need assistance to ambulate.

Supportive care is important in patients who have diabetic amyotrophy as most will recover fully. However, when a patient has significant weight loss as in this case, then insulin should be started not only to improve glycemic control but also as an anabolic agent to promote weight gain. Metformin does not need to be stopped in this patient (thus, Answer E is incorrect). He should continue metformin and start insulin (Answer A).

Gabapentin (Answer B) and pregabalin (Answer D) are anticonvulsant medications that are used to treat neuropathic pain associated with diabetes and other disorders. As the patient in this case was already started on duloxetine, it is redundant to add either gabapentin or pregabalin. Duloxetine is a selective serotonin and norepinephrine reuptake inhibitor that can be used to treat depression and diabetic neuropathy pain. None of these medications will alter the root cause of the diabetic proximal neuropathy and are used to relieve symptoms.

Chronic inflammatory demyelinating polyradiculopathy should be considered in the differential diagnosis in cases of diabetic proximal neuropathy. However, patients with chronic inflammatory demyelinating polyradiculopathy have symmetric involvement of the extremities and there is greater motor than sensory involvement. In addition, affected patients typically do not lose weight. Patients with chronic inflammatory demyelinating polyradiculopathy are often treated with intravenous immunoglobulins or plasma exchange, usually combined with high-dosage pulse glucocorticoids.

No randomized controlled trials have been conducted to assess effective treatment of diabetic amyotrophy. There are limited and conflicting data on the effectiveness of immunoglobulin treatment, plasma exchange, cyclophosphamide, or glucocorticoids (Answer C). A randomized, double-blind study of patients with diabetic lumbosacral radiculopathy failed to demonstrate improvement in the primary study end point, a neuropathy impairment score, with intravenous methylprednisolone compared with placebo.

The patient in this vignette would benefit from physical therapy to improve strength and balance. Fall prevention is important. He should be evaluated for devices to assist ambulation such as a cane, a walker, or even a wheelchair until he recovers.

Educational Objective

Diagnose the syndrome of diabetic neuropathic cachexia and recommend appropriate treatment.

UpToDate Topic Review(s)
Epidemiology and classification of diabetic neuropathy

Reference(s)

Barohn RJ, Sahenk Z, Warmolts JR, Mendell JR. The Bruns-Garland syndrome (diabetic amyotrophy). Revisited 100 years later. *Arch Neurol.* 1991;48(11):1130-1135. PMID: 1953396

Bastron JA, Thomas JE. Diabetic polyradiculopathy: clinical and electromyographic findings in 105 patients. *Mayo Clin Proc.* 1981;56(12):725-732. PMID: 7311600

Dyck PJ, Norell JE, Dyck PJ. Microvasculitis and ischemia in diabetic lumbosacral radiculoplexus neuropathy. *Neurology.* 1999;53(9):2113-2121. PMID: 10599791

Zochodne DW, Isaac D, Jones C. Failure of immunotherapy to prevent, arrest or reverse diabetic lumbosacral plexopathy. *Acta Neurol Scand.* 2003;107(4):299-301. PMID: 12675705

Van den Bergh PY, Hadden RD, Bouche P, et al; European Federation of Neurological Societies; Peripheral Nerve Society. European Federation of Neurological Societies/Peripheral Nerve Society guideline on management of chronic inflammatory demyelinating polyradiculopathy: report of a joint task force of the European Federation of Neurological Societies and the Peripheral Nerve Society - first revision [published correction appears in *Eur J Neurol.* 2011;18(5):796]. *Eur J Neurol.* 2010;17(3):356-363. PMID: 20456730

Thaisetthawatkul P, Dyck PJ. Treatment of diabetic and nondiabetic lumbosacral radiculoplexus neuropathy. *Curr Treat Options Neurol.* 2010;12(2):95-99. PMID: 20842573

114 ANSWER: D) Administer hydrocortisone

This patient presents with relative primary adrenal insufficiency and treatment with hydrocortisone (Answer D)—and very possibly fludrocortisone—is warranted. He has symptoms of adrenal insufficiency, mild hyponatremia, and hyperkalemia. Although his morning cortisol level is deceptively normal, the markedly elevated ACTH suggests that a cortisol value of 14 µg/dL (386.2 nmol/L) is the maximum adrenal reserve. This constellation of findings suggests relative primary adrenal failure.

Mitotane can induce adrenal insufficiency and other endocrinopathies via multiple mechanisms. Mitotane is adrenolytic and/or adrenostatic and therefore impairs adrenal steroidogenesis from the remaining right adrenal gland. Further, mitotane induces hepatic synthesis of cortisol-binding globulin, which results in reduced bioavailability of free cortisol. For these reasons, patients treated with mitotane need concomitant glucocorticoid therapy (and often mineralocorticoids as adrenal function decreases). Lastly, mitotane also substantially increases hepatic CYP3A4 activity and therefore the metabolism of exogenous glucocorticoids is accelerated. Thus, patients taking mitotane not only require glucocorticoid therapy but often require much higher dosages than usual to maintain adequate adrenal function. It is generally recommended that patients on mitotane be treated with glucocorticoid supplementation, and increasing these doses to supraphysiologic levels should occur based on the detection of signs and symptoms of relative adrenal insufficiency (such as fatigue, weakness, low blood pressure).

Mitotane similarly induces other notable endocrinopathies. It causes secondary hypothyroidism via unknown mechanisms and increases thyroxine-binding globulin resulting in decreased free thyroid hormone availability. The increase in CYP3A4 activity accelerates the metabolism of exogenous levothyroxine. Therefore, patients treated with mitotane often need much larger levothyroxine dosages to maintain a euthyroid state.

Mitotane induces secondary hypogonadism via unknown mechanisms, increases sex hormone–binding globulin to decrease free testosterone availability, increases the metabolism of exogenous testosterone by inducing CYP3A4, and may also inhibit 5α-reductase activity and thereby the generation of dihydrotestosterone. Therefore, male patients treated with mitotane often need much higher testosterone dosages to maintain a eugonadal state.

Even after mitotane has been stopped (Answer A), it may take many weeks to months for it to be cleared from the body. Further, stopping mitotane would not reverse the primary adrenal insufficiency. Although the administration of sodium chloride tablets (Answer B) or ondansetron (Answer C) might make the patient feel better temporarily, neither would address the underlying cortisol insufficiency. Metyrapone (Answer E) would further decrease cortisol and would potentially make the patient more ill.

Educational Objective

Manage mitotane-induced adrenal insufficiency and other endocrinopathies.

Reference(s)

Else T, Kim AC, Sabolch A, et al. Adrenocortical carcinoma. *Endocr Rev.* 2014;35(2):282-326. PMID: 24423978

Fay AP, Elfiky A, Telo GH, et al. Adrenocortical carcinoma: the management of metastatic disease. *Crit Rev Oncol Hematol.* 2014;92(2):123-132. PMID: 24958272

115 ANSWER: A) Valproic acid

When prescribing medications to overweight or obese patients, clinicians should avoid, when possible, drugs that are known to cause weight gain. This adverse effect interfered with the patient's treatment adherence. The initial anticonvulsant drug most likely prescribed to this patient was valproic acid (Answer A), an agent known to cause weight gain. A retrospective study of valproic acid documented that after starting the drug, 71% of patients gained more than 5% of their initial body weight and 47% gained more than 10%. Valproic acid also causes a clinical picture similar to that of polycystic ovary syndrome. Other anticonvulsant agents known to cause weight gain are gabapentin, pregabalin, and vigabatrin. Topiramate and zonisamide (Answer E) are both anticonvulsant drugs associated with weight loss. A randomized placebo-controlled trial of patients with refractory partial-onset seizures documented a weight loss of more than 5 lb (2.3 kg) in 21.6% of participants who took zonisamide compared with 10.4% in the placebo group. Levetiracetam (Answer B), phenytoin (Answer C), and lamotrigine (Answer D) are considered to be weight-neutral anticonvulsant drugs.

Educational Objective
Identify medications associated with weight gain.

Reference(s)

Apovian CM, Aronne LJ, Bessesen DH, et al; Endocrine Society. Pharmacological management of obesity: an Endocrine Society clinical practice guideline. *J Clin Endocrinol Metab.* 2015;100(2):342-362. PMID: 25590212

Corman CL, Leung NM, Guberman AH. Weight gain in epileptic patients during treatment with valproic acid: a retrospective study. *Can J Neurol Sci.* 1997;24(3):240-244. PMID: 9276111

Ben-Menachem E. Weight issues for people with epilepsy--a review. *Epilepsia.* 2007;48(Suppl 9):42-45. PMID: 18047602

Faught E, Ayala R, Montouris GG, Leppik IE, Zonisamide 922 Trial Group. Randomized controlled trial of zonisamide for the treatment of refractory partial-onset seizures. *Neurology.* 2001;57(10):1774-1779. PMID: 11723262

116 ANSWER: D) Ipilimumab/nivolumab–induced hypothyroidism

Immune checkpoint inhibitors represent a new and effective class of cancer therapies that have revolutionized the management of advanced metastatic melanoma. Their mechanism of action is through boosting the negative immunoregulatory receptors on the T-cell surface to enhance the host immunity against tumor cells. Several agents have been shown to improve overall patient survival in this setting. For the management of unresectable metastatic malignant melanoma, the US FDA has approved the use of ipilimumab, which blocks the cytotoxic T-lymphocyte antigen 4 (CTLA4) on activated T cells, and pembrolizumab and nivolumab, which are antibody-derived immune regulators, blocking the activation of the antiprogrammed cell death 1 (PDCD1, also called PD1) receptor. In addition there are various similar agents under investigation in clinical trials. Not unexpectedly, altering immune signaling pathways results in immune-related adverse events, which include dermatologic, gastrointestinal, and endocrine toxicities. The different endocrine adverse effects seen with use of immune checkpoint inhibitors include hypophysitis with or without hypopituitarism, thyroid dysfunction, and adrenalitis with associated hypoadrenalism.

The pattern of primary thyroid disturbances reported with immune checkpoint inhibitors includes transient thyrotoxicosis, transient or longstanding hypothyroidism, thyroid eye disease, painless thyroiditis, and occasionally severe forms of thyroid disease such as thyroid storm. Thyroid disorders or abnormalities in thyroid function tests are seen in 1% to 6% of patients treated with ipilimumab. Similar incidence rates have been reported with the use of nivolumab and tremelimumab, but a much higher incidence of thyroid dysfunction was observed when combination therapy with ipilimumab and nivolumab was used (9% to 22%, respectively). The patient in this vignette has developed primary hypothyroidism, which is most likely secondary to combination therapy with ipilimumab and nivolumab (Answer D).

Hypophysitis is a rare condition occurring in less than 1% of surgically treated pituitary lesions. In contrast, review of the trial data of immune checkpoint-induced hypophysitis for CTLA-4 drugs showed an incidence of hypophysitis for ipilimumab of 0% to 17%, while the incidence was less than 1% for nivolumab and pembrolizumab. It is unclear whether combination therapy with ipilimumab and nivolumab results in higher rates of drug-induced hypophysitis. The finding of primary hypothyroidism in this patient and the absence of clinical and biochemical parameters indicating evidence of pituitary insufficiency do not support ipilimumab-induced hypophysitis (Answer C) as the cause of the observed thyroid dysfunction.

Lithium (Answer A) can be associated with a variety of thyroidal adverse effects, including the induction of goiter, primary hypothyroidism, primary hyperthyroidism, and thyroiditis. While the timing that lithium-induced thyroid dysfunction onsets is variable, it usually occurs within the first 12 months of treatment. This patient has been on lithium for 5 years, and it is unlikely that this drug is the cause of his hypothyroidism.

Hashimoto thyroiditis (Answer E) is a possible explanation for the abnormal biochemical findings in this vignette, but this is a less plausible etiology in view of the well-documented association between immune checkpoint inhibitors and induction of hypothyroidism.

Euthyroid sick syndrome (Answer B) is a state of adaptation or dysregulation of thyrotrophic feedback in which biochemical tests are abnormal, but the thyroid gland is not dysfunctional. This is often seen in starvation, critical illness, or patients in the intensive care unit. The most common hormone pattern is low total T_3 (and free T_3) with normal free T_4 and low or normal TSH with normal concentrations of TPO antibodies. The findings of an elevated serum TSH value in conjunction with low free T_3 and free T_4 concentrations and raised TPO antibodies are not consistent with this diagnosis.

Educational Objective
Identify novel immune checkpoint inhibitors as the cause of primary hypothyroidism.

UpToDate Topic Review(s)
Disorders that cause hypothyroidism

Reference(s)

Ryder M, Callahan M, Postow MA, Wolchok J, Fagin JA. Endocrine-related adverse events following ipilimumab in patients with advanced melanoma: a comprehensive retrospective review from a single institution. *Endocr Relat Cancer* 2014;21(2):371-381. PMID: 24610577

Joshi MN, Whitelaw BC, Palomar MT, Wu Y, Carroll PV. Immune checkpoint inhibitor-related hypophysitis and endocrine dysfunction: clinical review. *Clin Endocrinol (Oxf)*. 2016;85(3):331-339. PMID: 26998595

Dadu R, Zobniw C, Diab A. Managing adverse events with immune checkpoint agents. *Cancer J*. 2016;22(2):121-129. PMID: 27111908

117 ANSWER: D) Greater longevity of the transplanted pancreas
Diabetic nephropathy is the leading cause of end-stage renal disease in adults in the United States. Renal transplant in these patients leads to improved survival when compared with outcomes of patients who stay on dialysis. Pancreas transplant offers patients improved quality of life, freeing them of the burden of insulin replacement therapy and the associated risk of hypoglycemia, and it can arrest—if not improve—microvascular diabetes complications. However, lifelong immunosuppression is required to prevent pancreas graft rejection and recurrence of autoimmune islet-cell destruction. Because of the multiple potential adverse effects of immunosuppressive therapy, pancreas transplant alone is reserved for those patients with dangerously uncontrolled hyperglycemia or recurrent severe hypoglycemia despite aggressive medical care.

Patients with type 1 diabetes who require kidney transplant for end-stage renal disease and who will already be subjected to immunosuppressive therapy are candidates for either a simultaneous kidney-pancreas transplant or pancreas after kidney transplant. While both can normalize glucose levels, there are drawbacks to pancreas after kidney transplant, including increased mortality, mostly due to cardiovascular events in the first year after pancreas transplant (thus, Answers A and E are incorrect) in a patient population at high risk for cardiovascular disease. Pancreas graft survival is longer in those patients transplanted simultaneously with a kidney than with a pancreas transplant alone or pancreas after kidney transplant (thus, Answer D is correct). Mechanisms for better pancreas graft survival include earlier detection of dual organ rejection with serial creatinine monitoring in those receiving simultaneous kidney and pancreas transplants, and the dissimilar antigenic stimulation coming from genetically different pancreas and kidney transplants in pancreas after kidney transplant recipients. Simultaneous rejection of both organs is the most common scenario in simultaneous kidney-pancreas transplant. Hyperglycemia is a relatively late manifestation of pancreas rejection.

Successful pancreas transplant normalizes glucose levels. It also appears to improve both patient survival in those with a functioning pancreas after 1 year and survival of the transplanted kidney over kidney transplant alone. No differential effects on rates of kidney rejection or diabetes-related microvascular complications have been demonstrated among patients receiving simultaneous kidney-pancreas transplant or pancreas after kidney transplant (thus, Answers B and C are incorrect).

Educational Objective
Compare outcomes of simultaneous kidney-pancreas transplant vs pancreas after kidney transplant in patients with type 1 diabetes and end-stage renal disease.

UpToDate Topic Review(s)
Benefits and complications associated with kidney-pancreas transplantation in diabetes mellitus

Reference(s)

Gruessner AC. 2011 update on pancreas transplantation: comprehensive trend analysis of 25,000 cases followed up over the course of twenty-four years at the International Pancreas Transplant Registry (IPTR). *Rev Diabet Stud.* 2011;8(1):6-16. PMID: 21720668

Robertson RP, Davis C, Larsen J, Stratta R, Sutherland DE; American Diabetes Association. Pancreas and islet transplantation in type 1 diabetes. *Diabetes Care.* 2006;29(4):935. PMID: 16567844

Maffi P, Scavini M, Socci C, et al. Risks and benefits of transplantation in the cure of type 1 diabetes: whole pancreas versus islet transplantation. A single center study. *Rev Diabet Stud.* 2011;8(1):44-50. PMID: 21720672

118 ANSWER: B) Norethindrone

In a breastfeeding mother who does not desire pregnancy, hormonal contraception can be used. It is often initiated at the 6-week postpartum visit to avoid unwanted pregnancy. However, older studies demonstrate that combined hormonal contraception (ethinyl estradiol and a progestin) (Answer C) can decrease breast milk production and it is therefore not the contraception of choice. Hormonal contraception containing only a progestin (Answer B) does not appear to decrease breast milk volume and is the best choice for hormonal birth control in a breastfeeding mother. Other options include nonhormonal contraceptive devices or levonorgestrel-coated intrauterine devices, which do not appear to have an adverse effect on lactation.

Prolactin rises as high as 300 ng/mL (13.0 nmol/L) during the third trimester of pregnancy and remains elevated while breastfeeding. Although baseline prolactin can normalize after approximately 6 months of breastfeeding, it increases during and just after suckling and can remain slightly high for the duration of breastfeeding. There is no need to measure prolactin in a breastfeeding mother such as this one. A microprolactinoma is not expected to undergo symptomatic growth (ie, affect vision or cause other neurologic symptoms) during pregnancy or breastfeeding. Further, hyperprolactinemia is often mitigated after a pregnancy, and breastfeeding does not increase the likelihood of hyperprolactinemia or tumor expansion after pregnancy. Therefore, treatment of the prolactinoma with dopaminergic agents during pregnancy and lactation is not recommended. Further, dopamine agonists decrease physiologic prolactin and abolish breast milk production. Therefore, bromocriptine (Answer A) and cabergoline (Answer D) should not be used in a woman with a microprolactinoma who desires to breastfeed. The normal physiologic increase in prolactin after delivery results in the rise in prolactin that promotes breast milk production. Therefore, metoclopramide (Answer E) is not necessary.

Educational Objective
Choose the most appropriate contraceptive medication for a breastfeeding mother.

UpToDate Topic Review(s)
Management of lactotroph adenoma (prolactinoma) during pregnancy

Reference(s)

Melmed S, Casanueva FF, Hoffman AR, Kleinberg DL, Montori VM, Schlechte JA, Wass JA; Endocrine Society. Diagnosis and treatment of hyperprolactinemia: an Endocrine Society clinical practice guideline. *J Clin Endocrinol Metab.* 2011;96(2):273-288. PMID: 21296991

Auriemma RS, Perone Y, Di Samo A, et al. Results of a single-center observational 10-year survey study on recurrence of hyperprolactinemia after pregnancy and lactation. *J Clin Endocrinol Metab.* 2013;98(1):372-379. PMID: 23162092

Lopez LM, Grey TW, Stuebe AM, Chen M, Truitt ST, Gallo MF. Combined hormonal versus nonhormonal versus progestin-only contraception in lactation. *Cochrane Database Syst Rev.* 2015;(3):CD003988. PMID: 25793657

119 ANSWER: A) Continue the 2 antihyperglycemic medications and start basal insulin in the evening

Diabetes that occurs in patients with cystic fibrosis (CF) is an important secondary form of diabetes. The prevalence of cystic fibrosis–related diabetes (CFRD) has increased because patients with CF are surviving longer because of improved medical and nutritional care. The diabetes in CF is rather unique and has features of both type 1 and type 2 diabetes. Affected patients are generally of normal body weight but do not have an autoimmune form of diabetes. Insulin resistance may be present but is milder than in patients with typical type 2 diabetes. The primary defect is impaired insulin secretion, which occurs due to destruction of pancreatic tissue. The chloride channel dysfunction seen in CF contributes to excess viscous secretions that lead to fibrosis and fatty infiltration of pancreatic tissue. Over time, there is a loss of β, α, and pancreatic polypeptide mass. However, patients with CF do not usually develop complete insulinopenia, so ketosis is rare.

Patients who develop CFRD generally have poorer lung function, worse nutritional status, and a higher rate of death than patients with CF without diabetes. CFRD occurs most often in patients with pancreatic exocrine insufficiency. The prevalence of the disease increases with age and 25% to 50% of patients aged 30 years and older have CFRD. Women tend to develop CFRD at higher rates than men. Impaired glucose tolerance usually develops first without accompanying fasting hyperglycemia. There is progression to impaired glucose tolerance with elevated fasting glucose levels and finally to frank diabetes. The screening method of choice for patients with CF is the 2-hour 75-g oral glucose tolerance test. Hemoglobin A_{1c} testing is not sensitive and should not be used for screening or diagnosis of CFRD. Consensus guidelines recommend screening for CFRD starting at age 10 years, although some CF centers start screening at younger ages. The oral glucose tolerance test should be obtained during baseline health and not during an exacerbation of CF or while the patient is being treated with antibiotics or glucocorticoids. The cutpoints for diagnosis of impaired glucose tolerance and CFRD are the same as in conventional diabetes.

Other important facets of CFRD include malnutrition, malabsorption, gastroparesis, and glucagon insufficiency. Glucocorticoids used to treat CF exacerbation can, of course, worsen hyperglycemia. Patients with CFRD develop microvascular complications as frequently as patients with conventional diabetes.

Treatment of CFRD should include initiation of insulin early in the disease course not only to lower glucose levels but also to improve appetite, which may help lead to weight gain. Two nonrandomized 12-month trials in children and adolescents with either impaired glucose tolerance or CFRD demonstrated that basal insulin treatment led to weight gain and improved lung function.

The patient in this vignette has CFRD and suboptimal glycemic control. In addition, she has lost weight. The best step now is the addition of basal insulin to the treatment regimen of glyburide and sitagliptin (Answer A). She does not need to start basal-bolus insulin (Answer B) at this time as this may lead to an increased risk of hypoglycemia. Her hyperglycemia is modest and should respond well to the addition of basal insulin alone. Basal insulin should not be substituted for the 2 oral antihyperglycemic agents (Answer C). The glyburide and sitagliptin should be continued. Doubling her glyburide dosage (Answer E) would lead to minimal improvement in glucose control. Finally, there are no data on treatment of CFRD with glucagonlike peptide 1 analogues (Answer D). In addition, use of such an agent may contribute to further weight loss, which would be detrimental in this case.

Educational Objective
Manage cystic fibrosis–related diabetes mellitus.

Reference(s)

Ode KL, Moran A. New insights into cystic-fibrosis related diabetes in children. *Lancet Diabetes Endocrinol.* 2013;1(1):52-58. PMID: 24622267

Moran A, Dunitz J, Nathan B, Saeed A, Holme B, Thomas W. Cystic fibrosis-related diabetes: current trends in prevalence, incidence, and mortality. *Diabetes Care.* 2009;32(9):1626-1631. PMID: 19542209

Scheuing N, Holl RW, Dockter G, et al. Diabetes in cystic fibrosis: multicenter screening results based on current guidelines. *PloS One.* 2013;8(12):e81545. PMID: 24324701

Moran A, Brunzell C, Cohen RC, et al; CFRD Guidelines Committee. Clinical care guidelines for cystic fibrosis-related diabetes: a position statement of the American Diabetes Association and a clinical practice guideline of the Cystic Fibrosis Foundation, endorsed by the Pediatric Endocrine Society. *Diabetes Care.* 2010;33(12):2697-2708. PMID: 21115772

Mozzillo E, Franzese A, Valerio G, et al. One-year glargine treatment can improve the course of lung disease in children and adolescents with cystic fibrosis and early glucose derangements. *Pediatr Diabetes.* 2009;10(3):162-167. PMID: 19207231

Hameed S, Morton JR, Field PI, et al. Once daily insulin detemir in cystic fibrosis with insulin deficiency. *Arch Dis Child.* 2012;97(5):464-467. PMID: 21493664

120 ANSWER: B) Surgical resection of the right adrenal gland

This patient presents with a clinical syndrome that is suspicious for excessive mineralocorticoid receptor activation. The biochemical test results are highly suggestive of primary aldosteronism as they demonstrate suppressed plasma renin activity and a relatively high serum aldosterone level such that the aldosterone-to-renin ratio is 41. In the context of hypertension and hypokalemia, this is almost certainly confirmatory for primary aldosteronism. To be certain, an oral sodium loading test or a saline infusion test would confirm autonomous aldosterone secretion and the diagnosis of primary aldosteronism.

The treatment of primary aldosteronism depends on patient preference, disease severity, and eligibility for medical or surgical therapy. Generally, unilateral primary aldosteronism is treated with surgery when desired and possible, whereas mineralocorticoid receptor antagonist therapy is often preferred for bilateral primary aldosteronism. This patient has evidence of bilateral adrenal adenomas, which suggests either bilateral primary aldosteronism or unilateral primary aldosteronism with a nonfunctional adenoma on the contralateral side. Adrenal venous sampling is the most certain method to decipher the source of aldosterone autonomy.

Interpreting the results of adrenal venous sampling should be systematic. The first step involves confirming appropriate catheterization of the adrenal veins to ensure adequate sampling. This is confirmed when the ratio of the cortisol concentration in the adrenal vein to the cortisol concentration in the peripheral vein or inferior vena cava is greater than 2 (also referred to as the selectivity index). The selectivity index can be further evaluated following a dose of exogenous ACTH, where a marked rise in adrenal venous cortisol confirms accurate catheter placement. This patient had a baseline selectivity index greater than 2 in each adrenal vein and also demonstrated a robust response to ACTH in each vein, providing reassurance that subsequent sampling is reliable. Thus, repeated adrenal venous sampling (Answers D and E) is unnecessary. The next step involves assessing the aldosterone-to-cortisol (A/C) ratio in each adrenal vein and determining the lateralization ratio. The lateralization ratio is calculated by dividing the larger A/C ratio by the smaller one—a ratio greater than 4 is generally considered highly suggestive of a unilateral source of autonomous aldosterone secretion. In this case, the lateralization ratio is greater than 18 favoring the right adrenal vein, suggesting that the right adrenal adenoma is the culprit. Importantly, the serum aldosterone concentration in the left adrenal vein is almost the same as it is in the inferior vena cava, and the A/C ratio on the left (0.25-0.30) is even lower than that in the inferior vena cava (1.7), suggesting that aldosterone secretion from the left adrenal gland is suppressed. Together, these findings strongly support a unilateral source of aldosterone autonomy from the right adrenal gland that may be cured with a right adrenalectomy (thus, Answer B is correct and Answers A and C are incorrect).

Educational Objective

Interpret adrenal venous sampling results in the evaluation of primary aldosteronism.

UpToDate Topic Review(s)
Diagnosis of primary aldosteronism

Reference(s)

Funder JW, Carey RM, Mantero F, et al. The management of primary aldosteronism: case detection, diagnosis, and treatment: an Endocrine Society Clinical Practice Guideline. *J Clin Endocrinol Metab.* 2016;101(5):1889-1916. PMID: 26934393

Rossi GP, Auchus RJ, Brown M, et al. An expert consensus statement on use of adrenal vein sampling for the subtyping of primary aldosteronism. *Hypertension.* 2013;63(1):151-160. PMID: 24218436

Lethielleux G, Amar L, Raynaud A, Plouin PF, Steichen O. Influence of diagnostic criteria on the interpretation of adrenal vein sampling. *Hypertension.* 2015;65(4):849-854. PMID: 25646291

ENDOCRINE SELF-ASSESSMENT PROGRAM 2018

Part III

This question-mapping index groups question topics according to the 8 umbrella sections of ESAP (Adrenal, Bone-Calcium, Diabetes, Lipid-Obesity, Pituitary, Reproduction [Female], Reproduction [Male], and Thyroid). Relevant **question numbers** follow each topic.

ADRENAL

Adrenal incidentaloma: **20**
Adrenal insufficiency: **79, 114**
Adrenal venous sampling: **120**
Adrenocortical carcinoma: **2, 114**
Autoimmune diseases: **79**
Bilateral macronodular adrenal hyperplasia: **93**
Carbamazepine: **65**
Catecholamine-secreting tumors: **97, 102**
Cushing syndrome: **11, 29, 65, 93**
Cushing syndrome, iatrogenic: Glycyrrhizic acid: **43**
Hypercortisolism: **11, 29, 65, 93**
Hypertension: **43, 97, 102, 120**
Hypokalemia: **43**
Mifepristone: **11**
Mitotane: **114**
Non–islet-cell hypoglycemia: **2**
Paraganglioma: **102**
Pheochromocytoma: **97, 102**
Primary aldosteronism: **120**
Succinate dehydrogenase genes: **102**

CALCIUM-BONE

Albers-Schonberg disease: **60**
ALPL gene: **24**
Androgen-deprivation therapy: **8**
Atypical femoral fractures: **57**
Barakat syndrome: **3**
Bisphosphonates: **40, 51, 57, 63, 101**
Bisphosphonate holiday: **63**
CYP24A1 gene: **15**
Familial hypocalciuric hypercalcemia: **85**
Fanconi syndrome: **47**
Fibroblast growth factor 23: **96**
HDR syndrome: **3**
Hypercalcemia: **10, 15, 28, 77, 85**
Hypercalcemia, non–PTH-mediated: **10, 15**
Hypercalcemia of malignancy: **77**
Hyperparathyroidism: **107**
Hyperparathyroidism, primary: **28, 85**
Hypocalcemia: **3, 40**
Hypoparathyroidism: **3**

Hypophosphatemia: **24, 47, 96**
Inflammatory bowel disease: **72**
Ketoconazole: **40**
Nephrolithiasis: **15, 72**
Osteogenesis imperfecta: **51**
Osteomalacia: **47, 96**
Osteopetrosis: **60**
Osteoporosis: **8, 24, 47, 63**
Paget disease: **101**
Parathyroidectomy: **107**
Renal disease: **107**
Sarcoidosis: **10**
Teriparatide: **24**
Vitamin D deficiency: **40**

DIABETES

Bariatric surgery: **67**
Cardiovascular risk: **75**
Celiac disease: **104**
Continuous glucose monitoring: **70, 81**
Cystic fibrosis: **119**
Depression: **36**
Diabetic amyotrophy: **113**
Diabetic ketoacidosis: **7, 9, 25, 36**
Dipeptidyl-peptidase 4 inhibitors: **84**
Exercise: **23**
GCK gene: **94**
Gestational diabetes mellitus: **12**
Glucagonlike peptide 1 receptor agonists: **1**
Hemoglobin A1c: **64**
Hyperglycemia in hospitalized patients: **30, 64, 111**
Hypertension: **59**
Hypoglycemia: **17, 53, 70, 81**
Insulin pump therapy: **23, 81**
Insulin therapy: **7, 17, 23, 25, 50, 111**
Insulin, U500: **111**
Ketosis-prone diabetes mellitus: **9**
Kidney transplant: **117**
Maturity-onset diabetes of the young: **94**
Metformin: **108**
Monogenic diabetes: **94**
Nephropathy: **117**
Neuropathy: **113**

Octreotide: **53**
Pancreatic cancer: **45**
Pancreas transplant: **117**
Prediabetes: **99**
Preconception planning: **42, 67, 88**
Pregnancy: **12, 42, 67, 88**
Prevention: **99**
Psychological insulin resistance: **25**
Renal disease: **50, 84**
Secondary forms of diabetes: **56, 119**
Somatostatinoma: **56**
Type 1 diabetes mellitus: **7, 17, 23, 42, 70, 81, 104, 117**
Type 2 diabetes mellitus: **1, 12, 30, 36, 45, 50, 53, 56, 59, 64, 75, 84, 88, 108, 111, 113**

LIPID-OBESITY

Anticonvulsant drugs: **115**
Bariatric surgery: **4**
Cardiovascular disease: **13, 26, 39, 87**
Cholesteryl ester storage disease: **49**
Diabetes mellitus: **73**
Familial hypercholesterolemia: **39**
Glucagonlike peptide 1 receptor agonists: **33**
HDL cholesterol, low: **26**
Hypertriglyceridemia: **62, 73**
Inflammatory joint disease: **87**
Lipid-lowering therapy: **13, 26, 87**
Lysosomal acid lipase deficiency: **49**
Medication-associated weight gain: **115**
Naltrexone/bupropion: **100**
Obesity: **4, 16, 33, 52, 80, 100, 115**
Oral contraceptives: **62**
PCSK9 inhibitors: **39**
Phentermine: **33, 52**
Prader-Willi syndrome: **80**
Sleeve gastrectomy: **4**
Statin therapy: **13, 26, 87**
Very low-calorie diet: **16**

PITUITARY

Acromegaly: **82**
Adrenal insufficiency: **54, 68**
Checkpoint inhibitor immunotherapy: **89**

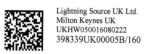